Great Discoveries in Medicine

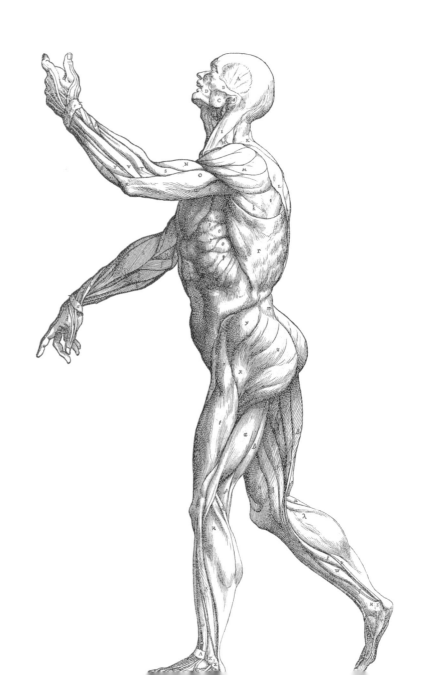

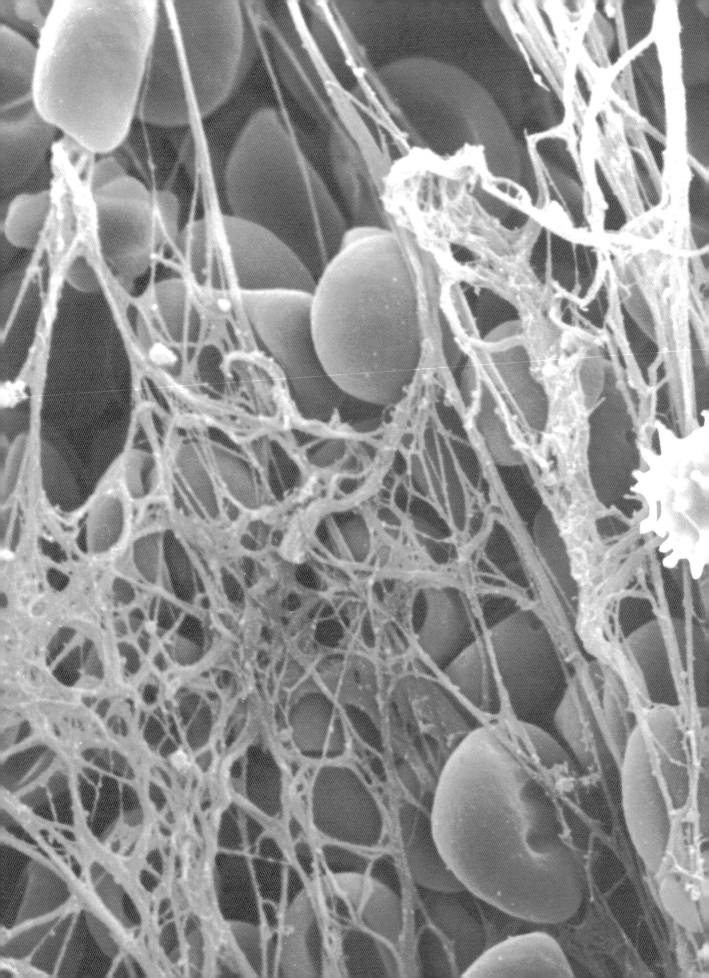

Great Discoveries in Medicine

Edited by **William & Helen Bynum**

With 382 illustrations, 342 in color

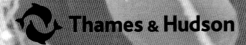
Thames & Hudson

Half-title: Detail of a plate from Andreas Vesalius, *De humani fabrica corporis* (On the Fabric of the Human Body), 1543.
Title-page: Electron micrograph of a blood clot.
Opposite (left to right): Detail from a plate illustrating the ear and the temple, after Duverney, Valsalva and Ruysch, engraving by Prevost, 1762; hand-coloured woodblock print of *duruo* plant (*Pollia japonica*) used in Chinese medicine, 1665; scanning electron microscope view of a breast cancer cell.
Page 6 (left to right): Ivory anatomical model with removable parts, German, 17th century; physician wearing a plague preventive costume, 17th century; modern tablets; the heart, detail from a plate from Matthew Baillie, *A series of engravings*, 1799.
Page 7 (left to right): Detail from a plate illustrating surgical instruments used in the American Civil War; Thomas Graham's apparatus used to determine the laws of diffusion; detail of a tobacco plant, from the frontispiece of Edward Brailsford, *An experimental dissertation on the chemical and medical properties of the* Nicotiana tabacum..., 1799.

First published in 2011 in hardcover in the United States of America by Thames & Hudson Inc., 500 Fifth Avenue, New York, New York 10110

thamesandhudsonusa.com

Library of Congress Catalog Card Number 2011922602

ISBN 978-0-500-25180-5

Printed and bound in China by Toppan Printing

CONTENTS

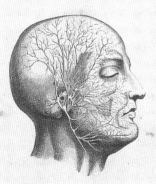
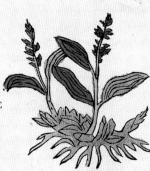
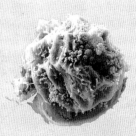

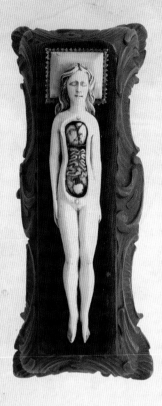

Nº 4.

BATTLING THE SCOURGES 142

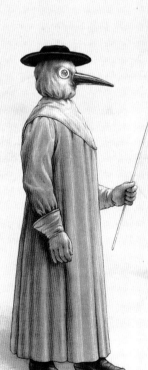

Nº 5.

'A PILL FOR EVERY ILL' 180

Nº 6.

SURGICAL BREAKTHROUGHS 214

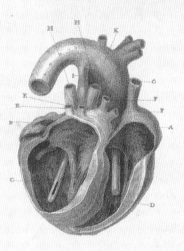

MEDICAL
TRIUMPHS 258

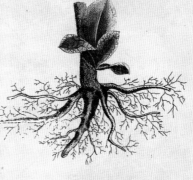

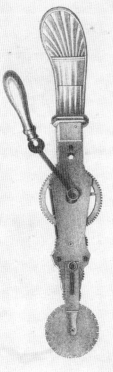

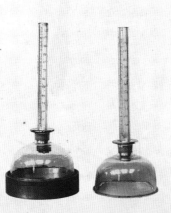

The SCIENCE &
Art of Medicine

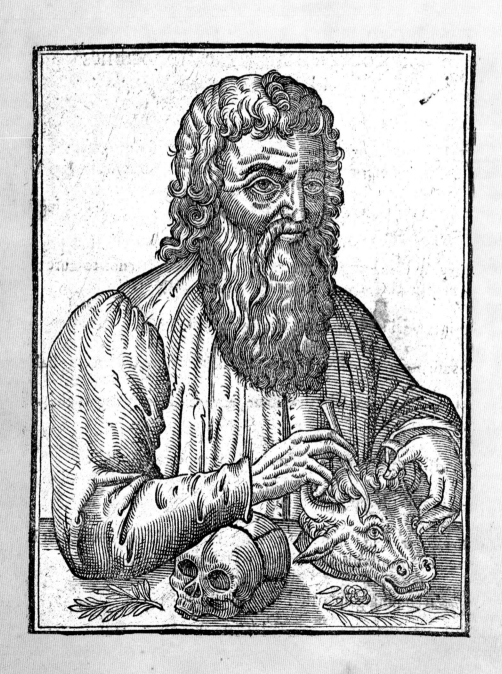

Health matters. When people fall ill, they want sympathy, and help, from family, neighbours or healers of whatever stripe. It has ever been thus. Consequently, medicine, if not necessarily the oldest profession, is of very ancient origin.

Medicine has also long been intimately linked with religion and supernatural interpretations of the world and everything in it. In the earliest descriptions of disease and healing in ancient Assyrian, Babylonian, Egyptian and other Near Eastern cultures, religious explanations of both the cause and cure of disease predominate. There were healing temples in ancient Egypt long before the more famous ones in classical Greece, and the physician-priest combination can be found in all ancient societies that have left written records.

From the 5th century BC, however, a new approach to medicine emerged in ancient Greece, associated with Hippocrates and his followers. The Hippocratics were not irreligious, but they can be said to have developed a secular medicine, one that sought to explain health and disease within a naturalistic framework. In this sense, Hippocrates deserves to be called 'the father of Western medicine'; he and his followers devoted themselves to the diagnosis and treatment of disease, and to advising their patients about how to maintain health, just as a modern doctor does.

Although health and disease have never been separated completely from religious and theological concerns, doctors for the most part want to understand their patients' afflictions in rational, scientific terms. Modern doctors employ a number of machines and instruments to diagnose and treat disease; they learn about physiology, biochemistry, microbiology and molecular biology in medical schools, and are encouraged to apply these disciplines at the bedside, when they are confronted with sick patients who need their help. This is the science of medicine, and much of this book is devoted to describing the individuals and insights that have gradually produced the medicine we have today.

But science has never been the whole story. There has always also been an art of medicine, as the Hippocratics recognized. Today, doctors are encouraged to use their subtle clinical skills, to listen carefully to their patients, and to treat them with empathy and compassion. The Hippocratics had as one of their goals, 'Always to aid, or at least do no harm'. This injunction, too rarely achieved in medicine's long past, does surface occasionally in the following pages, as we see doctors striving to understand why epidemics occur, or how it is that what we eat and drink, or whether we smoke or not, has implications for our life-chances. As modern societies become increasingly medicalized, the role of medicine has acquired many of the pastoral functions that were the job of the physician–priest of antiquity. We still have healing temples: we simply call them hospitals.

We do not know what Hippocrates looked like – there are descriptions, but no contemporary pictures. Such is his place in medicine's history and his evocation in contemporary practice, however, that there has been no shortage of imagined portraits.

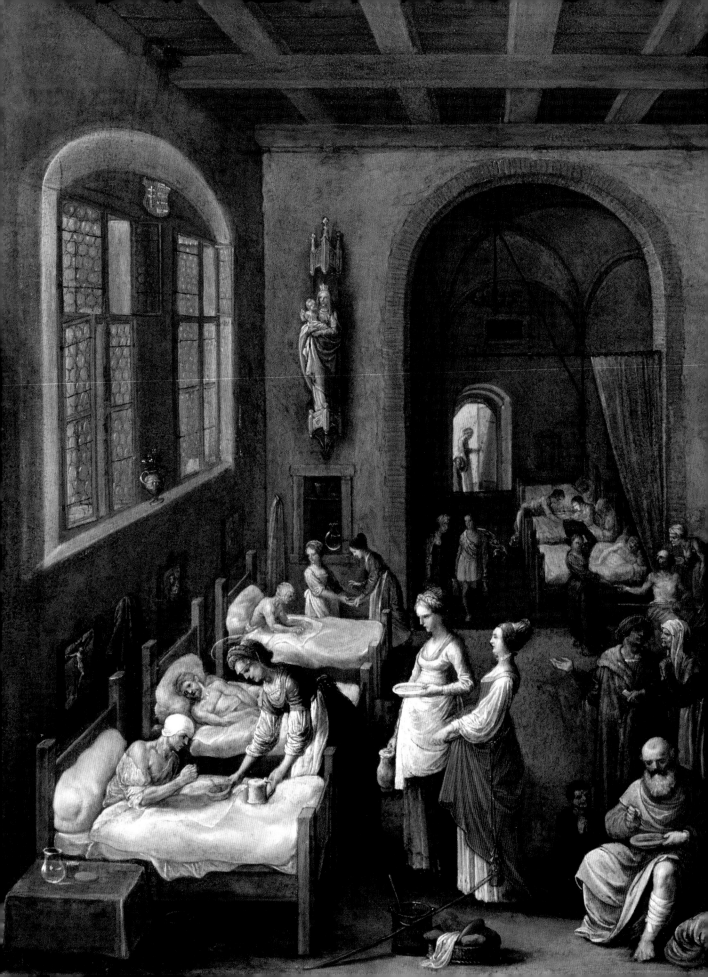

WAYS AND MEANS

Medicine's knowledge base has always involved understanding how the body works and how this is compromised in disease. Health and longevity can also be promoted by such understanding (although people tend not to bother with the doctor when they feel in the peak of health). The first two sections of the book, **Discovering the Body** and **Understanding Health & Disease**, look at how various cultures have regarded the healthy and sick body and mind. In the non-Western traditions an essential holism dominated. In Western medicine, on the other hand, ever smaller parts of the body – organs, cells, molecules – became the focus. The malfunctioning of these units and their faulty interactions explained much about sickness and offered new ways to treat and cure disease, but perhaps the patient slipped from view.

We know so much, and can do so much more now than in the past, because of the **Tools of the Trade**, the wonderfully simple and dazzlingly complex diagnostic and therapeutic technologies that feature in section three. In **Battling the Scourges** we meet the pantheon of microscopic organisms with which we share the planet and which have nagged away at our species over the millennia. The smoulder of endemic diseases may flare into epidemics – the scourges of the past and present – destroying individual lives and disrupting the fabric of society.

There are lots of ways that medicine has tried to help patients, and three key aspects form the final three sections of this book, broadening the emphasis beyond the infectious diseases. **'A Pill for Every Ill'** explores the diverse roles of medication – ingested, injected or inhaled – in killing pain, providing relief from mental illness and inducing a hormonal state in the body that prevents unwanted pregnancy. It used to be said that 'a chance to cut is a chance to cure', and **Surgical Breakthroughs** reveals the highs (and lows) of invasion by the knife and discusses some of the vital supporting techniques that make modern surgery possible. **Medical Triumphs** presents the wide range of methods we have developed to prevent illness and promote health. Doctors now have a better understanding of who gets sick and why, and have at their disposal vaccines and ways of keeping the body alive when key organs fail. We end with the Nobel Prize-winning discovery of the causative role of certain bacteria in stomach ulcers, some of which go on to develop into cancer if untreated. Joint prize-winner Barry Marshall reminds us in his own words of the persisting values of clear thought, questioning received wisdom and having the courage to act in the face of opposition. Along with the big science and high technology, we need these human qualities in medicine, as well as the ability always to care.

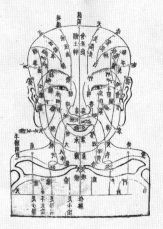

Above
An acupuncture chart of the front of the head, from a 17th-century Chinese woodcut. The lines indicate the energy channels, which run through the body, and the points – the places to apply needles or burn mugwort (moxibustion) to rebalance the flow of energy in this holistic understanding of the body.

Opposite
St Elizabeth offers a bowl of food and a tankard of drink to a male patient in the hospital in Marburg, Germany, in this 16th-century oil painting on copper by Adam Elsheimer. Early modern hospitals were intimately related with religious charity and care of the poor as well as healing.

Discovering
THE *Body*

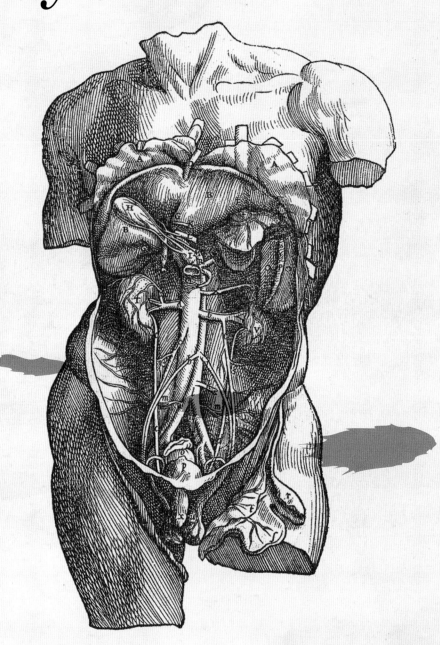

The ancient world saw the birth of several great medical traditions, including that in Egypt, but while these have largely disappeared, the systems that developed in China, India and Greece have proved remarkably resilient. They still have many adherents and practitioners, although each of them has changed over the centuries. The Chinese system, based on notions of *yin* and *yang*, of winds and energies, is still widely practised, in both China and the West. Its most visible Western manifestation is acupuncture, but many of its herbal remedies also have their devotees, and not just in China.

Ayurvedic medicine, the ancient Indian system, is also still in widespread use in India and beyond. It has as its rival within traditional Indian culture a second system, called yunani, a legacy of ancient Greek medicine as formalized and shaped by Islamic ideas. Yunani is still very popular in all Muslim societies and is thus one heir of Hippocrates. In the West, however, Hippocratic medicine provided the foundation of what has evolved into modern, scientific medicine. In their original frameworks, the Chinese, Indian and Greek medical systems shared much. Each emphasized the fluids (humours) within the body as the key to understanding health and disease. Each was holistic, seeing disease as something that happens in the whole patient, and each stressed the importance of balance in health. Each also had a range of therapies, including diet, exercise, drugs and what we now call 'lifestyle'.

Then, gradually in the European late Middle Ages and gathering pace during the Renaissance, the ancient Greek tradition of Hippocrates and Galen that was the cornerstone of medical understanding began to be modified. The process started with the systematic study of human anatomy, especially by Andreas Vesalius, whose great work of 1543 brought dissection to a new level. The role of the printing press and new techniques of illustrating books gave the anatomical tradition cultural as well as medical significance.

The title of Vesalius's work – *De humani fabrica corporis* (On the Fabric of the Human Body) – announces the shift in medical focus to the solid parts of our bodies, to the organs such as the heart, liver, spleen and brain, rather than on the humours (blood, yellow bile, black bile and phlegm). Vesalius was concerned primarily with normal, typical anatomy, but as doctors began to dissect the bodies of their dead patients, they soon discovered that diseases cause changes in the organs – what the English philosopher Francis Bacon described as 'footsteps of disease'. These 'lesions', as doctors called them, came increasingly to be identified with various diseases – types of fever, cancers, inflammations, ulcers, abscesses – offering a further way of understanding what happens when a person falls ill.

Beginning in the 19th century, the level of analysis was pushed ever further, from the organ to the tissue, from the cell to the molecule. As doctors and scientists sought to understand the mechanisms of health and disease at ever more minute levels, modern medicine became more powerful, and more inextricably intertwined with science and technology. At the same time, doctors are urged not to forget the whole patient, and therefore to retain some of the holism that was so essential to the ancient medical traditions.

The great 16th-century anatomist Andreas Vesalius sought to understand the structure of the body through his dissections in Padua. This torso, opened to reveal the viscera, comes from his monumental work, *De humani fabrica corporis* (On the Fabric of the Human Body) of 1543, an amalgam of Renaissance science and art.

01. # EGYPTIAN MEDICINE
Art, archaeology, papyri & human remains

A. Rosalie David

If any doctor, any wab *priest of Sekhmet or any magician places his two hands*
or his fingers … he measures the heart because of its vessels to all his limbs.
Ebers Papyrus (854a)

A page from the Edwin Smith Papyrus (*c.* 1570 BC), named after the American dealer who bought it in Egypt in the 19th century. Written in hieratic script from right to left, it is the first known account of surgery.

Ancient Egyptian medical practice combined both 'rational' and 'irrational' treatments, utilizing objective, scientific methods and magical procedures. Where the cause of an illness was outward and visible, rational treatments were usually employed, but a hidden agency, perhaps attributable to punishment by the gods or the vengeance of the dead or an enemy, was often addressed with spells and magical rites. Both routes were apparently considered to be equally effective, although modern scientific studies are now demonstrating that the Egyptians had a more pragmatic approach than previously supposed.

Our evidence about Egyptian medicine is derived from art, archaeology, papyri and human remains, but there is great variation in its quantity and accuracy. For example, whereas tomb art usually shows the elite with perfect, idealized bodies, free from disease or deformity, and only limited sources of archaeological and inscriptional material have survived, studies of human remains can provide extensive, unbiased information about disease, lifestyle and medical treatment.

DOCTORS' HANDBOOKS

Only 12 medical papyri have been found, presumably survivors of a much larger original corpus. Perhaps doctors' handbooks or manuals of instruction, they provide important information about the Egyptian concept of physiology, and describe the symptoms, diagnosis and treatments of a wide range of diseases. However, they pose many difficulties of translation, and the precise meaning and significance of many words remain obscure.

The Kahun Papyrus (*c.* 1825 BC), the earliest extant treatise on gynaecology, includes prescriptions for contraception and pregnancy testing. The Edwin Smith Papyrus (*c.* 1570 BC), the world's first account of surgery, demonstrates that some significant advances usually attributed to the Greeks actually occurred much earlier in Egypt. For example, symptoms are already considered here in groups (syndromes) rather than individually, and there is some indication that the Egyptians could count the pulse; they also understood localization of function within the brain.

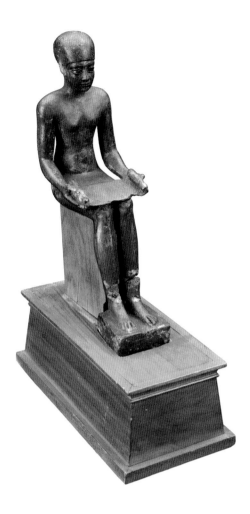

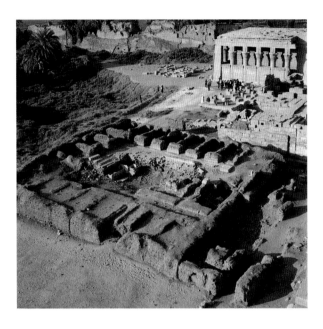

THE DIVINE DIMENSION

A range of practitioners used methods and treatments that included surgery, pharmacy and magic. While some practised locally in towns and villages, others – such as priests of Sekhmet, goddess of medicine – combined roles as temple ritualists and doctors. Several deities were associated with medicine and healing. Imhotep was a royal architect and probably king's physician who was deified after his death and credited as the founder of medical science; he was later identified with Asclepius, Greek god of medicine.

The temple played a significant role in healing. As well as possibly accommodating medical training, some temples were renowned as centres where treatments for patients included cleansing with sacred water and incubation ('temple sleep'). The patient, isolated in a small dark room, and induced into a trance-like state, was believed to encounter the gods and subsequently experience healing. Inscriptional evidence indicates that the Egyptians used this type of treatment long before the Greeks. However, only one such building has yet been excavated and identified in Egypt: adjacent to the temple at Denderah, it probably dates to the Ptolemaic period (332–30 BC).

EGYPT'S CONTRIBUTION

The Egyptian tradition, transmitted through Greek and Arabic sources, formed part of the medicine and pharmacy of Europe and the Near East. Egyptian innovations included observations in anatomy and experiments in surgery; anatomical and medical vocabulary; a reproducible and therapeutically efficacious pharmacy; use of splints, bandages and prostheses; and sanatoria where the mentally and physically sick were treated. However, despite these considerable contributions, the retention of irrational alongside rational treatments was a hindrance to further development.

02. CHINESE MEDICINE
Understanding the whole

Linda L. Barnes

By fully developing one's heart-mind, one knows one's nature,
and by knowing one's nature, one knows Heaven.
Mencius, 4th century BC

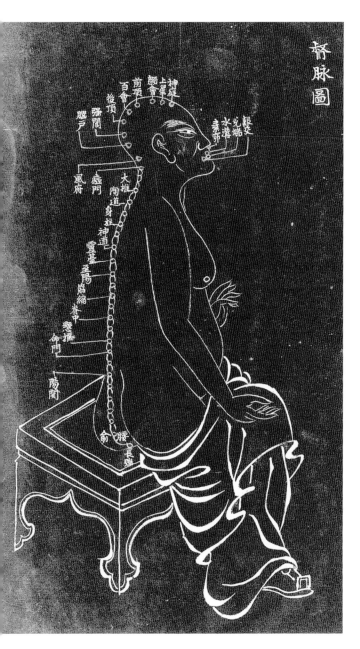

Over the course of Chinese history, Chinese thinkers and practitioners have explored the nature of change. Their pursuit grew out of the observation that everything has an inherent disposition to transform in patterned ways. The investigators discovered ways to apply their findings to the arts of healing, and developed conceptual frameworks with which to do so. They examined these frameworks over time, sometimes emphasizing one aspect, sometimes others, building up complex layers of interpretation.

QI, YIN AND YANG, AND WUXING

As early as the Neolithic period in China (beginning around 10,000 BC and ending with the introduction of metallurgy some 8,000 years later), no absolute boundaries were perceived as dividing the living from the dead. Instead, a dynamic cosmic vapour, *qi* (pronounced 'chee'), was experienced and recognized as the stuff of all reality. The conditions of being alive, ailing or dead came to be understood as variations on *qi*. This is possible because, on the one hand, *qi* can be as fine and subtle as steam rising from cooking rice, while on the other, it can be as dense as rock. Indeed, steam or breath can transform into substances as solid as rock. Since everything is *qi*, all change, whether at the level of person, natural world or cosmos, is an expression of *qi* in its endless patterned metamorphoses.

One such pattern involved the concepts of *yin* and *yang*, the former originally referring to the cool, shadowed, moist side of a mountain, and the latter to the hot, bright, dry side. As the sun moved across the sky, the shadowed side transformed into the sunlit one, indicating a relationship of two complementary phenomena – darkness and light – linked by a continuum of variations. Hence a

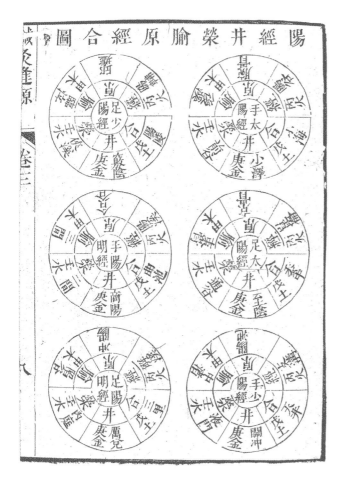

diagram in which *yin* always contains the seed of *yang*
and vice versa.

A second such pattern is expressed as the Five
Phases (*wuxing*). Sometimes translated as 'Five
Elements', because the Chinese terms are fire (*huo*),
earth (*tu*), metal (*jin*), water (*shui*) and wood (*mu*),
these concepts represent the properties and qualities
of five types of change, or *qi*. Each arises, combines
and recombines, and transmutes into the next. Each
has the capacity to influence and be influenced by
the others in patterned ways.

DAO

Chinese thinkers and practitioners identified a
dynamic principle that both characterized and
governed these patterns of change – the concept of *dao*.
Sometimes translated as 'way' or 'path', the *dao* is also
characterized as 'nameless', because words can never
fully explain it. The *dao* precedes everything else, but

is also reflected in all manifestations of nature
and the world. This underlying principle produces
a network of interwoven, reflective patterns and
processes at work in phenomena that may initially
appear unrelated. For this reason, the teacher Mengzi
(Latinized as Mencius; 372–289 BC) could suggest that,
through self-cultivation, one develops a deep awareness
both of one's capacity to feel, think and know, and,
especially, of the movement of the *dao* through one's
own life and in the unfolding processes at work in
the world.

As they are manifestations of the *dao*, *qi*, *yin*, *yang*
and the *wuxing* can be discerned at work both *in* the
human system and *as* the human system. As such, a
person can learn to detect, experience and, particularly,
harmonize with each aspect not only internally, but
also with others and in the world around. The human
system, as a result, resonates deeply with all natural
and cosmic processes.

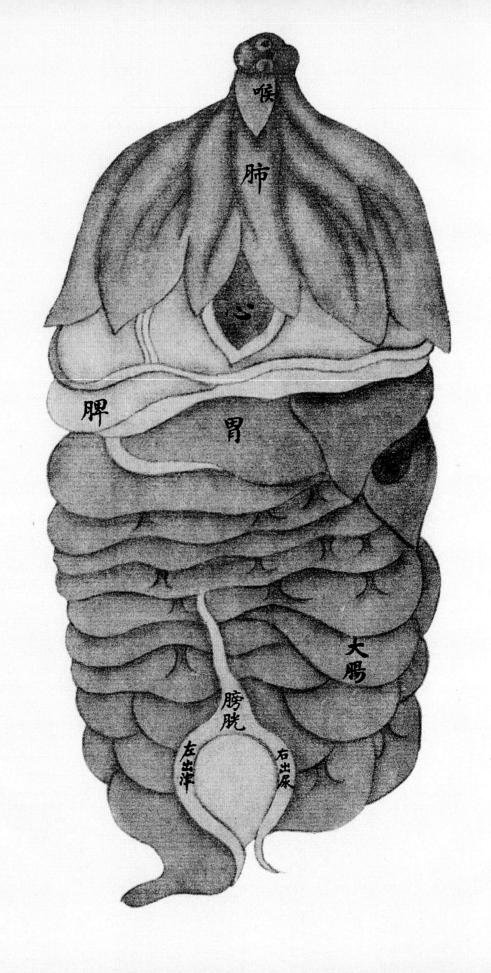

THE CHANNELS

One form of resonance involves currents, or connecting channels (*jingluo*), of *qi*, sometimes translated as meridians. Although many currents traverse the body, over time 20 achieved wide recognition. Twelve were associated with 12 organs – the lungs, large intestine, stomach, spleen, heart, small intestine, urinary bladder, kidney, pericardium, gall bladder, liver and what is known as the Triple Burner (*sanjiao*). The other 'Eight Extraordinary Channels' largely connect points on the first 12.

Just as the term 'elements' refers not to concrete phenomena but to processes, so 'organs' or 'viscera' refer to functions and processes associated with each physical body part. An 'organ' is thus the *doing* of certain kinds of things, as well as the relationships between them. The Triple Burner, for example, refers to the movements of heat and fluids throughout the body. Each organ function also corresponds to particular emotions, and has a unique spirit with its own form and attributes.

If the *dao* represents a profound dynamic balance both within and between things and their parts, as well as the free flow of the different currents and channels, then imbalance and obstruction compromise a person's wellness, and can transmute into sickness and disease. For example, because the dead represent the transformation of *qi* from one expression into another, they and the living continue to interact. The living must express their ongoing appreciation for the departed, just as they would for a living family member. Should they fail to do so, the dead can become angry and, as ghosts, afflict the living to get their attention. The neglected ghosts from other families may also inflict suffering. Remedies can involve offerings, symbolic restitution or, in extreme cases, exorcism.

EFFECTS OF THE EXTERNAL AND INTERNAL ON THE WHOLE

External natural forces – heat, cold, dampness, dryness, wind and fire – can adversely influence the body, either singly or in combination. Resulting excesses or deficiencies in the balance of one's *qi* can be further exacerbated through such mundane events as the consumption of certain foods or engagement in certain activities. Internal factors include the over- or under-functioning of the organ processes and their related emotions – the lungs are linked to sadness or grief, for example, the liver to anger or resentment,

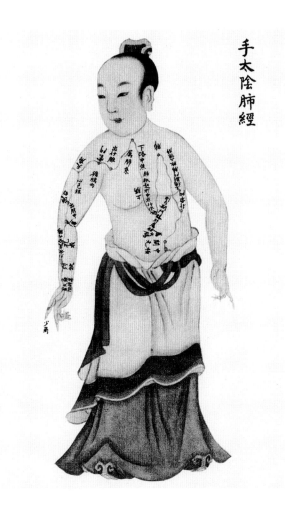

手太陰肺經

Above
Taken from *Renti jingmai tu* (Illustrations of the Channels of the Human Body), a manuscript of the early Qing dynasty, this figure illustrates the path and points of the *taiyin* or lung channel of the arm.

Opposite
An anatomical drawing of the front view of the abdominal viscera from the same manuscript as the illustration above, which included 24 colour paintings.

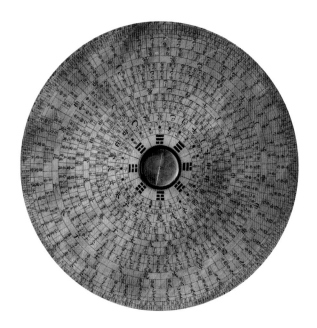

Left
A wooden geomantic compass and perpetual calendar. In the divination art of *fengshui*, compasses such as this are used to determine the healthiest position to build a house, ensuring that the forces of *yin* and *yang* are balanced and the risk of illness minimized.

Below
A selection of Chinese surgical instruments, including acupuncture needles and knives.

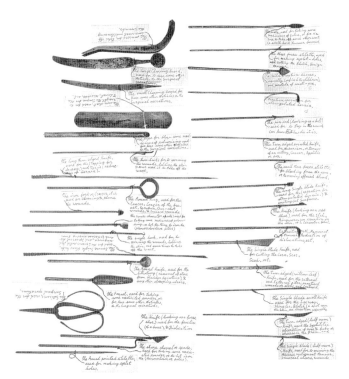

the kidneys to fear or insecurity, and the spleen to excessive worry.

Chinese medicine has also, historically, functioned as a system whose different branches address the impact of imbalanced diet, internal and external pathogens, the blocked flow of *qi*, bruises and broken bones, the effects of ageing, and the influence of one's surroundings. This led to the development of food and dietary therapies; herbal medicines; movement-based practices such as *taijiquan*; bone setting and therapeutic massage (*tuina*); self-cultivation practices for extending one's life (*qigong*); divination practices ranging from face-reading to assessing the *qi* involved in the placement of things and their relationship to each other (*fengshui*); and the interventions of moxibustion (burning mugwort, moxa, on or over the body) and acupuncture, the latter originally involving not only needles, but also implements for minor surgery. Petitions to figures such as the Medicine Buddha may complement these other approaches.

Practitioners assessing obstructions or blockages of *qi* developed diagnostic methods grounded in the senses – looking (observation), smelling, touching, listening, and asking questions to discern the specific nature of the imbalance. Touching refers in particular to highly sophisticated approaches to taking a patient's pulse. The detection of imbalances at the social or cosmic level requires analogous strategies, such as special compasses to discern the flows of *qi* in the ground.

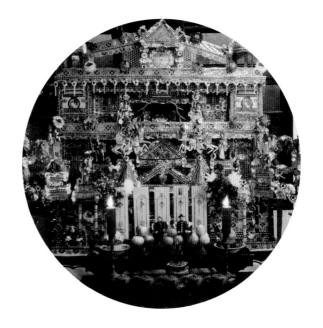

LIVING TRADITIONS

All these practices persist not only in Mainland China, Taiwan, Hong Kong and throughout the Chinese Diaspora, but they have also been adopted by cultures throughout the world. Each modality has undergone variations over time, leading to diverse lineages, schools of practices and traditions of transmission, with little apparent need to merge them into a systematized approach. Acupuncture has become perhaps the best known practice since the 1970s (see also [21]), particularly the standardized version referred to as 'Traditional Chinese Medicine', or 'TCM', produced by the People's Republic of China. However, since the more recent opening of the medical marketplace in Mainland China, older approaches have resurfaced, even as they continue to flourish in other parts of the world alongside TCM.

These practices are linked as different facets of Chinese medicine by the underlying focus on *qi*. One phenomenon is therefore connected to every other expression of the *dao*, providing a window on to another. Although individual practitioners may employ only a subset of this larger repertoire, and the different scientific communities have focused on even fewer of them, it is in the whole that one finds the full expression of Chinese medicine's ideas about body and personhood.

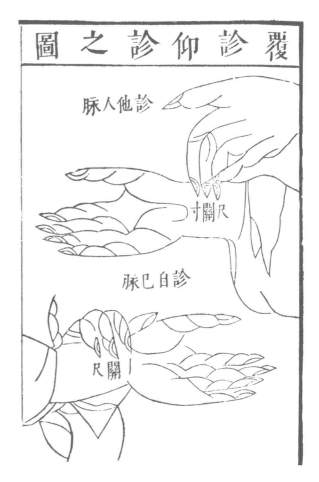

03. MEDICINE IN INDIA
Ayurveda in context

Guy Attewell

It is called 'ayurveda' because it tells us which substances,
qualities and actions are life enhancing, and which are not.
Charaka-samhita 1.30.23

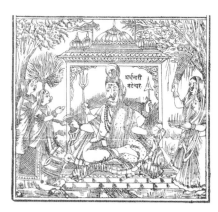

The Indian subcontinent is heir to a complex variety
of healing cultures, which exhibit significant local
and regional variations and marked changes over time,
as well as transregional interpenetration through the
mobility of people, materials and textual knowledge.
Of the state-supported Indian systems of medicine
– ayurveda, yunani tibb, siddha and yoga – ayurveda
has been the most widely practised and the most
successfully projected as Indian medicine.

Ayurveda is understood to be grounded in a
Sanskrit textual tradition, especially in a triad of
medical compendia inscribed between 200 BC and AD
600 – the *Susruta-samhita*, *Charaka-samhita* and the
Astangahridaya-samhita of Vaghbata. The precise
dating and authorship of the *Astangahridaya-
samhita* have been variously interpreted, but its
abundance in manuscript libraries dating from 1400
in many parts of India is an indication of the importance
of this synthetic work. Less attention has been paid
to regional traditions of healing and their vernacular
texts, some of which were translations from the
Sanskrit, or to knowledge transmitted within localized
oral traditions, which have had limited political
resources and influence.

THE BODY IN IMBALANCE

The complex historical layering of ayurveda precludes
a straightforward discussion of its foundational
concepts. However, the principle of *tridosha*, or the
three humours (literally 'faults': *vata*, *pitta* and *kapha*)
of the human body, runs through the fabric of much of
textual ayurveda and has been regarded as an essential
component of ayurvedic theory and practice. *Tridosha*
correspond to concepts of humoral theory found in
Indo-Muslim traditions and elaborated in Persia –
with Arabic antecedents – from the 14th century
(see [04] and [05]).

Sanskrit texts describe the *doshas* in material forms,
each having particular sensory attributes; thus in the
Charaka-samhita, *vata* is dry, cold and light, *pitta* is
hot, sour and pungent, and *kapha* is cold, unctuous,
heavy and sweet. The *doshas* become pathogenic when
they are displaced from their seats within the body, or
if they accumulate or diminish to excessive degrees. In
the *Astangahridaya-samhita* the *doshas* are considered
one of three fundamental constituents of the body, along
with body tissues (*dhatus*) and waste products (*mala*).
In their uncorrupted and balanced state, the *doshas*
are vital for the proper functioning of the body: *vata*
supports physical dynamism, movement; *pitta* supports

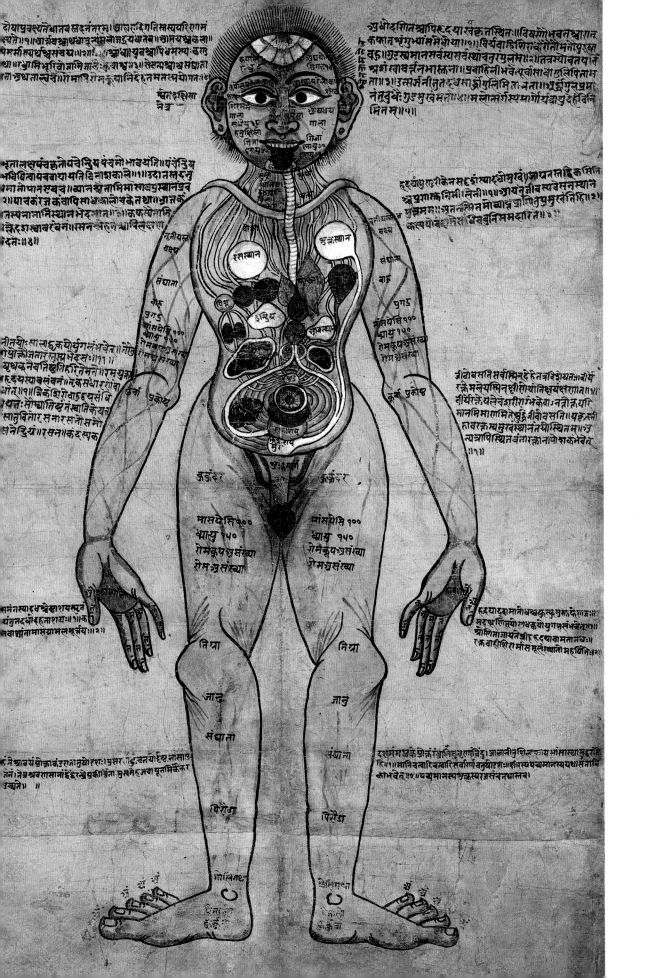

digestive fire, intelligence, good looks; *kapha* supports the body through unctuousness, steadiness, patience. However, if increased, *vata* causes emaciation, constipation, blackening and a weakening of the senses; *pitta* causes yellowing, hunger, thirst and insomnia; *kapha* stills the digestive fire, causing whiteness, debility, slackening and heaviness.

The writer Vaghbata emphasizes that disequilibrium transforms the *doshas* from supportive to destructive aspects. These states may be brought about by such things as 'crimes against wisdom', seasonal changes, inappropriate consumption (in quantity or kind), immoderation in sexual activity, and everyday habits. While later views of the *doshas* may agree with some of these general formulations, the contextual meaning of the *doshas* is an area of continued debate. The interpretation of *tridosha* in biomedical terms (such as endocrinology) is characteristic of formulations of ayurvedic theory from the early 20th century on.

DIAGNOSING THE BODY

Diagnostic and prognostic procedures in ayurveda have varied a great deal over time. The *Astangahridaya-samhita* sets out three parameters, which were prescriptive and were not necessarily followed in practice: *darsana* (inspection of all parts of the patient, with especial attention to the tongue); *sparsana* (palpation, feeling with the hands); and *prasna* (interrogation). The 14th-century text *Sarnagadhara-samhita* outlines a systematic procedure for pulse examination, which was not found in the earlier texts but subsequently becomes iconic of certain kinds of ayurvedic practice. These practices may have been introduced through tibb (Persian-Galenic medicine), long-established contacts with China or through the mediation of traditions of tantric alchemy. Some scholars, evidently averse to ideas of the cross-fertilizing of healing cultures, maintain that such practices were originally ayurvedic but were then lost prior to the three major medical compendia discussed here.

TREATING THE BODY

Therapy in ayurveda has included a vast array of different techniques. The *Susruta-samhita* is known for its emphasis on surgical procedures, though these do not figure prominently in subsequent Sanskrit texts and appear to have been the domain of lower-caste occupation groups in later times. Birth attendants,

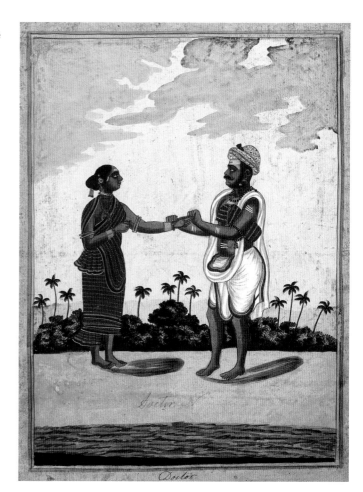

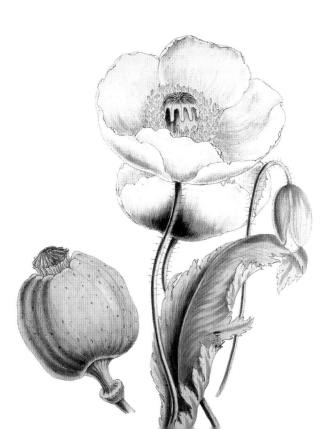

oculists, bone-setters, blood-letters, snake-bite healers, itinerant herbalists, veterinary healers and those who treated possession are among the specialist groups of healers whose skills may have intersected with elite textual knowledge, and who have all been part of the stratified and diverse sphere of Indian medicine.

A standard feature of Sanskrit compendia is *bhutavidya* (the knowledge of spirits), but strong emphasis was also placed on materia medica of vegetable, mineral or animal origin, and a sophisticated systematization of pharmacy (*dravyaguna*). One element of *dravyaguna* is *prabhava* (specific action), which points to the incorporation of direct, empirical observation of the actions of ingested substances on the body. From the 10th century there is a marked mention in texts of calcined metals (especially mercury) in compound remedies, and this has been a consistent feature of pharmacopoeia across the different 'systems' (ayurveda, yunani, siddha).

While most compound remedies in the pharmacopoeia would have been beyond the reach of all but the wealthy, the flourishing trade in and discussion of materia medica are indications of transregional linkages through trade and migration. Opium, sarsaparilla and China root, noted for the treatment of syphilis from the 16th century, are evidence of intra-Asian and indeed American contact, and such connections may call into question the idea of discrete 'systems' of medicine at the level of practice.

Above
A page of the *Susruta-samhita*, one of the three most important medical compendia of the ayurvedic tradition. The text presents itself as the teachings of the god Dhanvantari to his pupil Susruta. It contains instructions for surgical procedures, including the reconstruction of the nose with skin grafts, or rhinoplasty.

Opposite below
An ayurvedic practitioner takes the pulse of his female patient in this mid-19th century gouache drawing. Systematic pulse examination appears in texts from the 14th century onwards and may be part of the rich fluidity of medical systems in Asia.

Left
Papaver somniferum or the white opium poppy. The inclusion of the juice of this plant in the ayurvedic pharmacopoeia is another example of the interchange of medical products and ideas in the Asian region.

04. HUMOURS & PNEUMAS
The Hippocratic tradition

Vivian Nutton

He knew the cause of every malady,
Were it of hot or cold, of moist or dry,
And where engendered, and of what humour;
He was a very good practitioner.
Chaucer, *The Canterbury Tales*, Prologue, 14th century

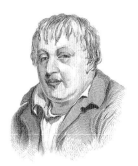 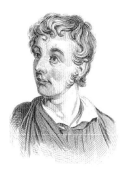 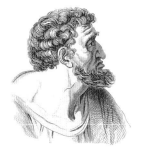 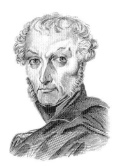

Although many others, including some groups in India [04] and the Babylonians, saw health and disease as a balance or imbalance of bodily fluids, it was the ancient Greeks who developed what Western physicians later called the theory of humours, literally 'juices'.

FROM CLASSICAL GREECE TO GALEN

By 450 BC many Greek authors laid particular stress on bile and phlegm, while others added water, blood and other fluids. Yet others disputed whether bile and phlegm were naturally present in the body or were derived from harmful changes in the blood. Although the theory of the four humours is traditionally ascribed to Hippocrates of Cos (*c.* 460–*c.* 370 BC), it was his son-in-law Polybus who added black bile ('melancholy') to blood, bile and phlegm in his tract *On Human Nature*. He also correlated his four fluids with the four seasons, and with the four elemental qualities – hot, cold, wet and dry – and with four ages. A perfect balance was constantly under threat from variations in climate, seasons, diet, lifestyle and so on, but, armed with this schema, the doctor could predict possible changes and protect against them or bring the patient back to health.

This 'Hippocratic' notion quickly developed other correlations, although it was perhaps the authority of Galen of Pergamum (AD 129–*c.* 216) that established the four humours as the dominant theory among the Greeks. Rather than health being one perfect balance between the humours and the qualities, Galen argued that a slight natural imbalance of one or two humours was not in itself unhealthy, but merely predisposed an individual to diseases of a particular type. Galen's arguments, learning and practical skills convinced many of his contemporaries, and his views were later translated into Syriac, the language of the Christian Near East, and then into Arabic, Hebrew, Armenian and eventually into Latin, to become by 1250 the sole medical theory espoused by the new universities.

Galen was also a philosopher and anatomist. Following one of his heroes, Plato (428–347 BC), he believed that the body depended on three major organs, brain, heart and liver, that communicated with the rest of the body through separate channels, nerves, arteries and veins. Venous blood from the liver, the source of bodily nutriment, was turned in the heart into a mixture of arterial blood and *pneuma* (or spirit), the

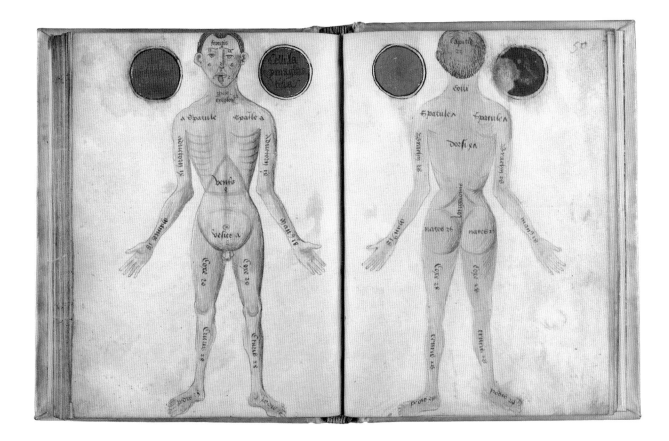

source of what might be termed energy, and this in turn was transformed in an arterial plexus, the *rete mirabile* (an organ not found in humans), into psychic *pneuma*, which was carried in the nerves and which in some way was involved in the processes of thought and sensation.

This strong link between body and mind (or soul) also allowed Galen, and many predecessors going back to the 5th-century BC author of *The Sacred Disease*, to explain human psychology in terms of changes in the humours. An excess of melancholy was considered responsible for both what today might be termed depression and also creative genius; likewise one of blood for both courage and cheerfulness. It was a two-way process. Just as excess drink could lead to obvious changes in behaviour, so anger or fear could have an effect on the body's humoral balance and produce illness.

FROM GALEN TO GALENISM

Galen was never a systematic thinker, and it was his successors in late antique Alexandria and in the Middle East, such as Ibn Sina (Avicenna; see [05]), and his medieval Latin interpreters, who conceived of the body

Above
This mid-15th-century copy of an *Anathomia* ascribed to Galen and translated into Middle English included eight coloured drawings. It is an example of Galenism – the enduring tradition of Galen's codified works passed on through the Islamic translation movement before reappearing in the West first in Latin and then in vernacular languages. These anatomical renditions depict anatomy as expounded by Galen but never illustrated by him. The four circles represent the ventricles in the brain.

Opposite
The four humoral temperaments as depicted in an early 19th-century engraving. From left to right these are lymphatic (phlegm), sanguine (blood), bilious (yellow bile) and nervous (black bile). The dominant humour was thought to shape an individual's appearance, personality and health. Here the influence of the 18th-century knowledge of the solid parts of the body, especially the nerves, has been incorporated into that of the historic bodily fluids.

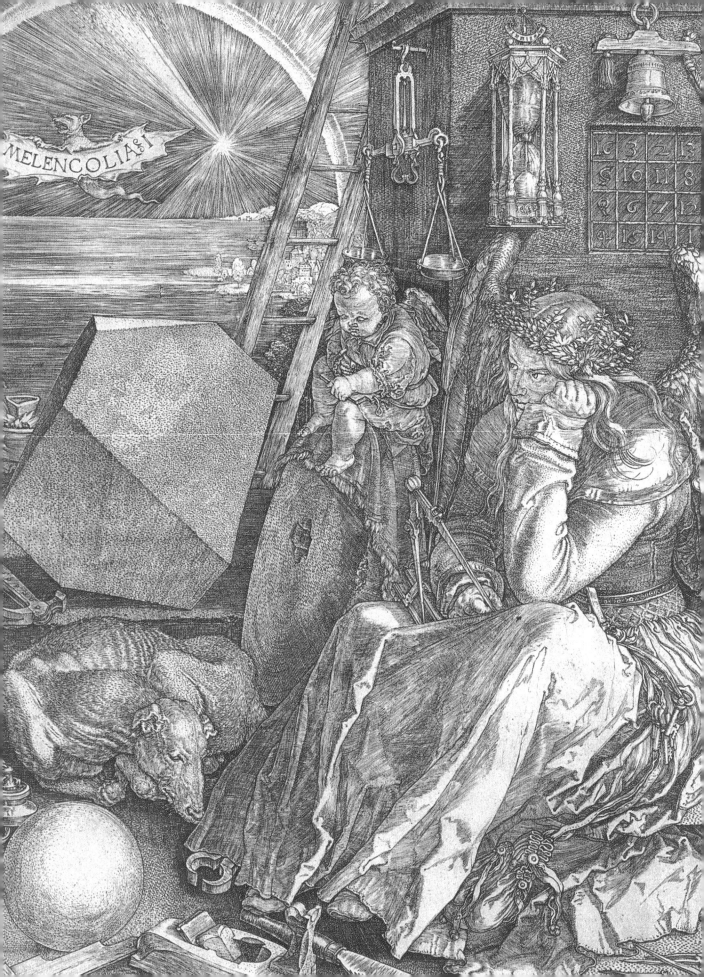

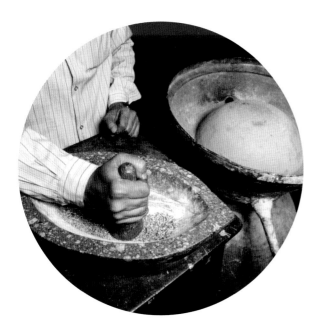

Left
In the pharmacies of yunani hospitals, such as the Nizamia Yunani
Hospital and Medical College in Hyderabad, India, prescriptions for the
patients are prepared daily by pharmacists trained in accordance with
the yunani traditions of the humours and spirits.

Opposite
Albrecht Dürer's *Melancholia* (1514). The despondent winged female
holds a compass and is surrounded by other symbols of the pursuit of
learning, particularly alchemy. Alchemists were given to despondency,
but all students or others who sought knowledge had a tendency to
melancholy.

in terms of three parallel sets of organs and spirits,
and who organized all diagnosis and treatment in terms
of the patient's humoral balance. This schema was
now extended to cover the influence of the stars, and of
musical tones, and allowed the doctor to claim to be able
to prescribe in accordance with the individual nature
of each patient, a selling point for the learned doctor.

Galenism was also made compatible with Christian
(and Aristotelian) belief in a unitary soul by insisting
that the three spirits, psychic, vital and natural, were
merely tools of the single soul. The Renaissance
rediscovery of Galen in the original Greek only
strengthened further the hold of the theory of humours,
which, in some form or other, held sway among Western
learned doctors into the 19th century, despite the major
changes that occurred in the understanding of the
body's anatomy and physiology.

MODERN SURVIVALS

Even in the 20th century, endocrinologists could set
out their theories in terms of an individual's natural
balance that could not easily be detected by mechanical
means. Popular views of illness still talk in terms of
an imbalance brought about by some of the factors that
Galen, and Polybus, had singled out for attention. In the
Islamic world, and particularly in India and Pakistan,
humoral medicine continues to flourish today with
official state support as yunani (i.e. Greek) medicine.
While the notion of spirits survives in yunani medicine,
it has faded entirely from Western medicine, although it
appears as a metaphor in such phrases as 'high spirited'
or 'raising one's spirits'.

By contrast, some modern psychologists have
revived Galenic somaticism as a valid explanation
for child development, and for different psychological
types. In this they are going beyond the notion, familiar
at all levels of society today, of using metaphors derived
from humoralism to describe and explain physical
and mental types. Indeed, it is in discussions of
behaviour and appearance that one meets most often
today such concepts as the phlegmatic or melancholic
temperament, originally a mixture of humours.

05

ISLAMIC MEDICINE
Transmission & innovation

Cristina Álvarez Millán

The Art of Medicine is based on the assessment of practical experience.
Abu Marwan Ibn Zuhr, 12th century

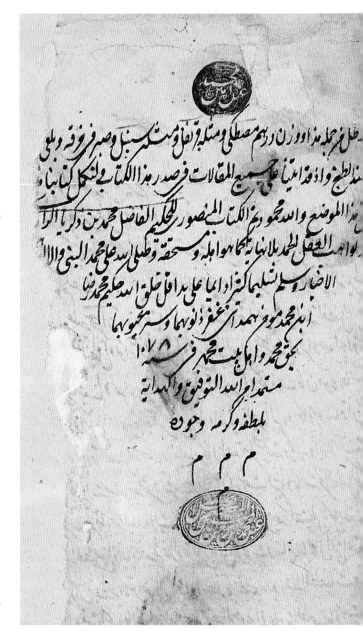

What we conventionally call Islamic or Arabic medicine in fact consists primarily of an elaborate systematization and synthesis of ancient Greco-Roman medical sources. Huge political expansion brought the Islamic empire into contact with philosophical and scientific knowledge from India in the east, through Byzantium to North Africa and Spain in the west. However, although elements from other conquered lands were assimilated, and (more importantly) although scholarly medicine also coexisted with popular and magical practices, it was the Classical and Hellenistic (Greek) medical tradition that set the agenda for later medical theory and practice in medieval Islam. From around AD 750 to 1000, almost all the scientific and philosophical works available throughout the eastern Byzantine empire and the Near East were rendered into Arabic, in an unprecedented programme of translation. Islamic medicine was not developed exclusively by Arab or Muslim physicians, since Jews, Christians and Muslims of diverse ethnic origin also contributed to its development, with Arabic as the *lingua franca*. Nevertheless, the continuity of theories inherited from the Greco-Roman world never ceased to be a driving force.

SYSTEMATIZATION

The concept of disease in scholarly Islamic medicine was based on the Hippocratic–Galenic theory of humours [04]. Anatomical and physiological knowledge likewise mirrored Greco-Roman lore. A major contribution of medieval Islamic medical authors was their bringing together of the dispersed and fragmentary legacy of their predecessors (especially Galen) into a systematic and comprehensive format, so that their efforts in synthesizing and elaborating earlier medical literature resulted in original masterpieces of their own. The most famous and most influential in European medical universities was the *Canon of Medicine* by Ibn Sina (Avicenna; 980–1037).

INNOVATION

Although a number of the discoveries and therapeutic procedures attributed to medieval Islamic physicians now require critical reassessment, Islamic medicine did undoubtedly contribute to clinical developments. The careful observation of symptoms and use of logic both improved knowledge of traditional diseases and also led to the description of new ones. For example, Ibn Masawayh (*c.* 777–*c.* 857) gave details of *pannus*, an eye condition previously unidentified in the available Greek sources. Although already described by Thabit ibn Qurra (*c.* 836–901), it is al-Razi (*c.* 865–*c.* 925) who has traditionally been credited with providing a detailed account of smallpox and measles.

Dissection was not explicitly forbidden in Islam, but seems not to have been practised by medieval Islamic physicians. Nevertheless, intellectual speculation and personal observation did result in anatomical innovations. In an extensive commentary aimed at illuminating some of the obscure points of Ibn Sina's *Canon*, Ibn al-Nafis (*c.* 1213–88) described the lesser or pulmonary circulation of blood for the first time. However, this discovery came about through logical deduction derived from the knowledge of the impenetrability of the cardiac septum. Also, as a consequence of the number of skeletons left by famine in Egypt, 'Abd al-Latif al-Bagdadi (1162–1231) was able to provide an accurate description of the bones of the lower jaw and the sacrum.

While such anatomical contributions passed largely unnoticed, those relating to pharmacology subsequently had major relevance. Greco-Roman pharmacology, mainly from Dioscorides (fl. *c.* 40–80), was expanded with the incorporation of a vast number of new drugs from all around the Islamic world. Substances such as sweet flag, sandalwood, pepper and cloves, camphor, musk, nenuphar (white water lily), sal ammoniac or tamarind, among many others, were incorporated into the pharmacological arsenal. More familiar products such as the orange tree were introduced into Spain, and cotton and sugar cane found their way to the West. A large number of simple and compound medicines entered early European pharmacopoeias, which also inherited Arabic terminology (often of Greek, Indian and Persian origin).

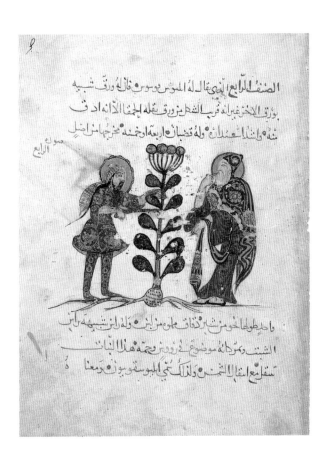

Opposite
Colophon of the *Book for al-Mansur* of al-Razi. Al-Razi (Rhazes) was one of the most influential medieval Islamic physicians and a noted polymath.

Above
A 13th-century translation of Dioscorides' *De Materia Medica*, which formed the original core of the Islamic pharmacopoeia before its expansion with drugs from the growing empire and beyond. Dioscorides (right) collects herbs with his assistant.

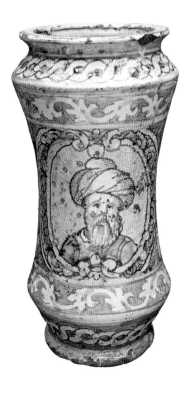

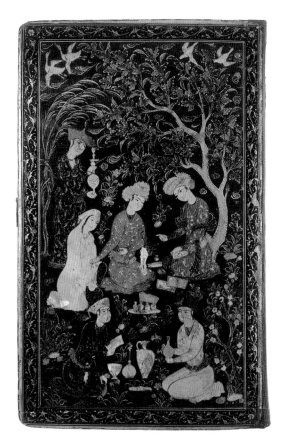

Medieval Islamic physicians also described a number of invasive surgical operations. The most celebrated text is that by the Cordoban surgeon, al-Zahrawi (*c.* 936–*c.* 1013), which had a major impact on Western tradition. It includes copious descriptions and illustrations of a range of traditional surgical instruments, as well as some innovative ones. However, the Islamic surgical material was drawn from Greek sources, and there is little evidence that such operations were performed by learned Islamic doctors. Surgery, it seems, was restricted to bone-setting, blood-letting, cupping, removal of tonsils, circumcision, cautery and the excision of haemorrhoids and growths. No explicit mention of the use of drugs such as opium or henbane as anaesthetics is found in medieval Islamic medical literature, although they do appear in the composition of pharmacological recipes for the treatment of varied conditions.

Noteworthy achievements were the establishment of hospitals (*bimaristan*) and public health regulations against fraudulent practices among pharmacists, surgeons and medical practitioners in the marketplace. General examinations of physicians were also sometimes carried out.

A LASTING LEGACY

The history of Western medicine cannot be fully understood without an appreciation of medieval Islamic medicine. Through its translations, commentaries, summaries, refutations, expansions and reformulations of earlier Greco-Roman sources, Islamic culture preserved the Classical heritage and became its custodian and transmitter to medieval Europe. The Islamic medical tradition also provided the intellectual framework for professional medical practice in western Europe, since through Latin translations it became the source of European philosophical and scientific ideas, from which modern medicine eventually arose.

Although treatises written in the Ottoman period from 1600 onwards included aspects of Western medical knowledge, such as syphilis, the Islamic scholarly medical tradition prevailed. Under the name of yunani ('Greek') medicine, it continues to survive today as a formal medical practice in some Asian countries, notably India and Pakistan, alongside modern Western medicine and the ayurvedic tradition [03].

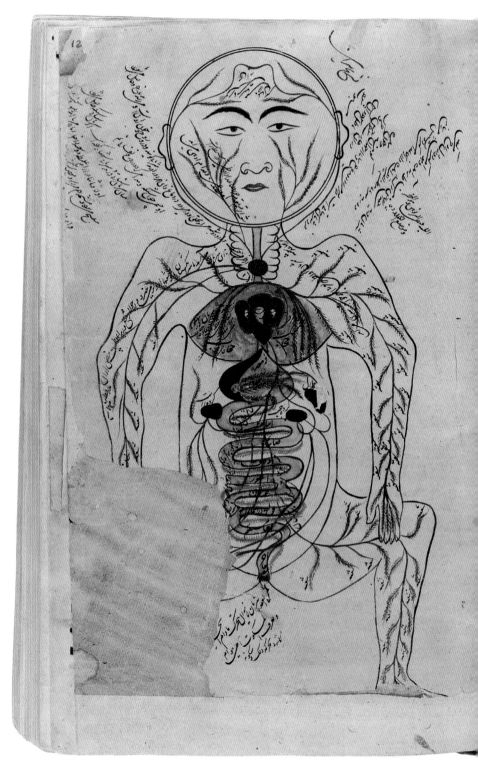

Opposite left
A maiolica stoneware albarello, 1640. Albarelli were the medicinal jars of apothecaries' shops and pharmacies, used for ointments and dry drugs. These jars were brought into Europe from the Middle East and manufactured in Italy from the 15th to 18th centuries.

Opposite right
Persian lacquered binding from an early 17th-century copy of Ibn Sina's *Canon of Medicine*, showing a physician talking to his female patient. This work of Ibn Sina (Avicenna) epitomized the Islamic systematization of medical knowledge and practice.

Above
Drawings of the ventricles and arteries by Tashrih-i Mansuri included in a copy of Ibn Sina's *Canon of Medicine* from 1632. The frog-like pose and highly stylized depiction – based on a reading of a text rather than direct observation from life – are characteristic of early representations of the body.

06

DISSECTING THE BODY
Laying bare the flesh

Simon Chaplin

I think it my duty to entreat you, to dissect as much as you can.
William Hunter, 1784

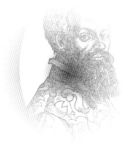

Dissection is the act of physically opening up the
body in order to understand its structures. Between
the 15th century and the mid-19th century, anatomical
dissection of the human body went from being an
occasional and often highly ritualized performance,
limited to a small number of elite practitioners, to a
routine act conducted by many (if not most) doctors at
some stage in their careers. Laid bare in the flesh, on
the page and as anatomical specimens, the dissected
body – a thing simultaneously attractive and repulsive
– became a defining emblem of medical authority.

DISSECTION AS RITUAL

Early modern dissections were as much about
showmanship as scholarship. Conducted in churches
before crowds of onlookers, public dissection not
only celebrated the divine wonder of the body, but
also provided a chance for self-promotion. In Padua,
Andreas Vesalius (1514–64) openly criticized Galen's
anatomical knowledge and in doing so propelled
himself to fame (or infamy, in the eyes of his critics).
In his wake the dissected body became the ground on
which medical battles were fought. Like explorers,

anatomists such as Gabriele Falloppio (1523–62) and
Bartolomeo Eustachi (d. 1574) laid claim to the body's
landmarks.

Within the great universities of Italy, France and the
Low Countries, anatomical dissection was pursued as
a form of philosophical inquiry rather than as an aid to
the physician or surgeon. Its importance was reflected
in the construction of purpose-built anatomical
theatres, such as those in Padua and Leiden (both
completed in 1594). In Britain – where the universities
of Oxford and Cambridge were anatomical backwaters
– it had a more direct application. The surgeon John
Banister (1532/3–99?) conducted dissections at the
Barber-Surgeons' Company in London for audiences
of his peers in the 1580s. In doing so he earned elevation
to the status of physician – one of many anatomists
who climbed up through society on the corpses of
their subjects.

EXPERIMENTAL ANATOMY

By the beginning of the 17th century interest in
dissection had shifted north and east. Leiden,
Amsterdam, Paris and Copenhagen became major

IOANNIS MEVRSI

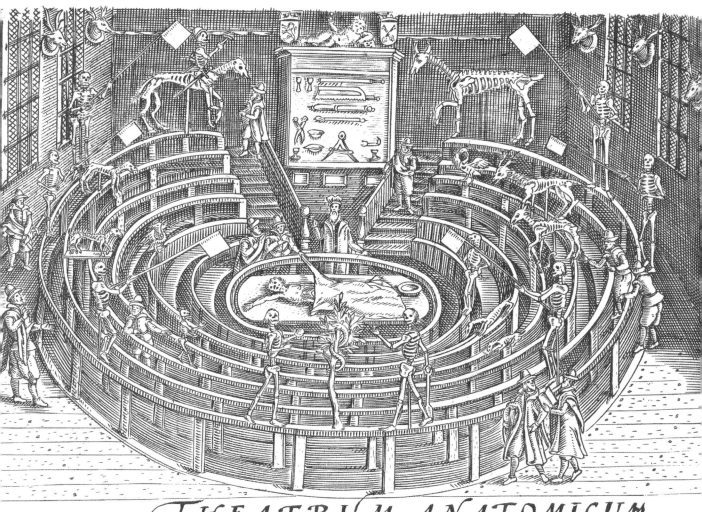

THEATRVM ANATOMICVM.

centres for research. Dissection became a tool of the experimental natural philosopher: a means to understand the body as machine. In London the physician William Harvey (1578–1657) used dissection and vivisection (the dissection of live animals) to develop new insights into the workings of the body, rather than its mere structure. Across the North Sea, Dutch anatomists such as Jan Swammerdam (1637–80) and Frederick Ruysch (1638–1731) pioneered new techniques for injecting and preserving body parts. Using mercury and coloured waxes they traced the path of fine vessels, and kept the evidence of their research as preparations 'put up' in oil of turpentine or alcohol.

Disputes over anatomical science translated into attacks on its methods. The English physician Thomas Sydenham (1624–89) claimed knowledge gained by dissection was 'acquired easily … by men whose wit is limited'. In response, proponents of dissection lambasted the lily-livered and effeminate physicians who could not stomach the sight of blood. Increasingly seen as a secular rather than sacred operation,

dissection became more closely allied with the practice of surgery – the 'cutting trade'.

DIDACTIC DISSECTION

The decline of formal public dissections was accompanied by a rise in the number of dissections carried out not just for research, but for teaching. It was no longer enough to observe an anatomized body: being a good anatomist now meant mastering the practical skills of dissection for oneself. In Paris in the 1720s, surgical students dissected dead patients at the Hôtel-Dieu and the Charité hospitals, and anatomists such as Jacques Winslow and Antoine Ferrein offered 'extramural' dissection classes in private premises. The dissolution of the Barber-Surgeons' Company of London in 1745 coincided with a dramatic increase in the number of hands-on anatomy courses. One of the first to seize the opportunity was William Hunter (1718–83), a Scottish-born and Paris-trained surgeon and man-midwife (like Banister, he too later rose through the ranks to become a physician).

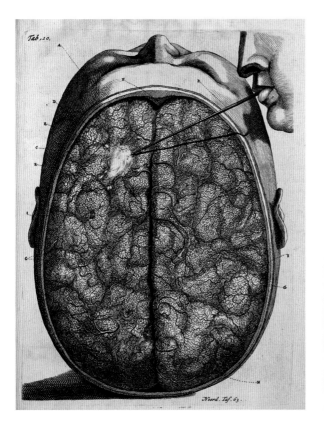

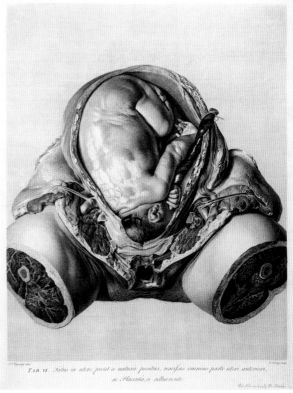

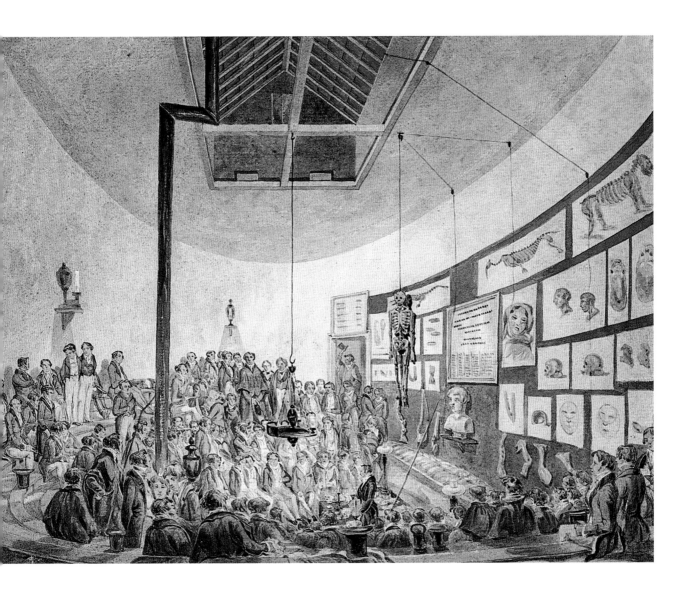

Opposite left
A plate from Frederick Ruysch's *Epistola anatomica* (Anatomical Letters) of 1744, showing his new technique of injecting wax into the blood vessels in the arachnoid and pia mater, the inner two of the three meninges or membranes surrounding the brain.

Opposite right
'The child in the womb, in its natural situation' from William Hunter's *Anatomia uteri humani gravidi* (The Anatomy of the Human Gravid Uterus) of 1774. Hunter's book, with its fine engravings by Jan van Rymsdyk, illustrated the anatomy of pregnancy. A detailed text, prepared before Hunter's death, was subsequently added posthumously in 1794.

Above
Watercolour (by Robert Blemmel Schnebbelie) of an anatomical lecture at the Hunterian Anatomy School, Great Windmill Street, London, 1830. The legacy of John Hunter's interest in comparative anatomy is in evidence on the back wall.

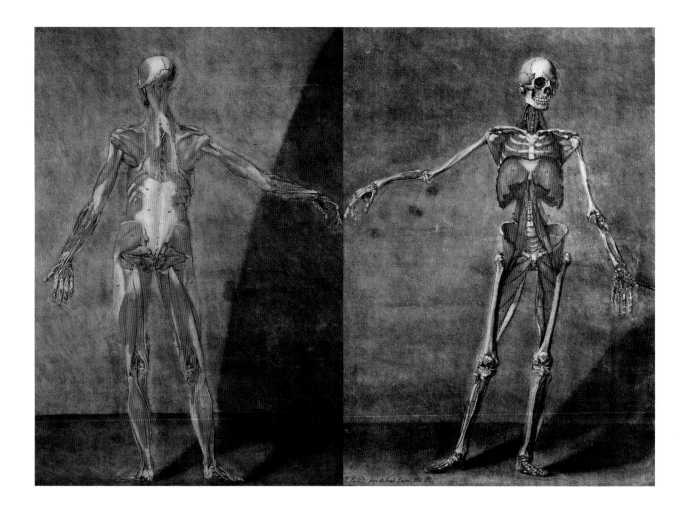

Originally marketed by William Hunter and others as the 'Parisian' method, this kind of teaching became firmly associated with London from the 1750s onwards. By the end of the century it was increasingly common for physicians, as well as surgeons, to take at least one course of anatomical dissections. What they gained was not simply knowledge, but a shared experience. Dissection was physically unpleasant. And, working on decomposing bodies, at constant risk of infection from a carelessly wielded blade, it was also dangerous. To its adherents dissection was not simply a way of learning anatomy, but a process of physical and moral tempering that taught doctors how to ply the knife with confidence and dispassion.

Pupils of the Hunterian schools such as William Shippen Jr (1736–1808) spread the practice across the Atlantic, while in Edinburgh the Monro dynasty and their successors sought to emulate their expatriate brethren. Dissection classes demanded much greater numbers of bodies, and in Britain and America there

Above
'The muscles of the human body, second layer, seen from the back' and 'The muscles of the human body, fourth layer, seen from the front': coloured mezzotints by Arnaud-Éloi Gautier d'Agoty, one of the sons of Jacques Fabien Gautier d'Agoty, who exploited this technique in anatomical depictions. The figures are posed as if in a life class to make this text appealing to artists as well as anatomists.

Opposite
A plate from Jacques Fabien Gautier d'Agoty's *Anatomie des parties de la génération de l'homme et de la femme*, 1773. Of almost the same date as William Hunter's book on the anatomy of pregnancy (see p. 37), it shows the contrasting styles of 18th-century anatomical illustration.

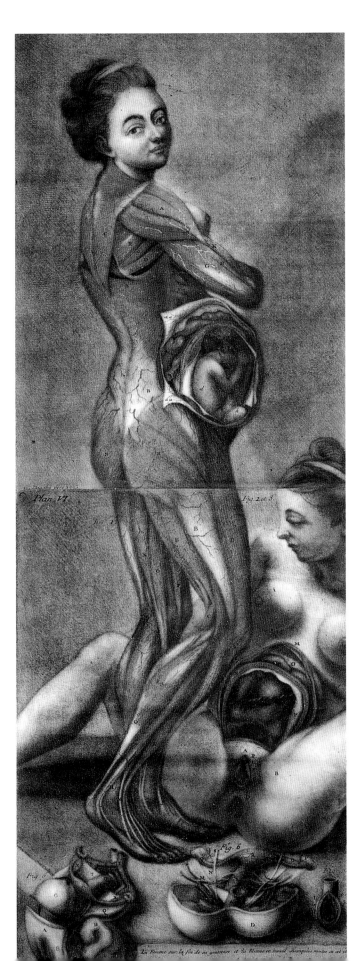

were periodic outcries against the illicit removal of corpses from burial grounds – though for the most part, the authorities appear to have echoed William Hunter's belief in the 'necessary inhumanity' of dissection. The passage of legislation governing the supply of bodies (such as the Massachusetts Anatomy Act of 1831 and the British Anatomy Act of 1832) was both a response to the problem of grave-robbing, and a formal recognition of the importance of anatomical dissection in the medical curriculum.

DISSECTION ILLUSTRATED

Like public dissections, illustrated anatomical atlases were a means of promoting one's work as well as sharing knowledge. They remained a constant presence, from Vesalius's groundbreaking *On the Fabric of the Human Body* (1543), to William Hunter's *Anatomia uteri humani gravidi* (The Anatomy of the Human Gravid Uterus; 1774). These were books designed to impress: hefty folios, painstakingly crafted and, above all, beautifully illustrated. They were also ruinously expensive to produce and to buy.

While physical form and political function remained constant, however, the techniques and style of illustration did not. Woodcuts gave way to engraving and etching. William Chesleden (1688–1752) encouraged his artists to use the camera obscura to make more precise drawings, while in Leiden Bernhard Albinus (1697–1770) worked with Jan Wandelaar to render perspective in minute detail. In Paris, Jacques Fabien Gautier d'Agoty (1717–85) used coloured mezzotints to create a more painterly effect. Allegorical symbolism also gave way to a deliberately spartan, but no less artful, naturalism. If today the illustrations in Hunter's atlas appear more realistic than those of Vesalius, or even of Albinus, it is because we are still accustomed to the idea that science eschews decoration.

The graphic emphasis on the detached, disembodied body part found parallels in a new form of visual representation: the anatomical specimen. William Hunter's brother John (1728–93) amassed over 13,000 specimens of normal, abnormal and comparative anatomy in a purpose-built museum in his home-cum-anatomy school in London. With dissection now conducted behind closed doors, away from the public eye, anatomical museums became a visible reminder of the art of dissection, and its centrality to medical science.

07. PATHOLOGICAL ANATOMY
Cutting the corpse

Malcolm Nicolson

Open up a few corpses: you will dissipate at once the darkness that observation alone could not dissipate.
Marie-François-Xavier Bichat, 1801

ORGAN PATHOLOGY

During the 15th century, the study of anatomy became an important and progressive enterprise [06]. While research generally focused on normal structure, it was inevitable that pathological lesions would occasionally be found and taken note of. Thus in 1557, Andreas Vesalius (1514–64) described aortic aneurysm, explaining the symptoms he had observed in his living patient by reference to the pathological alterations revealed post-mortem. The Genevan physician Théophile Bonet (1620–89) was the first to gather such observations together in a systematic manner, in his *Prodromus anatomiae practicae* (1675) and later in the vast *Sepulchretum* (1679). Bonet undertook dissection himself, but most of the post-mortem accounts in these two books were not his own. A formidable scholar, he had surveyed works by more than 400 authors to compile a total of 2,934 cases in which a structural relationship could be discerned between symptoms complained of in life and pathological lesions revealed after death. An experienced practitioner, Bonet was often able to generalize clinical principles from the individual cases.

In 1707, in Bologna, Giovanni Morgagni (1682–1771), outlined the possibility of basing diagnosis 'on the anatomies of morbid cadavers'. This clinico-pathological project, as it became known, dominated his career, culminating in the publication of his great work, *The Seats and Causes of Diseases Investigated by Anatomy* (1761), in which around 700 post-mortem examinations are described. Morgagni had conducted the majority himself, although he also drew on the investigations of his teacher Antonio Valsalva (1666–1723).

Morgagni's objective was to identify the precise lesion which had produced the symptoms he had

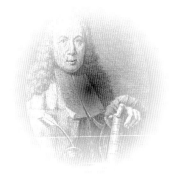

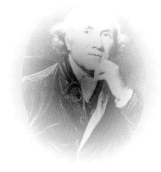

Top
Portrait of Giovanni Morgagni from the frontispiece of his *The Seats and Causes of Diseases* – the only illustration in this massive, erudite text of pathological anatomy, published in 1761.

Above
John Hunter, engraving after a painting by the great 18th-century artist Sir Joshua Reynolds That Hunter should have been the subject of a Reynolds portrait is testimony to his social standing despite being involved in the grisly business of pathological anatomy.

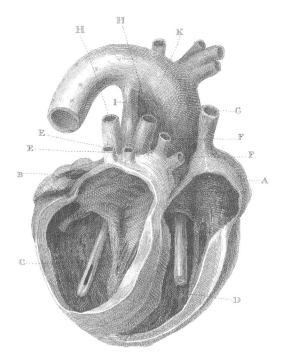

Above
Matthew Baillie brought the study of pathological anatomy to new heights in his *Morbid Anatomy of Some of the Most Important Parts of the Human Body*. A series of engravings helped the reader appreciate the changes he described in the text; here the heart is cut open to reveal the chambers.

Below
Baillie's post-mortem investigation of the author and lexicographer Samuel Johnson (1709–84) revealed the characteristic signs of emphysema in the tissue of the lungs.

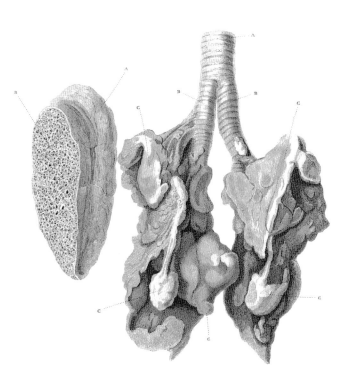

observed in his patients while they were alive. Disorders of all the major organ systems were surveyed in *The Seats*, and many of Morgagni's descriptions were of lasting value. For instance, his demonstration that much intracranial disease originated in the middle ear vividly illustrated the value of an anatomical understanding of disease processes. He also established the validity of Valsalva's observation that stroke lesions impair function on the opposite side of the body. After Morgagni, the importance of pathological anatomy could not be reasonably doubted.

TISSUE PATHOLOGY

In the later 18th century, knowledge of the fine structure of the body in both health and disease considerably improved, and the pathological museum became an essential adjunct to medical research and education. The museum of John Hunter (1728–93) contained almost a thousand diseased human organs, arranged to illustrate not merely the effects of disease, but also the processes of healing and the restoration of function. Hunter insisted that knowledge of pathology could assist the improvement of surgery. In *A Treatise on the Blood, Inflammation and Gunshot Wounds* (1794) he argued that disease processes were best understood not as acting uniformly upon whole organs but rather as affecting particular 'surfaces' or 'textures' – what were later to be termed 'tissues'.

In 1793, Matthew Baillie (1761–1823), Hunter's nephew, published *The Morbid Anatomy of Some of the Most Important Parts of the Human Body*. Baillie was indebted to Morgagni, but was also greatly influenced by his uncle's investigations into human and comparative anatomy. Whereas Morgagni had laboured to record the details of each case he discussed, from initial presentation through clinical treatment to post-mortem appearances, *Morbid Anatomy* provided concise descriptions of the most common pathological alterations of structure.

Baillie's work expressed a novel conception of pathological anatomy as a scientific pursuit in its own right, a form of inquiry that, while relevant to clinical practice, was not wholly encompassed within it. Baillie was sufficiently experienced as a practitioner to be able to distinguish between pathological changes that were clinically significant and structural alterations that were trivial or within normal variation. He could also confidently differentiate between changes that had occurred during life and those that followed death, such

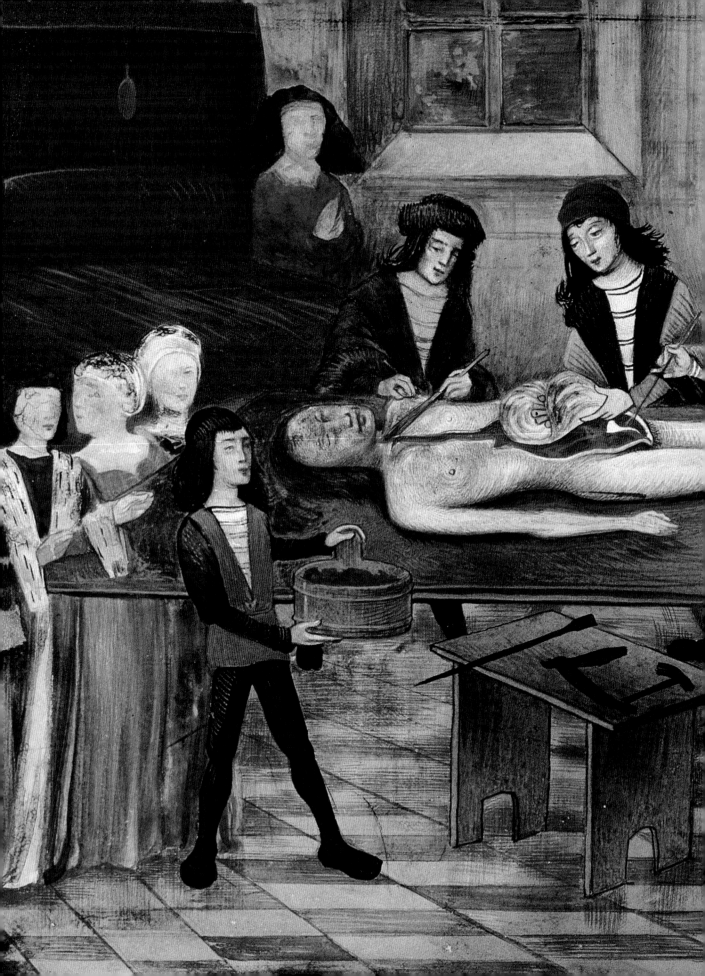

as the formation of large blood clots in the chambers of the heart.

The example set by Hunter and Baillie was taken up in Britain and, even more enthusiastically, in France. In Paris, Marie-François-Xavier Bichat (1771–1802) further developed the tissue theory, making it the basis of a comprehensive conception of disease processes. In France, systematic correlation between ante- and post-mortem observation developed into a routine feature of hospital medicine. This provided an important impetus to physical diagnosis. The invention of the stethoscope [22] by René Laennec (1781–1826) enabled pathological changes in the thoracic organs to be accurately discerned in the living patient. Laennec's major text, *On Mediate Auscultation* (1819), was firmly based on post-mortem dissection and tissue pathology. In Vienna, Carl Rokitansky (1804–78) showed the value of pathologist and clinician working together to improve the understanding of the information about underlying structure that could be gained from the entire living body by skilled physical examination.

CELLULAR PATHOLOGY

The late 19th century saw the microscope [23] systematically applied to pathological phenomena and the development of cellular pathologies. It became possible to characterize disease from small tissue samples (biopsies) taken from living patients. Surgeons began to pause in the course of operations to await the pathologist's opinion on biopsied material, particularly when malignancy was suspected.

Nevertheless, gross, naked-eye, pathology still played a major role in hospital medicine and medical education. In many teaching hospitals, the post-mortem conference, in which a pathologist would open a body in front of an audience of clinicians and students, commenting upon and amending the clinical diagnosis, remained a daily event, well into the 20th century. Doubtless these encounters provided salutary lessons for many a young doctor, an experience they would have shared with Morgagni's students and colleagues.

Opposite
A medieval post-mortem shown in a 15th-century manuscript illustration. Cutting open the body to determine the cause of death might occur when foul play was suspected or early in an epidemic; it is a public event.

Right
A magnified image of a biopsy sample obtained by fine needle aspiration (suction) from a cancerous lymph node in the neck. The patient has metastatic malignant melanoma – a tumour of the melanin-forming cells in the skin, hence the black pigmentation. Such pathological techniques aid diagnosis during life and can assist with assessing the results of treatment.

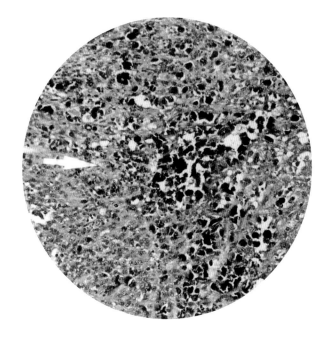

08. CELL THEORY
Units of life

Ariane Dröscher

I could exceedingly plainly perceive [the piece of cork] to be all perforated and porous, much like a Honey-comb, but that the pores of it were not regular; yet it was not unlike a Honey-comb in these particularities.
Robert Hooke, 1665

Robert Hooke's 'little boxes' or cells: cut sections (longitudinal on the left; transverse on the right) of a bottle-cork seen though a microscope, illustrated in Hooke's *Micrographia* (1665) – one of the great books of 17th-century science.

Cell theory was the first synthetic and comprehensive theory of modern life sciences. Its history is intimately linked with the microscope [23], but it was only in the 19th century that cells became central to explanations of physiological and pathological phenomena.

Soon after the invention of the microscope, the 'armed eye' was directed to fine anatomy. Not surprisingly, the first cells were observed in plants, although they were not cells as we think of them today. Rather, the 'cells' and 'little boxes' described by Robert Hooke (1635–1703), the 'bubbles' of Nehemiah Grew (1641–1712) and the 'utriculi' and 'sacculi' of Marcello Malpighi (1628–94) were in fact cell walls enclosing empty holes or spaces filled with juices. Shortly afterwards, single animal cells, namely blood corpuscles and spermatozoa, were independently described by Malpighi, Antoni van Leeuwenhoek (1632–1723) and others; yet no analogy was made between these structures in animals and in plants.

Though often seen and described, it was only in the early 19th century that the cell itself became an object of inquiry. When microscopists began to investigate the embryological origin of tissues, and physiologists started to search for the sites of biochemical action, attention was drawn to internal organization and its dynamics. In 1759 Johann Christian Wolff (1734–94) demonstrated that development starts with an unformed mass of microscopic 'globules'. The first mention of 'cell' in its singular meaning was made in 1792 by physiologist Stefano Gallini (1756–1836). Fifteen years later, Heinrich Friedrich Link (1767–1851) noted a 'double line' between neighbouring cells in the pith of the devil's trumpet plant. This meant that every cell has its own membrane. Another five years passed until Jakob Paul Moldenhawer (1766–1827) succeeded in separating a series of single cells from fresh plant tissues, each of them enclosed by a proper membrane.

THE FIRST UNIFYING CONCEPT OF THE LIFE SCIENCES
The following years saw several conceptualizations of the role of cells for living bodies, but it was the *Zellenlehre* (cytology) of Matthias Jakob Schleiden

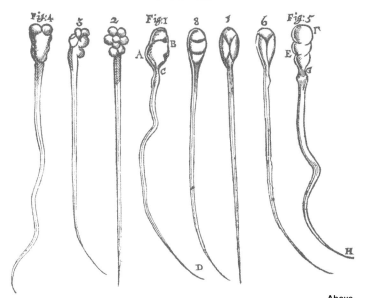

Above
In 1677 the Dutch draper and part-time lens grinder and microscopist Antoni van Leeuwenhoek published these observations of animal cells in the Royal Society of London's journal the *Philosophical Transactions*. On the left are four spermatozoa of rabbits and on the right four from a dog.

Left
Nehemiah Grew's profusely illustrated *The Anatomy of Plants* (1682) included this drawing of a transversely cut vine branch as seen under the microscope, which showed how the cellular structure formed its complex anatomy. However, like Robert Hooke, Grew saw the cell as an empty box – an understanding of its contents would come later.

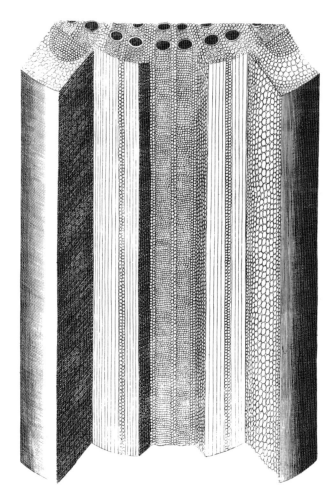

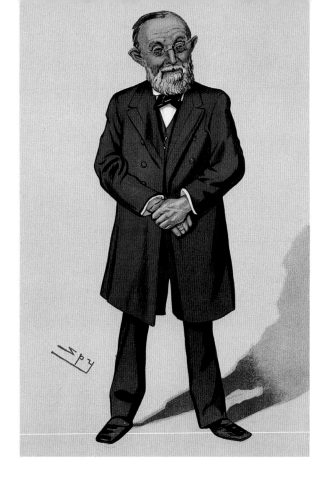

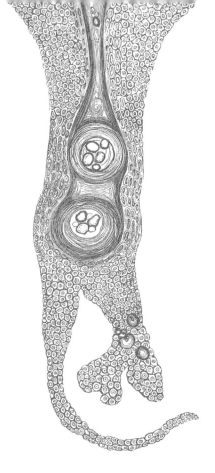

(1804–81) and Theodor Schwann (1810–82), formulated in 1838 and 1839, that received the most attention and support. This directed focus on to the central role of the cell and its nucleus for development, its anatomical and physiological autonomy, and its function as the elementary building block of all living organisms. Within a few years, cell theory developed considerably and its great investigative potential in other fields of biological research was realized. Many scholars made cells the basis of their studies in histology, physiology, embryology, microbiology and even zoological systematics and Darwinism. Based on cell theory, Rudolf Virchow (1821–1902) developed a new concept of pathology in the 1850s, attributing the origin of diseases such as tumours not to the condition of the entire body but to single cells.

In 1836 Robert Brown (1773–1858) had clearly identified the cell nucleus as a general constituent of cells. Jan Evangelista Purkinje (1787–1869) called the rest of the cell's contents 'protoplasm' in 1839. The term, established by Hugo von Mohl (1805–72) in 1846, took the centre stage of cytological inquiry with the declaration in 1861 by Thomas Huxley (1825–95)

that protoplasm was the 'physical basis of life'. In the following decades several cell organelles were distinctly described, including chloroplasts (1883), the part of a plant cell holding the chlorophyll, hence its greenness, where photosynthesis (conversion of sunlight into energy) takes place, and mitochondria (1886), where energy production in animal cells occurs. Chromosomes were first clearly described in 1873 by Anton Schneider (1831–90).

Division as the exclusive process of cell multiplication was clearly stated in the 1840s, mainly by Robert Remak (1815–65) and John Goodsir (1814–67), and definitively established by Virchow's famous aphorism *omnis cellula e cellula* ('all cells from cells'). In 1883 Édouard van Beneden (1846–1910) unveiled the stages of chromosome change during cell division.

THE CRISIS AND THE RENAISSANCE OF CELL STUDIES
However, around the middle of the 20th century the idea of the cell as the essential key for the explanation of vital phenomena suffered a crisis. Though the study of cells went on apace, cutting-edge research now shifted to

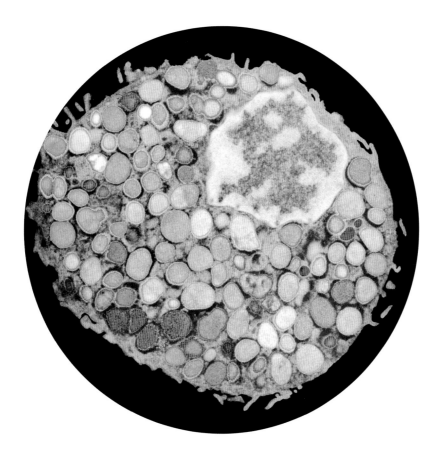

the subcellular level. For most biochemists, geneticists and molecular biologists now, the secret of life was to be revealed by investigating the molecular mechanisms.

In the 1940s a procedure called differential centrifugation was introduced, which separates the different cell contents according to their size and density. By purifying the single extracts, it was now possible to analyse the exact chemical composition of the organelles. Independently, from the early 1950s, with the new fixative of George Palade (1912–2008), the electron microscope began to penetrate into the ultrastructure of the cell.

Three fundamental concepts of the structure and function of membranes had been introduced in 1895 by Ernest Overton (1865–1933), but his contribution was appreciated only decades later when electron micrographs revealed a surprising abundance of membranes inside the cell. Soon, the cell was reconceived as a complex system of inner and outer membranes. In 1961 Peter Mitchell (1920–92) succeeded in localizing steps of the synthesis of ATP (adenosine triphosphate; see p. 51) – the production of the cell's most important source of chemical energy

– within the membranes of mitochondria, thus linking biochemical and structural research. From the 1980s molecular biologists became increasingly aware of the necessity to broaden their view to look at cell processes dynamically and three-dimensionally, and to focus on the interrelationships and more complex pathways of information and membrane traffic between different cell regions. All this converged into the renaissance in cell studies under the auspices of cell biology.

Opposite left
Rudolf Virchow was one of the great 19th-century exponents of cell theory. He joined an elite group of celebrities caricatured by 'Spy' (Sir Leslie Ward) in the magazine *Vanity Fair* in 1893.

Opposite right
An illustration of a carcinoma of the skin (at the cellular level) from Virchow's landmark publication *Cellular Pathology*, published in German in 1858 and translated into English in 1859.

Above
A colour-enhanced transmission electron micrograph of a mast cell, full of histamine granules (pink). The cell's nucleus is the large structure to the top right. Mast cells are part of the immune system and play an important role in allergy; histamine triggers the inflammatory response.

09. NEURON THEORY
The last cellular frontier

Ariane Dröscher

Thus a nerve-element exists (a 'nerve-unit' or 'neuron', as I have decided to name it).
Wilhelm von Waldeyer-Hartz, 1891

Although great advances had been made in cell theory [08], the question of whether the brain and nervous system were also composed of cells and how they related to each other remained uncertain. The brain, because of its softness, fragility and great structural complexity, was long precluded from fine anatomical analysis. It was not before the late 1880s that investigations paved the way for neuron theory and modern neuroscience.

THE RETICULAR THEORY
Significant pioneering observations in the study of nerve cells were made in the 1830s by Jan Evangelista Purkinje (1787–1869), and then in the 1860s by Otto Friedrich Karl Deiters (1834–63), who applied his microdissection technique. However, it was still impossible to distinguish clearly and correlate all the parts of the nerve cell: the cell body; the fibres, named axons in 1896; and the branching prolongations, called dendrites in 1889. Therefore, some of the leading neuroanatomists of the day advocated the reticular theory of the nervous system, which proposed that it was a continuous network of nerve cells. Albert von Koelliker (1817–1905) and Joseph von Gerlach (1820–96), for example, put forward the view that nerves were fused and thus formed an anatomical and functional continuum throughout the body.

THE 'BLACK REACTION'
A radical shift in theory came about by accident. In 1873, while experimenting with several staining and fixing solutions in the kitchen of his apartment in a hospital near Milan, Camillo Golgi (1843–1926) unintentionally poured some silver nitrate on brain tissue previously fixed with potassium dichromate. Before throwing it away he examined it under the microscope and to his

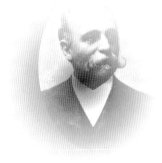

Above
A photograph of Camillo Golgi, who developed the important neurohistological staining technique known as the 'black reaction'.

Below
One of Santiago Ramón y Cajal's drawings of individual nerve cells, showing the cell body, axon and dendrites.

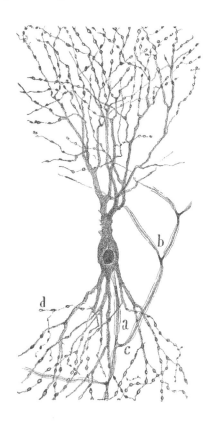

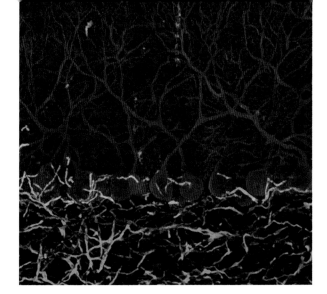

Above
Purkinje cells (shown in red) in the cerebellum, the part of the brain located at the back of the skull in vertebrates which is responsible for voluntary movements, motor skills, such as riding a bicycle, and orientation. Purkinje cells send out vast numbers of branches connecting to other cells in the cerebellum.

Below
A sensory neuron from an adult dorsal root ganglion (the part of the nervous system that communicates with the nerves in the spinal cord). This cell is growing in a culture dish in the presence of Nerve Growth Factor (a protein which sustains the cell *in vivo*) and stained with a fluorescent dye so it is visible with a special fluorescence microscope.

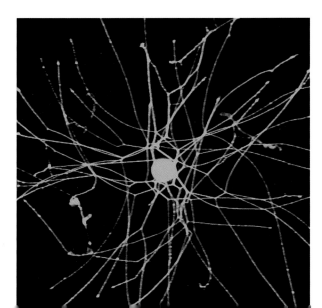

astonishment realized that the 'black reaction' had caused a precipitation that blackened a small number of nerve cells in their entirety, while others were completely spared. In this way it was finally possible to observe their silhouettes, with all their complex ramifications, and their position within the tissue. In the following years, Golgi published several important works on neurohistology. Although he discarded Gerlach's idea of fused dendrites, he did support the idea of a continuous axon network, which he identified as the transmitter of communication.

THE NEURON THEORY

In the late 1880s, Golgi's impregnation method became widely known and undermined the reticular theory. Embryologist Wilhelm His (1831–1904) and psychiatrist August Forel (1848–1931) conceived the nerve cell body and its prolongations as forming an independent unit. The strongest evidence came from the artistically gifted Spanish neurologist Santiago Ramón y Cajal (1852–1934), who slightly modified the Golgi technique in order to obtain more detailed images. Cajal systematically studied the nervous tissue of numerous different animal species, arriving at the idea of the individuality of nerve cells. Moreover, with Arthur von Gehuchten (1861–1914), he formulated the law of dynamic polarization, according to which information flows in one direction from the dendrites through the cell body to the axons. In 1906 he shared the Nobel Prize with Golgi.

Finally, anatomist Wilhelm von Waldeyer-Hartz (1836–1921) made these descriptions compatible with cell theory, and, in 1891, coined the term 'neuron' for nerve cells (from the Greek for 'sinew' or 'tendon'). Six years later Sir Charles Sherrington (1857–1952) proposed the concept of the synapse (the junction between two neurons), explaining how neighbouring neurons, though separated by a gap, can transmit the impulses (see also p. 210).

By 1900 the classic neuron theory was completed. Today, however, many exceptions are known, showing that the nervous system is anatomically and functionally more complex and diverse than previously thought. Moreover, the electron microscope has revealed that nerve cells use not just chemical synapses, but also electrical ones.

10. MOLECULES
The chemistry of life

David Weatherall

A living organism is nothing but a wonderful machine.
Claude Bernard, 1865

Despite having roots in many different fields, biochemistry – the chemistry of living organisms – was recognized as a scientific discipline only in the early 20th century. From the time of the ancient Egyptians and Greeks until the 16th century it was believed that the primary constituents of the world were air, water, earth and fire, and that health and disease reflected the balance or imbalance of the four humours constituting our bodies [04]. Paracelsus (1493–1541) rejected this view in the 16th century and, influenced by alchemy, suggested that living organisms do not just resemble the universe, but are composed of the same materials, thus stressing the importance of chemistry for understanding both normal and abnormal biological function.

During the next three centuries, though dogged by the argument that the life force is a separate entity designed by a divine being and hence not amenable to chemical exploration, the field continued to evolve. By the end of the 18th century, Antoine Lavoisier (1743–94) and Joseph Priestley (1733–1804) had demonstrated the importance of oxygen and its interactions with carbon in releasing energy. Some basic constituents of nutrients were identified and, from studies of yeast, enzymes – chemicals that can control various reactions without themselves being changed – were discovered. In the 19th century the recognition of the cell's central role in all biological systems [08], and the formulation by Claude Bernard (1813–78) of the key importance of the constancy of an organism's internal environment [13], profoundly influenced the development of physiology and biochemistry.

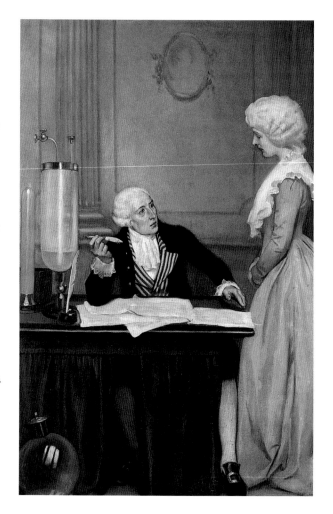

Above right
A painting of Antoine Lavoisier and his wife and assistant Marie-Anne Pierrette Paulze, by Ernest Board; she learned English, which Lavoisier did not read, and, as a fine draftsman and engraver, illustrated his texts.

Opposite left
The frontispiece from Joseph Priestley's *Experiments and Observations on Different Kinds of Air* (1775), illustrating the work discussed in the book on the importance of oxygen.

Opposite right
Linus Pauling was one of several people working on an understanding of the structure of DNA. He suggested a triple helix, but it was Watson and Crick's double helix that proved to be correct.

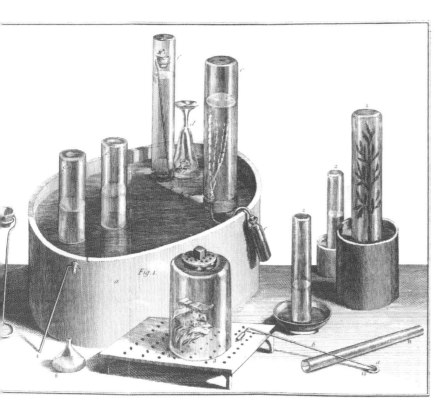

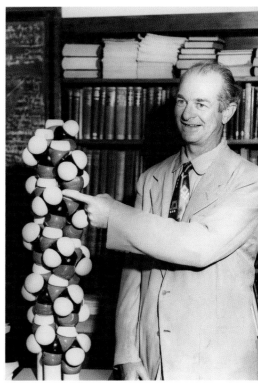

BIOCHEMISTRY: 'A UNITARY SCIENCE'

At the beginning of the 20th century, biochemistry evolved in many different directions. It was found that energy transfer is mediated by compounds, including adenosine triphosphate (ATP), either by mitochondria – 'factories in cells' – or through a related variety of enzyme-controlled pathways, some of which degrade molecules like sugars, fats and amino acids with the formation of ATP, while others synthesize vital agents such as glucose, glycogen, fats and proteins.

The unravelling of these complex pathways (such as the Krebs cycle, named after its discoverer, Hans Krebs (1900–81)), was later to have an important impact on many branches of medicine. For example, between 1920 and 1935 Otto Warburg (1883–1970), Gustav Embden (1874–1933) and Otto Meyerhof (1884–1951) described every step by which glucose is metabolized in the red blood cell, and how these pathways both yield energy and provide fail-safe mechanisms that protect the cell against damage from the by-products of its chemical factory. Later, defects of the enzymes involved were found to be the cause of many different forms of inherited anaemia.

THE STRUCTURE AND FUNCTION OF PROTEINS

Spectacular progress during the 19th century also followed the discovery of the structure of proteins, how they function and how their production is regulated. Emil Fischer (1852–1919) found that proteins are made up of strings of amino acids, later called peptide chains. Remarkably, there are only about 20 amino acids, which are shared by all living organisms, and the differences in the properties of individual proteins reflect the order in which they exist in their constituent chains.

In the 1930s Linus Pauling (1901–94) and others characterized the chemical bonds and configuration of the peptide chains responsible for protein structure, and X-ray defraction studies enabled it to be analysed in three dimensions. In the early 1950s Frederick Sanger (1918–) described the structure of insulin [65] and Max Perutz (1914–2002) that of haemoglobin; both won Nobel Prizes. It was Pauling again, with others, who in 1949 reported that an inherited form of anaemia – sickle cell disease – which affects thousands of patients worldwide, results from a structural change in haemoglobin. Many other haemoglobin variants associated with different forms of anaemia or other

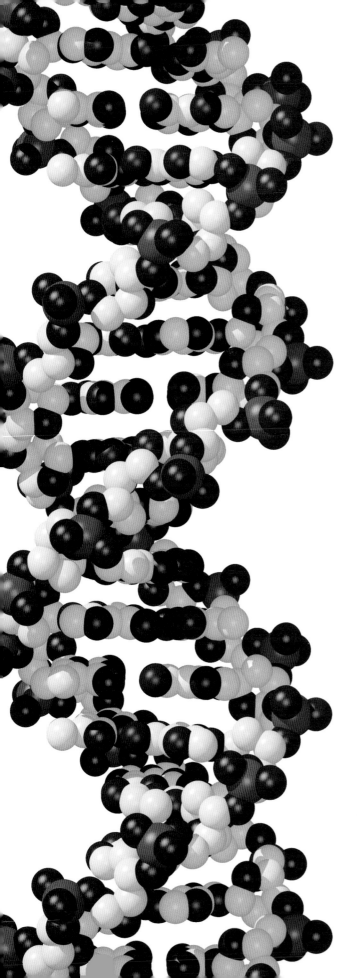

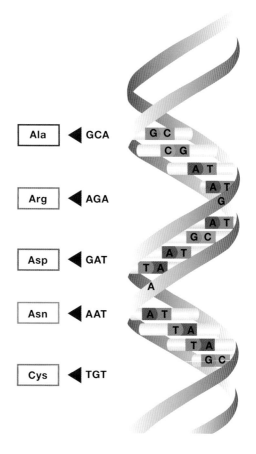

Ala	◀ GCA
Arg	◀ AGA
Asp	◀ GAT
Asn	◀ AAT
Cys	◀ TGT

Left
The DNA double helix in a model of a short length of a DNA molecule, approximately 12 base pairs in length. The oxygen atoms are shown in red, nitrogen in blue, phosphorus in purple and carbon in white. In life DNA can be millions of base pairs long.

Above
DNA is a double helix consisting of two chains of the four bases – adenine (A), guanine (G), cytosine (C) and thymine (T) – wrapped round each other. Because of the rules of base pairing, A always pairs with T and C with G. The bases form the rungs of the double helix. Each amino acid (left column) is produced from a sequence of three bases or codons (middle column). Individual amino acids combine to form proteins.

Opposite left
Francis Crick's pencil sketch of the DNA double helix from 1953, the year he and Watson announced their discovery. It shows a right-handed helix and the nucleotide bases of the two-anti parallel strands.

Opposite right
Another sketch (dated 19 January 1954) by Francis Crick, from his notebook, as he continued to work further on DNA. He eventually decoded the genetic or triplet code with colleagues.

clinical disorders were subsequently discovered, and numerous abnormalities of enzyme structure were found to be the basis for different inherited diseases.

During the 20th century biochemistry also made major contributions to other disciplines, for instance in nutrition the discovery and characterization of vitamins [64], and in endocrinology [17] the structure and function of hormones. And it also helped to explain the wide range of metabolic abnormalities in diseases ranging from diabetes [65] to renal failure.

DNA AND MOLECULAR BIOLOGY

The related science of genetics [19] evolved alongside biochemistry. Work on fruitflies and other organisms showed how genes can mutate, and suggested that there is a direct relationship between a gene and the structure of an enzyme. It was originally thought that genetic information was passed from person to person and cell to cell by particular proteins, but in 1944 Oswald Avery (1877–1955) and others proved that the genetic material is nucleic acid, first discovered by Friedrich Miescher (1844–95) in 1869. One form – DNA (deoxyribonucleic acid) – consists of a sugar, deoxyribose, combined with four bases.

In 1953 James Watson (1928–) and Francis Crick (1916–2004) described its structure: a double helix consisting of two chains of the four bases wrapped round each other. When the two strands come apart during cell division, each acts as a template for the synthesis of an identical DNA molecule – it is a self-replicator. It was later discovered that the order of these bases is responsible for the order of amino acids in individual peptide chains; that is, DNA carries genes, various lengths of bases that code for the precise structure of every protein. Using technology developed from what was now called molecular biology, the mechanism and control of protein synthesis was subsequently described, the cause of numerous genetic diseases determined, and a start made in analysing diseases such as cancer at the molecular level.

WHAT HAPPENS NEXT?

In little over a hundred years our understanding of the chemistry of life has moved from physiological chemistry, through biochemistry to molecular biology, with important developments for medical practice at each stage. The big question for the 21st century is what will be the next discipline that integrates the extreme complexities unearthed by the study of living processes at the chemical and molecular level, and tells us more precisely why we are what we are, both in health and disease.

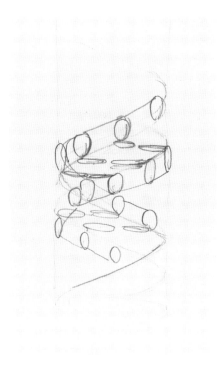

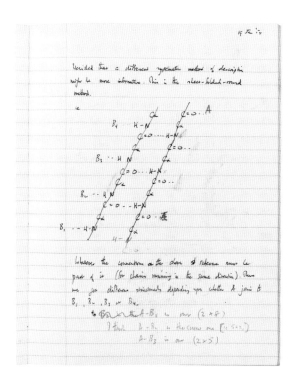

Understanding
HEALTH & *Disease*

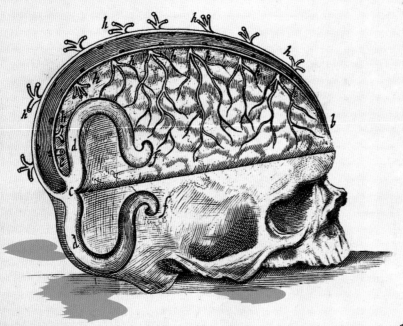

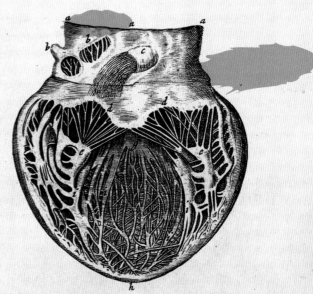

Nº 2.

In all cultures, the notion of disease (dis-ease) presupposes one of health. We hardly notice health; only when something is wrong do we become aware that things were formerly right. It is this logic that orders the education of doctors: they first learn about the normal, about how bodies function, before they study the abnormal, about how bodies become diseased.

This section explores how the normal/abnormal continuum has been formulated within Western societies. Sometimes the focus is almost exclusively on the normal: the circulation of the blood is so 'natural' to our way of thinking that it is hard to imagine that alternative explanations of the heart's role persisted for 2,000 years after Hippocrates. Formulations of body regulation (the *milieu intérieur* in Claude Bernard's phrase) and of hormones came even later; both expressed truths about how the body operates, guessed at by earlier doctors. Our modern understandings rely on a central pillar of health and disease – the range of the normal and pathological.

Such a notion of ranges and averages bears little resemblance to the way of thinking about disease that underlay the germ theory. This fundamental discovery of medical science offered a new conception of disease: as an invasion, or something external to the body itself. Germs encouraged doctors to separate the patient and his or her illness and to see disease as a battle. Warfare imagery has a long history ('fighting for one's life', 'struggling against disease'), but 'germs' encouraged doctors to understand the ways in which our bodies cope with the reality of nasty invading organisms – bacteria, viruses, worms. The nuances of infections, their spread and the body's coping mechanisms are further explored in the discussions of parasites and immunology. The body can also turn against itself and employ the benefits of the immune system in a negative way.

Modern understanding of why different people respond differently to similar kinds of disease challenges often falls back on our individual genetic makeup. The 'genome' is big news nowadays, as a new gene associated with some particular disease or disorder is regularly announced. We remain at the beginning of the 'genetic revolution', and it still promises more than it can currently deliver. But there is no doubt that the medicine of the future will be more intimately informed by personal genetic considerations. So, it seems certain, will our understanding of cancer and its evolution. Cancer has become one of the major fears of modernity, and both its prevention and treatment are high on medicine's contemporary agenda.

Psychiatry has been described as 50 per cent of medicine. What this means is that a large number of visits to the doctor have causes that can be called 'mental': feeling down, sleeping badly, unexplained pains, tiredness and anxiety. To these can also be added more dramatic symptoms – hearing voices, feelings of paranoia or grossly confused thinking. The talking cures can treat the less severe ('neurotic') cluster of symptoms. More seriously disturbed individuals ('psychotic') who pose a threat to themselves or others have generally been confined in special hospitals, of which 'Bedlam' was the most famous.

Alternative ways of understanding health and disease are also widespread in the West. Homeopathy, chiropractic, osteopathy and naturopathy are described today as 'complementary', and they have many adherents.

Two illustrations (blood vessels in the head and the heart's interior structure) from Richard Lower's *Tractatus de corde* (A Treatise on the Heart) of 1669. Lower extended William Harvey's work on the circulation of the blood – such basic knowledge of how the body functioned was crucial to understanding health and disease.

11. CIRCULATION
What goes round comes round

John Ford

The motion of the heart was only to be comprehended by God.
William Harvey, 1628

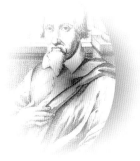

Above
Michael Servetus was one of a group of Renaissance thinkers
and investigators who questioned ancient ideas about how the blood
moved in the body.

Right
William Harvey, who proposed that blood circulates through the body
pumped by the heart, is seen here dissecting the body of Thomas Parr,
who was reputedly 152 years old at his death.

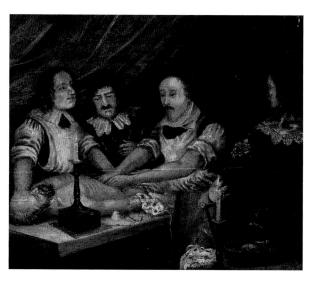

The idea that the heart is a pump propelling blood
through the body in a circular motion is a relatively
new concept. Throughout antiquity, blood was seen as
a nourishing humour [04]. Some theories held that it
contained a life-giving *pneuma*. Galen (AD 129–*c.* 216),
who was a prolific dissector of animals, proposed that
blood was produced, or 'concocted', in the liver and
moved through the body in a tidal fashion to the organs
which it nourished. According to this theory, the blood
was split into two streams: one went to the lungs, where
it was mixed with air; the other flowed through holes
in the septum dividing the ventricles of the heart in
half, and from there it was moved through the main
arteries of the body by the expansion of the heart and
blood vessels until it was consumed at the periphery.
The heart was thus not recognized as having a motive
power. This was the dogma of the Middle Ages.

THE PUZZLE OF THE PULSE
During the Renaissance ancient concepts were
questioned. People wondered about the nature of the
pulse, which they had felt in health and disease for
centuries, and they had noticed that blood spurted from
arterial wounds in a way different from the sluggish
flow when a vein was punctured. Michael Servetus
(1509–53) proposed a circulation from the right side
of the heart to the left through the lungs, which was
reiterated by Matteo Colombo (1516–59), who showed
that there were no holes in the heart's interventricular
septum. So Galen's views were not accurate.

In Padua, Andreas Vesalius (1514–64) performed
precise human dissections whose results he published
with elegant illustrations in 1543 [06]. Fabricius ab
Aquapendente (1537–1619) showed that veins had
one-way valves that allowed venous blood to flow only
towards the heart. In spite of knowing the accurate

anatomy of the heart and blood vessels, however, he did not proceed to a theory of circulation.

THE HEART AS PUMP

William Harvey (1578–1657) was a pupil of Fabricius in Padua from 1600 to 1602, and when he returned home, in addition to setting up practice in London, he continued his study of the heart with regular animal dissections. By 1619 he had a clear idea of the concept of circulation of the blood powered by the heart, but he continued his experiments to accumulate further evidence. This delayed publication of his treatise

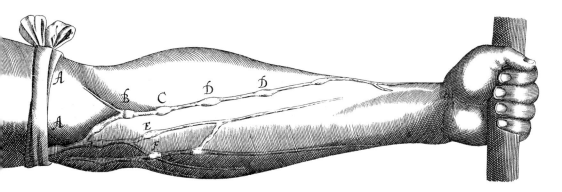

Above and below
Harvey relied upon both experiment and logical deduction in framing his theory of the circulation of the blood. In these illustrations from his 1628 treatise he demonstrated (above) how if a tourniquet is applied to the upper arm the circulation is impeded and no further blood enters or leaves this part of the blood system, and (below) how the valves in the veins allow the blood to move only towards the heart.

De motu cordis et sanguinis in animalibus (Concerning the Motion of the Heart and Blood in Animals) until 1628. His radical proposal was that the heart was the most important organ for the blood rather then the liver, and that it acted as a pump that circulated blood round the body: out through the arteries and back through the veins. Harvey dedicated the book to King Charles I, likening the heart to the king as 'the fountain whence all grace, all power doth flow'. As a royal physician and ardent royalist supporter during the English Civil

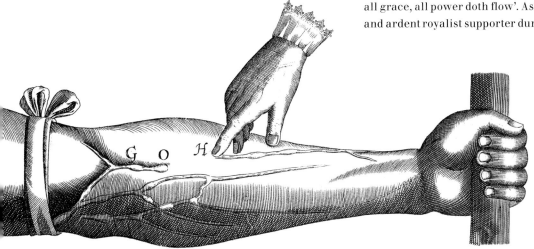

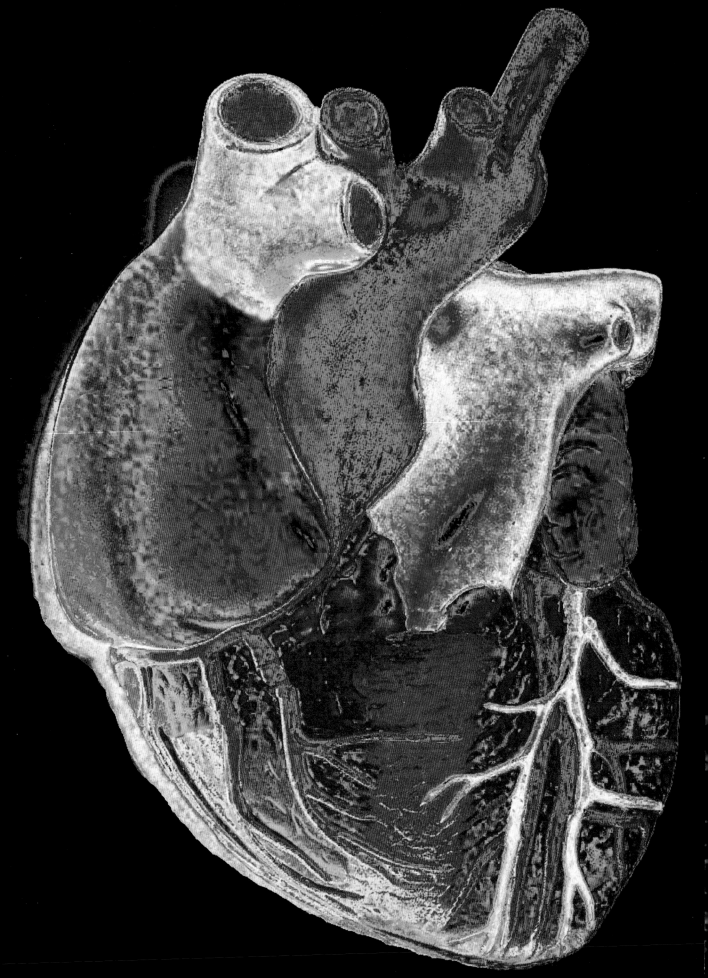

War, he had access to the court and demonstrated his findings before the king.

Harvey's experiments had shown that each ventricle held 2 ounces (56.7 g) of blood and that the heart beat roughly 72 times a minute. Therefore in an hour the heart would eject 8,640 ounces (244.9 kg), or about three times the weight of an average man, into the arteries. No liver could produce that amount of blood so quickly, nor could the periphery dissipate it at that speed. The only conclusion that Harvey could draw was that a constant volume of blood circulated out from the heart into the arteries and returned through the one-way valves in the veins. Unfortunately, he was unable to see where the two systems met. This was not understood until Marcello Malpighi (1628–94), using a microscope, demonstrated the peripheral capillaries in lung tissue in 1661 [23]. Although Harvey had demonstrated the circulation, he had little idea of its significance, writing that 'whether for the sake of nourishment or for the communication of heat is not certain'.

ESSENTIAL TO LIFE

The relevance of blood passing through the lesser circulation of the lungs was demonstrated by the experiments of Richard Lower (1631–91) and Robert Hooke (1635–1703). They showed that dark red venous blood entered the lungs from the right side of the heart and left them coloured bright red, just like that in the arteries, but they did not appreciate why. It was not recognized until the next century that the change of colour was produced by oxygenation of the blood in the lungs, which was then carried to the periphery. Oxygenated blood is essential for human metabolism.

In spite of Harvey's clear logical exposition of his experimental results and the conclusions that he had drawn from them, the concept of the circulation was not universally accepted for several years. In particular, the reactionary medical school in Paris, led by Jean Riolan (1580–1657), held to the Galenic ideas, and in spite of having many followers in England, Harvey complained that his medical practice declined.

However, others were looking at the mechanics of the circulatory system. Stephen Hales (1677–1761) connected a glass tube to a horse's artery and was able to measure the pressure in it [27], as well as estimate the volume of the capacity of the heart and the velocity of the blood. John Floyer (1649–1743) designed a watch with which to count the pulse and René Laennec (1781–1826) started listening to the heart sounds with his newly invented stethoscope in 1819 [22].

As the heart is now identified as a pump and the circulation of the blood as essential to life, it is not surprising that the 20th century saw the development of artificial hearts. Heart–lung machines are used to support the circulation temporarily during cardiac operations and work has been done on designing artificial hearts for use when the human one fails [59].

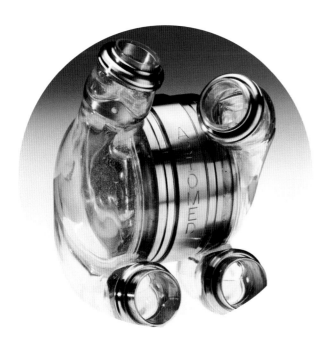

Opposite
A digitally enhanced image of a model human heart; this vital organ retains its hold on our imagination.

Left
An artificial heart: external machines that pump the blood around the body were developed in the mid-20th century, greatly facilitating heart surgery. An implantable artificial heart, other than those used temporarily to keep patients alive before a transplant organ becomes available, remains beyond reach.

12. **BEDLAM & BEYOND**
Confining the mad

Andrew Scull

Madmen appear to have been employed to torment other
madmen, in most of the places intended for their relief.
Samuel Tuke, 1813

THE ANCIEN RÉGIME

Bethlem Hospital, or Bedlam, in London, has long
been the most famous mental hospital in the English-
speaking world. From the 14th century to the late 17th
century, it was almost the only institution in England
specializing in the care of the mentally ill. As part of
the later commercialization of English society, other
'madhouses' began to appear, as growing affluence
permitted families to pay others to cope with the
troubles and difficulties serious mental illness brought
in its train. In the 18th century, this so-called trade
in lunacy expanded, and in England, as well as in
Europe and in North America, other asylums were
founded, often on a charitable basis. Many of these
establishments enjoyed a bleak reputation, their high
walls, barred windows and secrecy arousing suspicion
about the treatment being meted out to their inmates.

In truth, many patients were chained up and often
treated with cruelty or indifference, with 'therapy'
largely consisting of the routine bleedings, vomits,
purges and lowering diets with which 18th-century
medicine treated many kinds of disease. However,
the growing number of asylums, and their lax

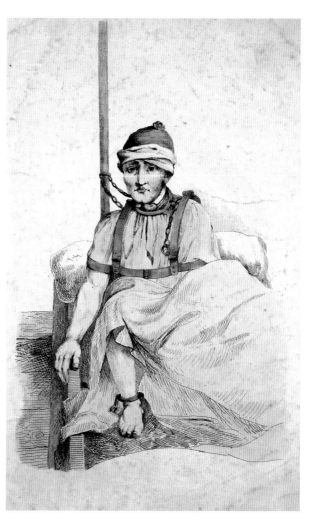

Above
James Norris, an American marine, was obliged to endure his
confinement in Bethlem in an iron harness chained to a post. Relief
of sorts came from reading and petting one of the asylum's many cats;
coloured etching by G. Arnald, 1815.

Opposite
In the 18th century, William Hogarth's 'Rake' ended his dissolute life
incarcerated in Bethlem. The inmates are 'performing' for the wealthy
voyeurs who come to gape at those who have lost their reason.

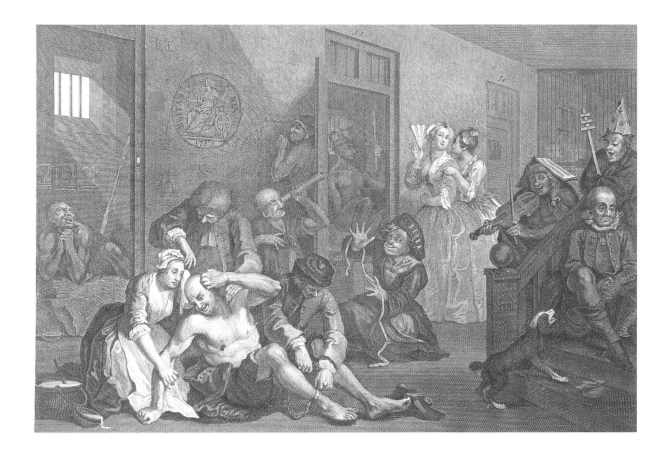

regulation, did encourage some degree of therapeutic experimentation, and the new institutions provided a social space within which some madhouse keepers – laymen and medical men alike – could develop experience in both handling the mad and applying empirically based treatments for improving their behaviours and mental states.

THE RISE OF MORAL TREATMENT

Almost simultaneously, and apparently independently, in France, England and Italy, a new approach to the management of mental illness began to appear in the late 18th century. Its proponents dubbed it 'moral treatment' to distinguish it from the more traditional medical regime of bleeding and purging. Indeed, this generation of asylum superintendents began to exhibit great scepticism, and often outright hostility, to the application of traditional 'heroic' medicine to the treatment of the mentally ill. Instead, theirs was an approach that emphasized the psycho-social elements in the therapeutics of mental disorder, and insisted that those still called 'lunatics' were best taken care of in reformed institutions run along moral treatment lines.

In its various national guises, moral treatment exhibited a number of common features. There was a growing conviction about the centrality of all aspects of the design of the physical spaces within which the mentally ill were confined, and an increasing optimism about the possibility of creating a curative environment for the mad. Architecture itself was moralized, reflecting the belief that in both obvious and subtle ways, the buildings themselves could contribute to, or help relieve, mental disturbance.

Bars, for instance, sent the wrong message to the inmates, and so at one of the pioneering institutions embodying the new approach, the York Retreat in northern England, the iron dividers between the panes of glass in the windows were painted to look like wood. No high wall separated the Retreat from the road, giving the impression to those who approached – mental patient, family, casual passer-by – that here was not a place of confinement, but a home. Built on a hill to secure fresh air and invigorating views, the Retreat's grounds sloped away from the buildings, and, as far as the eye could see, no barrier interposed itself between inmate and countryside (though in fact a hidden ditch,

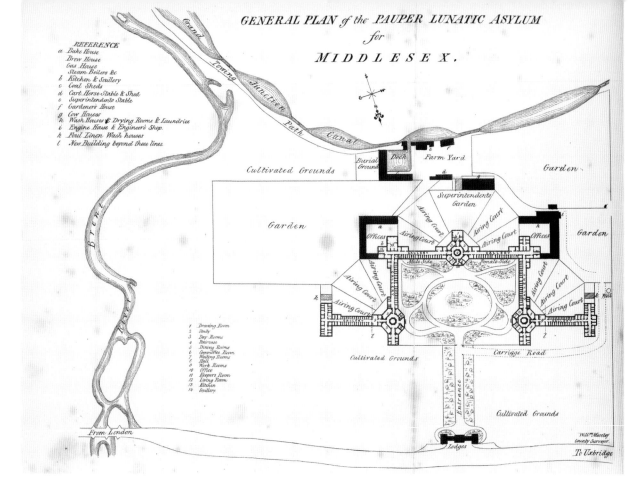

GENERAL PLAN of the PAUPER LUNATIC ASYLUM for MIDDLESEX.

REFERENCE
a Bake House
   Brew House
   Gas House
   Steam Boilers &c
b Kitchen & Scullery
c Coal Sheds
d Cart. Horse Stable & Shed
e Superintendents Stable
f Gardeners House
g Cow Houses
h Wash Houses & Drying Rooms & Laundries
i Engine House & Engineer's Shop
k Foul Linen Wash houses
l New Building beyond these lines

1   Drawing Room
2   Study
3   Day Rooms
4   Staircase
5   Dining Rooms
6   Committee Room
7   Waiting Rooms
8   Hall
9   Work Rooms
10 Office
11 Keepers Room
12 Living Room
13 Kitchen
14 Scullery

a 'ha-ha', presented a barrier to escape). Separate wards allowed the careful separation of the tranquil from the raving, the convalescent from the incurable, and this simultaneously gave those in charge a powerful weapon with which to encourage the patients to exercise self-control and self-restraint, vital – in the eyes of the proponents of moral treatment – to the recovery from insanity. Misbehaviour led to transfer to less desirable surroundings, and vice versa.

Moral treatment also emphasized the desirability of the least possible degree of external constraints and controls. Beating or assaulting patients, too common in *ancien régime* madhouses, were expressly forbidden, and physical restraints minimized. Staff were to treat their charges as individuals, and to turn the other cheek in the face of provocations that were deemed to be symptoms of mental illness, while praising and encouraging manifestations of more 'civilized' behaviours. The outrageous conduct exhibited by many mental patients, so it was now believed, was as much the product of mistreatment as of any underlying mental disorder.

MUSEUMS OF MADNESS

Initially, mental patients seem to have responded well to this radical shift in treatment. Though many proponents of moral treatment preferred to speak of 'recoveries' rather than 'cures', reflecting their belief that they were exploiting the healing powers of nature rather than obstructing them (as traditional approaches had), those recoveries appeared to be quite numerous. The contrast between the humane régime in the reformed establishments and the harshness of their predecessors encouraged an almost utopian optimism about what could now be achieved. Mental illness, many argued, was more curable than physical illness. In the United States, in particular, this cult of curability reached fantastic proportions, with claims that 70, 80 even 90 per cent of fresh cases could be cured, provided they were promptly removed to asylums.

Moral treatment thus contributed mightily to the Victorian fascination with the asylum as the solution to the problem of what to do with the mentally ill. On a wave of optimism, asylums, many built with public funds, soon became a familiar feature of the 19th-century landscape. But optimism faded. Moral

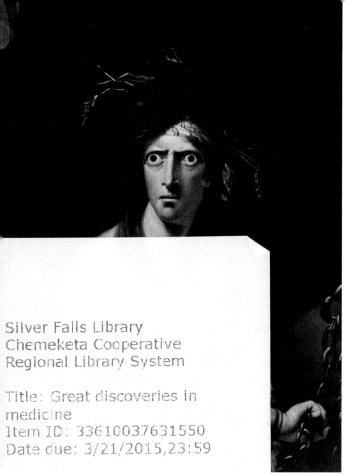

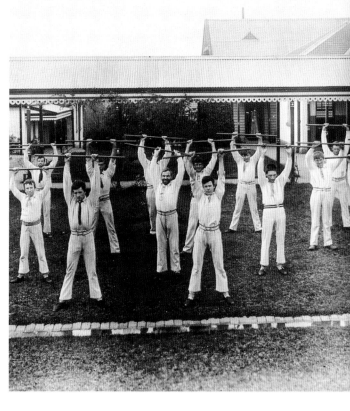

ıt. Cures
museums
small
supposed
d half of
on became
re rapidly
ndoned and
ish from the
munity.

Opposite
At the Middlesex County Asylum, also known as the Hanwell (after
the local village), the superintendent John Conolly pioneered the
abolition of mechanical restraint. Progress of sorts, but these vast,
self-contained units still became 'total institutions'.

Above left
An allegory of madness published in 1775: the partial nudity,
exaggerated, staring eyes, extravagant hat and chained wrists
conformed to 18th-century stereotypes of insanity and means
of restraint.

Above right
Physical drill for male patients at the Metropolitan Lunatic Asylum,
Kew, Victoria, Australia, in the early 20th century. The female patients
separately followed a similar routine, minus the sticks. This was one
of Australia's largest hospitals for the insane, with over 1,000 beds.

13. THE MILIEU INTÉRIEUR
The importance of equilibrium

Ana Cecilia Rodríguez de Romo

*Regulation in the organism is the
central problem of physiology.*
Walter B. Cannon, 1929

In 1850, the French physiologist Claude Bernard
(1813–78) postulated that multicellular organisms
remain alive because they possess an internal medium
that is capable of maintaining them in relatively
stable conditions, in spite of changes in the exterior
environment. In Bernard's view, for an organism to
survive it must be partially independent of that outer
environment, which means that the tissues of living
beings must somehow be shielded from direct
external influences.

Bernard summed up his studies of the higher
organisms in his celebrated phrase: 'The constancy of
the internal environment is the condition for the free
and independent life.' He used the term *milieu intérieur
physiologique* (internal physiological medium, or 'the
environment within') to refer to the series of chemical
substances and processes that constitute an organism,
and whose interrelations remain constant despite the
variations that may occur in the external environment.

This self-regulating aspect is of extraordinary
significance and is considered one of the most
important biological generalizations in the history of
science. Moreover, the concept of the stability of the
internal medium is one of the fundamental phenomena
that have guided the development of physiological
research. Physiology cannot be limited simply to
providing isolated descriptions of the functions of the
body's separate, individual organs and systems; rather,
they must all be studied in the broader context of their
participation in the common task of maintaining the
environment within.

HOMEOSTASIS
In the late 19th and early 20th centuries, Walter B.
Cannon (1871–1945) took Bernard's approach a step
further, with his description of the physiological

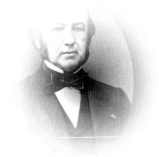

Above
Claude Bernard's multifaceted research career included work
on the internal environment of multicelled animals – what he
termed the *milieu intérieur physiologique*.

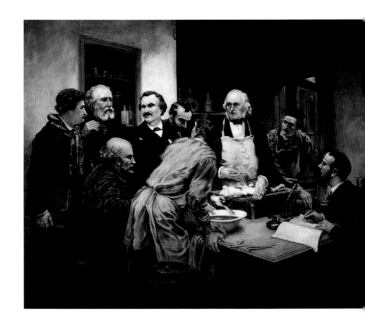

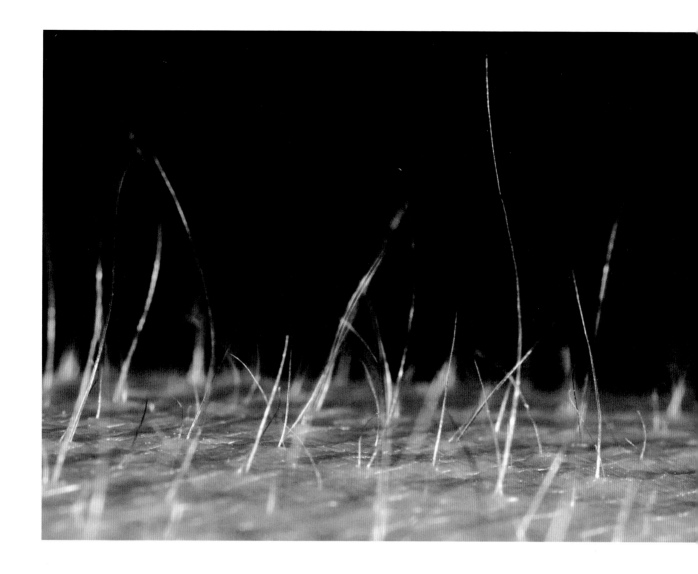

Opposite below
Bernard at work in his laboratory: an amanuensis takes notes and
blue-coated assistants help with the messier aspects of such research
involving animals, central to Bernard's studies, while he and his
colleagues and students discuss the experiment. Painting after Léon
Augustin L'Hermitte.

Above
Piloerection or hair 'standing on end' occurs as part of the body's
homeostasis mechanism. Nerves sensing a drop in temperature
stimulate hair follicles to contract and pull the hair erect. Erect
hairs trap warm air against the surface of the skin, thus creating
an insulation layer, to maintain a constant internal body temperature.
Today we do not benefit much from this evolutionary adaptation
because of a lack of body hair.

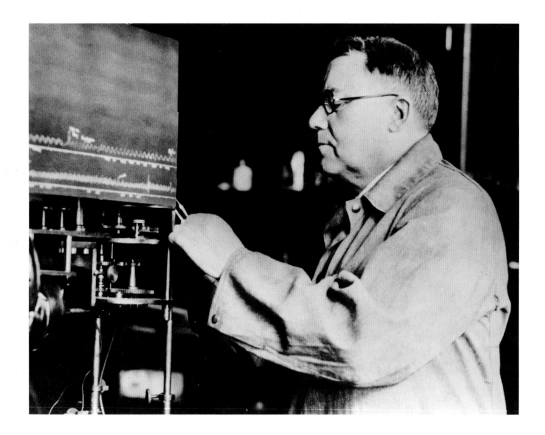

mechanisms that are involved in maintaining the body's essential physical-chemical equilibrium, an idea that he published in his masterwork, *The Wisdom of the Body* (1932). In 1929, this North American physiologist used the word homeostasis – from the Greek *homo*, 'equal', and *stasis*, 'standing' – to denote the 'state of equilibrium in which the internal corporal environment is maintained, owing to the continuous interaction of all the body's regulatory processes'.

In Cannon's usage, homeostasis referred to the sum total of the body's internal, structural and functional constancy. Thus the term suggests not only the condition of stability itself, but also the innumerable physiological processes required to maintain it. According to Cannon, homeostasis was the key to more highly evolved life forms, and he argued that the degree of evolution of living things was a function of their ability to increase their level of homeostasis.

Therefore, homeostasis constitutes a dynamic condition that responds to changing circumstances. But the body's equilibrium can be modified only within the narrow limits that are compatible with maintaining life. For example, the concentration of blood glucose does not

normally go below 70 mg per 100 ml of blood, nor rise above 110 mg/100 ml. Each one of the body's structures, from the cellular to the systems level, contributes in some way to conserving the internal environment within normal limits. Indeed, maintaining homeostasis requires many complex processes called homeostatic mechanisms to be generated and then triggered in response to some initial change in the internal medium. These reactions are called adaptive responses, and they allow the body to adapt to alterations in its environment in such a way as to preserve homeostasis and foster healthy survival.

Homeostasis resides in the corporal liquids located inside and outside the cells – all the substances required for preserving life are dissolved in those fluids, including oxygen, nutrients, proteins and a broad range of electrically charged chemical particles called ions. The extracellular liquid forms one-third of all biological fluids and is made up of the interstitial liquid – either plasma or lymph – that bathes the cells. It constitutes the organism's internal medium, and its usefulness lies in both providing the cells with a relatively constant environment and carrying substances to them. The

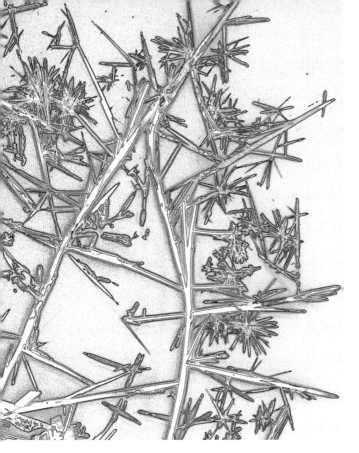

Left
Crystals of adrenaline viewed with a polarizing microscope.
Adrenaline increases the heart rate as well as increasing blood flow
to the muscles in preparation for the 'fight or flight' responses. Walter
Cannon's research on the way the body regulates itself through the
autonomic or involuntary nervous system helped elucidate processes
such as the adrenaline response.

Opposite
Walter B. Cannon at work with the equipment he used to explore
the physiological responses involved in homeostasis.

intracellular liquid represents the other two-thirds of all
organic liquids, and is an excellent solvent that facilitates
the chemical reactions necessary for life.

BEYOND THE MAMMALS

The concepts introduced by Bernard and Cannon have
had an enormous influence on the history of biology,
though many biologists think that they have sometimes
been extrapolated and used to excess. Throughout their
lives both Bernard and Cannon worked primarily with
mammals, an animal group with a particularly high
index of internal stability. In contrast, most fish and
amphibians do not stabilize their internal temperature
through physiological means, but instead allow it
to vary according to the temperature of the external
environment.

If Bernard and Cannon's models were applied to
these classes of animals (indeed, the latter did so), their
lack of internal thermal stability would appear as a
defect. In reality, however, there are benefits, because
in this way their internal temperature is permitted to
come into equilibrium with the external environment,
rather than being in conflict with the natural physical

tendency towards equilibrium. This mechanism yields
great energy savings. Since they do not produce heat,
such animals expend less energy and can subsequently
spend more time without eating. In order to reach the
temperature needed for their metabolism to work,
reptiles bask for lengthy periods in the sun.

In modern medicine, treating conditions including
dehydration, haemorrhages, metabolic imbalances
such as occur in diabetes, and the many other disorders
that so often appear in hospital emergency rooms,
intensive care units and in doctors' surgeries, would
be unthinkable without this understanding of the
physiological phenomenon of equilibrium. In fact, so
great is the importance of this principle that it has been
applied to the regulation of a variety of ecosystems and
even to the universe as a whole. The Gaia hypothesis
proposes that homeostasis on the earth is maintained by
feedback processes operated automatically by the biota.

14. GERMS
The greatest medical discovery?

Michael Worboys

The outstanding medical triumphs of the second half of the 19th century centre round the establishment of the doctrine of the germ origin of disease.
Charles Singer, 1950

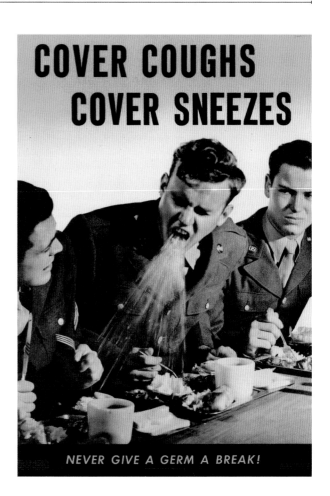

The late 19th-century discovery that germs cause infectious diseases has been described as one of the greatest medical discoveries of all time, if not the greatest. Not only did it help to explain the mystery of how major killer infections originated and spread, it also allowed doctors to develop better targeted methods of prevention and treatment. It changed the way doctors thought about all diseases, with a move from defining them largely by their signs and symptoms to identifying their specific causes.

The germ theory of disease was successful because it encompassed many ideas; indeed, it is more accurate to speak of germ theories of disease. There were numerous views on what germs were and how they caused different diseases. Germ *theories* rapidly became germ *facts*, as the microorganisms responsible for numerous infections were identified. It is often said that the arrival of germs in medicine was revolutionary, but it is important to remember that germ theorists drew on earlier ideas, and many doctors maintained already established views or adapted germ theories to suit these ideas.

Above
A Second World War poster reminding people to try to prevent the spread of coughs and colds by covering their mouths when coughing or sneezing; this crucial message is still advertised today, but was meaningless before the modern understanding of germs.

Opposite above
'The atmospheric germ theory': several early germ theorists including Pasteur and Lister believed that the air was full of germs; these drawings of air-borne germs illustrated a paper by another advocate, John Hughes Bennett, in 1868.

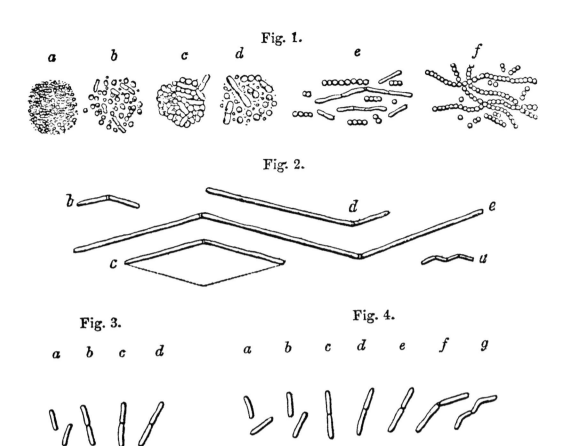

Fig. 1.

a   b   c   d   e   f

Fig. 2.

b   d   e

c   u

Fig. 3.   **Fig. 4.**

a   b   c   d   *a   b   c   d   e   f   g*

BEFORE THE REVOLUTION

The timeline of disease-germs has been traced back to
Avicenna (Ibn Sina; 980–1037), but more commonly to
Girolamo Fracastoro (1478–1553) and his claim that the
transmission of seed-like contagia caused epidemics.
Fracastoro proposed that diseases could spread in many
ways – directly, indirectly or remotely. His 'seeds' or
'seedlets' could be chemical or living, and arose from
sick bodies, spontaneously in the air or in decomposing
matter. His ideas had little impact until his elevation as
a precursor of germ theories in the late 19th century.

Antoni van Leeuwenhoek (1632–1723; see [23]) was
similarly promoted as a father of microbiology, while
yet other microscopists reported seeing worms and
foments (organisms associated with putrefaction and
decomposition) in diseased tissue, though whether
these were cause, consequence or concomitant of
disease was ambiguous. Agostino Bassi (1773–1856) has
also been credited as the creator of the germ theory of
disease through his finding, published in 1835, that the
growth of a microscopic fungus caused the silkworm
disease muscardine. However, the connection of this
work to human disease was not immediate, especially

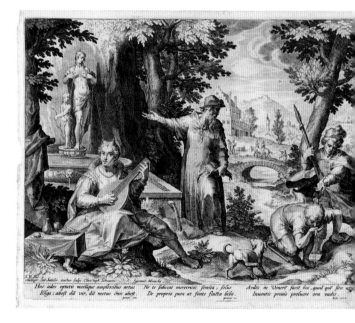

Above
A 16th-century engraving illustrating Fracastoro's poem *Syphilis*,
in which he warns the shepherd Syphilus (hence syphilis) against
casual sex, with its associated risk of infection. Syphilis was one of the
diseases Fracastoro thought could be spread by seed-like contagia;
these were not germs as we think of them today.

at a time when the dominant views on epidemic diseases, influenced by the experience of cholera, were anti-contagionist and chemically inclined.

PASTEURIAN DEVELOPMENTS

In the early 19th century infectious and contagious diseases were termed zymotic diseases, indicating a direct analogy with fermentation, then termed zymosis. Doctors went with the prevailing view that zymosis was due to chemical catalysts or ferments, assumed to be large, complex molecules that initiated powerful reactions. Another analogy was with poisoning. In highly contagious diseases such as smallpox, doctors spoke of the virus, by which they meant a particularly active poison. Zymotic models were also applied to septic infection – decomposition in damaged or dead tissue – where the process was known as putrefaction. In the late 1850s and early 1860s, Louis Pasteur (1822–95) began to change these views by proposing that fermentation and putrefaction were biological processes produced by microorganisms, rather than chemical reactions, persuading his fellow scientists as much by practical applications as by laboratory demonstrations. He found that heating wine to 50°C (122°F) killed the yeast cells responsible for its deterioration, and when applied to milk it stopped souring, a process still known as Pasteurization.

SURGERY AND INFECTIOUS DISEASES

The surgeon Joseph Lister (1827–1912) made the first and most famous medical use of Pasteur's germ theories by attempting to prevent and stop putrefaction in wounds by killing septic germs, either in the air before entry or directly by treating damaged and dead tissues [54]. The idea that germs could initiate putrefaction in tissue that had lost its vitality was novel and challenging to doctors. Yet it was easier to accept than the idea that these absolutely minuscule organisms produced major infectious diseases by entry into, and development within, living tissues. Furthermore, they were asked to believe that these organisms, seemingly impossible to differentiate under the microscope, were distinct species, each causing a different disease. When they turned their microscopes to look for disease-germs, scientists and doctors saw many microorganisms, but how these produced the severe bodily effects characteristic of infectious diseases was a major puzzle. Some doctors doubted that such powerful agents came from outside the body, proposing alternative theories

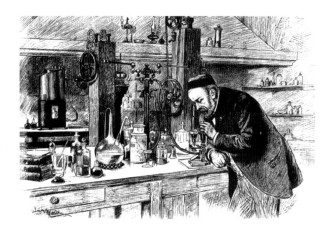

Above
Louis Pasteur at work with his microscope. Pasteur was a chemist not a doctor – he was one of the new laboratory scientists rather than clinicians who would come to dominate medical research.

Opposite
A photomicrograph by Andrew Pringle, author of *Practical Photomicrography* (1890), of tuberculosis bacilli (top), anthrax bacilli (centre), actinomyces (bottom left) and micrococci (bottom right). As the germ theory developed, scientists debated whether there was just one or many kinds of bacteria and whether they could mutate from one form into another, as well as whether specific bacteria caused specific diseases.

Below
The carbolic acid spray used by Joseph Lister (see also p. 222). During an operation the disinfectant carbolic acid or phenol was sprayed over the surgeons' hands and the patient's body to create an antiseptic environment. It was the least popular part of Lister's regime.

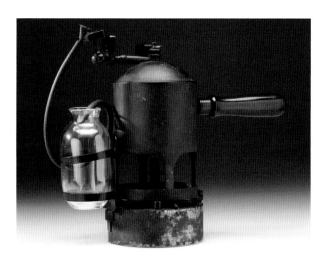

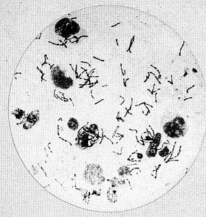

B. Tuberculosis. × 750.

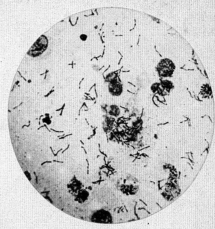

B. Tuberculosis. × 750

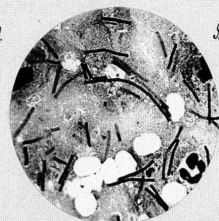

B. Anthracis. × 750.

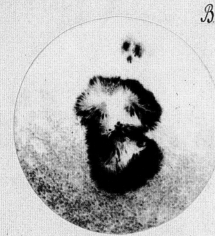

Actinomyces. × 150.

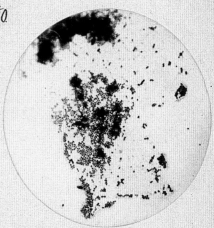

Micrococci, etc. × 750.

Micro organisms.

around the idea that disease-germs were damaged cells, or organisms that had arisen spontaneously in the body.

Anthrax provided the first widely accepted demonstration of a specific microorganism causing a specific disease. In 1876 Robert Koch (1843–1910), then a general practitioner in Wollstein, Germany, published details of the anthrax bacillus's life history – how it entered the body and reproduced in the blood, and how it caused disease by blocking blood vessels and secreting toxins. Koch was lucky in his choice of subject – the anthrax bacillus is relatively large and easy to work with – but he had invented innovative laboratory techniques of observing, staining, growing and manipulating bacteria that soon led to a rush of germ discoveries. Koch himself identified the bacterial causes with highest impact: tuberculosis [38] in 1882 and cholera [36] in 1883.

Despite these and other discoveries, germ theories remained controversial. Many laboratory findings were disputed, and the behaviour of germs in the clinic or environment was often at odds with laboratory observations. Moreover, the germs of many common infections, notably smallpox [40] and measles, seemed not to be bacteria and eluded investigators; none the less they confidently referred to their disease-agents as ultramicroscopic germs or viruses.

GERMS AND PUBLIC HEALTH

Bacteriological laboratory methods began to be used to diagnose individuals and map epidemic and endemic infections in populations. New impetus was given to the use of quarantine, isolation and disinfection in preventing and controlling infectious diseases by public health doctors. However, the most high-profile innovations were new vaccines, anti-sera and antitoxins. All were based on modified germs or germ products, and held the promise of extension to other infectious diseases [63].

Pasteur announced a vaccine against anthrax in 1881. Following the principle of smallpox vaccination – using a related, mild infection to protect against a more serious one – he reduced the bacillus's virulence by exposure to air and then inoculated sheep, allowing them to develop immunity. He used similar methods with great success against rabies in the mid-1880s. It was the germ theorists' greatest public relations triumph. In the 1890s diphtheria antitoxin followed. The neutralizing substances produced by animals that were not susceptible to the disease were harvested and given to sufferers, providing

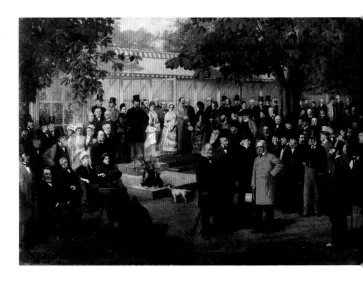

Above
Baroness Burdett-Coutts' garden party for members of the 1881 International Medical Congress, where the great men of medicine met. Among the 3,000 delegates from 70 countries were the architects of the germ theory Pasteur, Koch and Lister.

Opposite
Papier d'Arménie contains benzoin resin. Developed in France as part of the popular movement against germs, it purportedly disinfects a room when burnt, preventing infectious diseases such as cholera, typhoid, diphtheria and smallpox, as personified in this 1890 advertisement.

temporary immunity. Another high-profile medical breakthrough, this saved children from imminent death and encouraged public, private and philanthropic investment in biomedical research.

After 1900, doctors and the new specialists in bacteriology or microbiology referred to bacteria, viruses, fungi and cellular parasites, only using the word 'germ' as shorthand for all disease-causing organisms. However, germs remained in the public domain, in government health propaganda, commercial advertising and popular culture. Public health officials warned about the threat of disease germs lurking in water, food and the air, encouraging hygienic practices in the home, street and workplace. Awareness of germs changed public and personal behaviour: spitting in the street was prohibited; skirts were shortened to avoid picking up germs from pavements and floors; people slept with open windows to reduce the density of aerial germs; and house flies changed from innocent nuisances to deadly germ carriers. Popular versions of germs had strong continuities with the early medical and scientific views of disease-agents as invisible, protean and potentially very powerful.

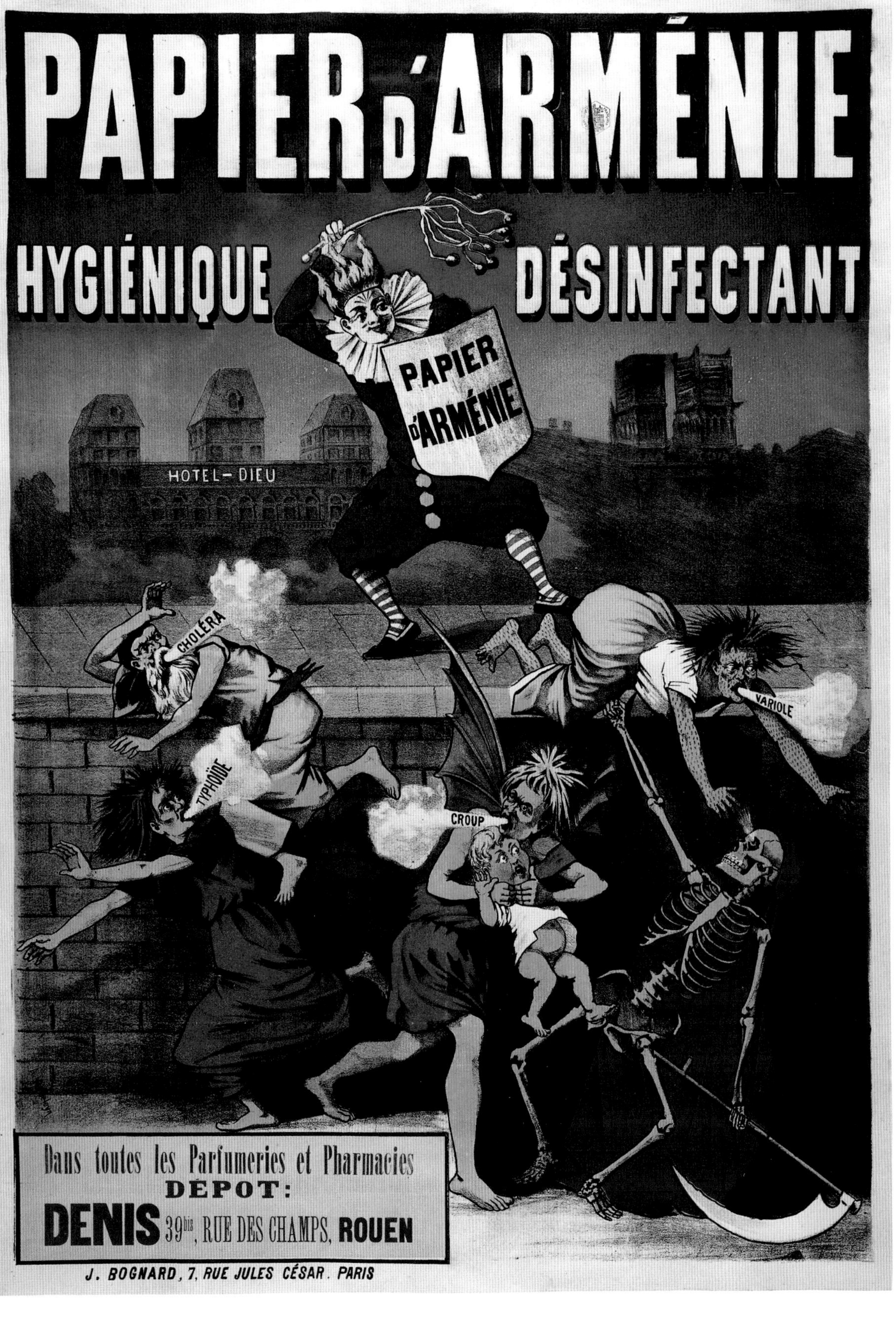
PAPIER D'ARMÉNIE
HYGIÉNIQUE
DÉSINFECTANT
PAPIER D'ARMÉNIE
HOTEL-DIEU
CHOLÉRA
VARIOLE
TYPHOÏDE
CROUP
Dans toutes les Parfumeries et Pharmacies
DÉPOT:
DENIS 39bis, RUE DES CHAMPS, ROUEN
J. BOGNARD, 7, RUE JULES CÉSAR. PARIS

15. PARASITES & VECTORS
Insects & disease

Gilberto Corbellini

*Our actual knowledge of the insect carriers of disease has all been acquired
during the last fifteen or twenty years, and marks as brilliant and successful
an epoch in the history of medicine as did the phenomenal development
of bacteriology in the years immediately preceding.*
Charles Chapin, 1910

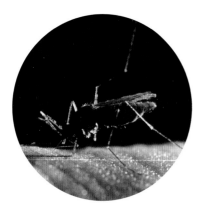

Left
A female anopheles mosquito: different anopheles species spread
the various malaria parasites from one person to the next when the
females (but not the males) take their blood meals.

Opposite left
Alphonse Laveran had described the malaria parasite in 1880; in this
cartoon by B. Moloch from 1909 he rides into battle against the insect
hordes after the mosquito's role in malaria's transmission had been
widely accepted.

Opposite right
A plate from the Italian malariologist Giovanni Battista Grassi's *Studi
di uno zoologo sulla malaria* ('Studies on the zoology of malaria'),
1901, which presented a comprehensive account of his extensive
research up to that point.

After it was established that infectious diseases are due
to the transmission of microbial agents, or germs [14],
attention turned to establishing 'the sources and modes
of infection', which included the concepts of healthy
or asymptomatic carriers, and insect vectors or hosts.
The knowledge that living microorganisms caused
contagious diseases could not sufficiently explain the
occurrence of new cases in individuals who had not had
any previous direct contact with infected subjects, or
the complete absence of new cases in groups of people
who had been in contact with the sick.

CARRIERS OF ALL KINDS
In 1884 Friedrich Loeffler (1852–1915) found the
diphtheria bacillus in the throat of a healthy person.
Five years later the bacillus was shown to persist in
the throats of convalescent cases. In 1893 the major
role played by asymptomatic carriers of diphtheria
was established, following epidemiological studies
among New York's population by Hermann M. Biggs and
William H. Parks. Also in 1893 Robert Koch (1843–1910)
determined that convalescent carriers were a source
of fresh cholera infections. Subsequently, convalescent

and healthy carriers of typhus and meningococcal
bacilli were discovered.

As, with a few exceptions, infectious agents
quickly die in non-living environments, they must
be transmitted by direct or indirect contact, food and
drink, or insects. The Russian Nikolai Mikhailovich
Melnikov provided the earliest description of an insect
acting as parasite's host, demonstrating in 1869 that the
cucumber tapeworm (*Dipylidium caninum*) develops
inside the dog louse *Trichodectes canis*. In 1878 the
Scottish tropical physician Patrick Manson (1844–1922),
working in China, discovered *Wuchereria bancrofti*
or filaria worms (which cause infections of the lymph
system) inside mosquitoes that had fed on human blood.
Manson observed the parasite develop to the larval
stage, but mistakenly believed the mosquitoes bit only
once and that humans were infected after drinking
water in which mosquitoes had laid their eggs. In 1900
George Carmichael Low (1872–1952) would show that
the bite of mosquitoes of the genus *Culex* transmits
filaria worms from person to person.

The active role of the host insect in the transmission of
infection was established by Theobald Smith (1859–1934)

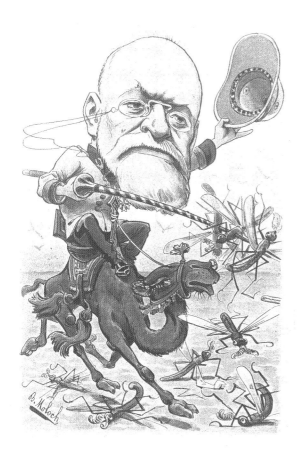

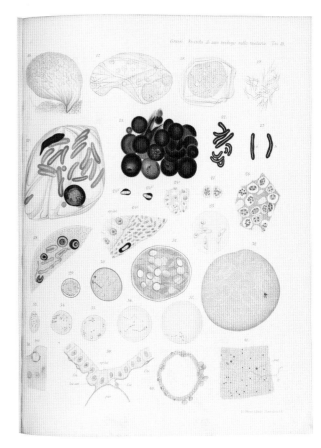

and Fred L. Kilbourne (1858–1936), between 1889 and 1892, when they demonstrated that Texas cattle fever was caused by *Pyrosoma bigeminum* (*Babesia bigemina*) and transmitted by tick bites. Between 1894 and 1897 David Bruce (1855–1931) applied the insect vector theory to nagana, a form of sleeping sickness of domestic animals in sub-Equatorial Africa, and demonstrated that the tsetse fly (*Glossina morsitans*) transmits the infection's causal agent, the microorganism *Trypanosoma brucei*. In 1903 it was discovered that human sleeping sickness was another form of trypanosomiasis, transmitted in the same way.

MALARIA AND MOSQUITOES

The most important example of insect vectors was the discovery of the transmission mechanism of human malaria. Alphonse Laveran (1845–1922) first described the human malaria parasite in 1880, and the mosquito-transmission hypothesis became widespread in the 1890s. Following suggestions by Patrick Manson, in 1897 Ronald Ross (1857–1932) observed the presence of pigmented cells – malaria parasites – in two mosquitoes fed on malarial blood. In 1898,

Ross described the development of the bird malaria parasite in mosquitoes, while Giovanni Battista Grassi (1854–1925), together with Amico Bignami (1862–1929) and Giuseppe Bastianelli (1862–1959), demonstrated that mosquitoes of the genus *Anopheles* transmit the human malaria parasite. Ross won the Nobel Prize in 1902. Study of the vectors of human malaria illuminates the disease's complex epidemiology. The different species of *Anopheles* vary in their efficiency as vectors; consequently specific environmental conditions that favour or disadvantage particular vector species can influence the disease's epidemiological dynamics.

YELLOW FEVER AND MOSQUITOES

Following the malaria-mosquito work came the discovery of the transmission mechanism of yellow fever. In 1881 the Cuban physician and researcher Carlos Finlay (1833–1915) had hypothesized that mosquitoes rather than direct human contact spread yellow fever. After the serious losses caused by this disease among the US troops occupying Cuba in the 1890s, Walter Reed (1851–1902) led a US Army commission (established in 1900) to study yellow

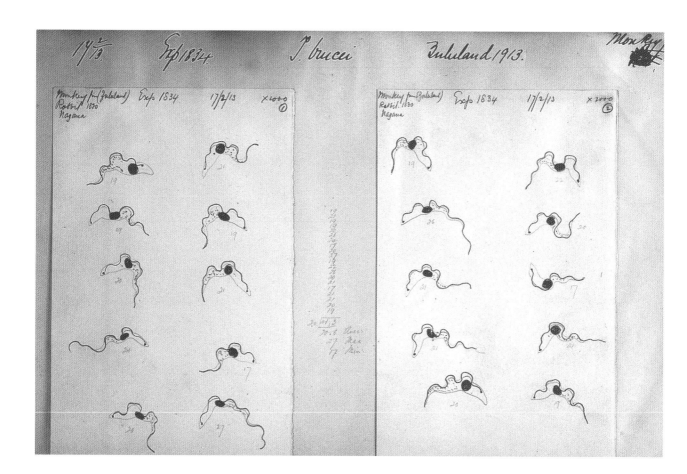

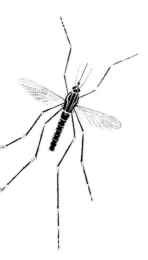

Above
Drawings of *Trypanosoma brucei* (named for its discoverer Sir David Bruce). These single-celled parasites, with their motile flagellum or tail-like structure, cause sleeping sickness in Africa, spread by the bite of the tsetse fly.

Left
A female *Aedes aegypti* mosquito. It is the females of this species of mosquito that transmit the viruses of yellow fever, dengue and other less well-known diseases.

Opposite left
In the 1950s and 1960s the World Health Organization attempted to eradicate malaria using the long-lasting insecticide DDT, as seen in this poster from India. Despite some success, the global campaign faltered as the mosquitoes developed resistance to DDT and the adverse environmental impact of the insecticide was realized.

Opposite right
After the discovery that mosquitoes transmit malaria, doctors advocated sleeping under a bed net. This poster from the Second World War reminded troops to protect their health. Today insecticide-impregnated bed nets are a key to the current 'Roll Back Malaria' campaign; unfortunately, they remain uncomfortable to sleep under.

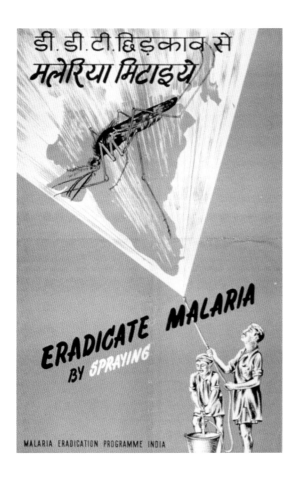

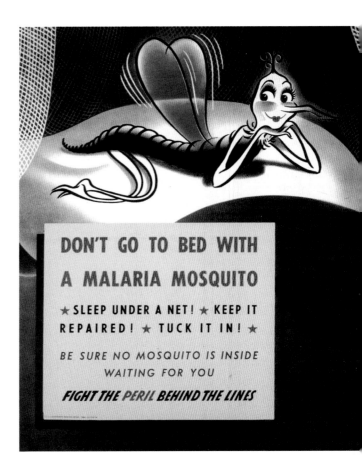

fever. Extending the malaria-mosquito hypothesis, Reed's experiments proved *Aedes aegypti* mosquitoes transmit yellow fever. This allowed William C. Gorgas (1854–1920) to apply stringent control methods and thus significantly reduce yellow fever and malaria cases in Cuba and later in Panama, making it possible to construct the Panama Canal. In 1916 John Burton Cleland (1878–1971) demonstrated that *Aedes aegypti* also transmits the dengue fever virus.

AND BEYOND

In the years that followed, the role of other important insect vectors was established. In 1908 an Indian commission published the famous report *The Etiology and Epidemiology of Plague*, which confirmed observations by Paul-Louis Simond (1858–1947) that rat fleas (*Xenopsylla cheopis*) transmit the bubonic plague bacterium *Yersinia pestis* to humans [34]. In 1909 Charles Nicolle (1866–1936) demonstrated that human lice spread epidemic typhus [35]. Also in 1909, the Brazilian physician Carlos Chagas (1879–1934) became the first person to describe the form of trypanosomiasis

known subsequently as Chagas disease. He observed a flagellate protozoa – a new species of the genus *Trypanosoma* – in the intestines of 'assassin bugs' (insects of the genus *Triatominae*) and proved it could be transmitted by marmoset monkeys previously bitten by the insect. Until 1925 Chagas incorrectly believed that the infection was transmitted by the insect's bite. Emile Brumpt proposed in 1915 that the insect's faeces were responsible – rubbed into the wound in response to the bite's irritation – which was proved in 1932 by Silveira Dias.

Other major parasitic diseases spread by insect vectors are Leishmaniasis, discovered in 1942 to be transmitted through the bite of female sandflies infected with the parasite *Leishmania donovani*, and Lyme disease, a borreliosis attributed to tick bites in the 1930s, whose specific bacterial cause and pathology were definitively established in 1975.

16. PSYCHOANALYSIS & PSYCHOTHERAPY
The talking cures

Andrew Scull

Psychotherapy is a most terrifying word, but we are forced to use it because there is no other which serves to distinguish us from Christian Scientists, the New Thought people, the faith healers, and the thousand and one other schools which have in common the disregard for medical science and the accumulated knowledge of the past.
Richard Cabot, 1908

In most respects, the closing decades of the 19th century were marked by a growing sense of pessimism about the prospects for the mentally ill. Cure rates in asylums, both public and private, were perceived as abysmal, and the psychiatric profession spoke of mental patients as degenerates, a biologically inferior lot best kept under lock and key lest they breed uncontrollably and further populate the world with mental defectives [12]. Madness, for many, was rooted in the body, and essentially beyond the reach of medicine.

Ironically, the very extremes of this pessimism helped to spawn a reaction. For psychiatrists, such doctrines protected them from accusations of failure, but offered little or nothing positive to do. For well-to-do patients and their families, such hopelessness and its accompanying stigma were distinctly unattractive. Affluent patients who experienced mental troubles were also desperate to avoid confinement in asylums increasingly seen as warehouses for the unwanted.

SEEKING ALTERNATIVES
Those on the borderlands of insanity looked anxiously for some other solution, and their milder, and perhaps therefore more treatable forms of mental disorder were attractive to an emerging group of 'nerve doctors'. Some of these were refugees from the world of the asylum, others were part of the emerging specialism of neurology, who sought alternatives to diagnosing and providing ineffective interventions geared to treating multiple sclerosis, neurosyphilis and other neurological problems that were their depressing stock in trade. Victims of hysteria, and of a newly fashionable weakness of the nerves dubbed neurasthenia, also constituted a potentially attractive market for the

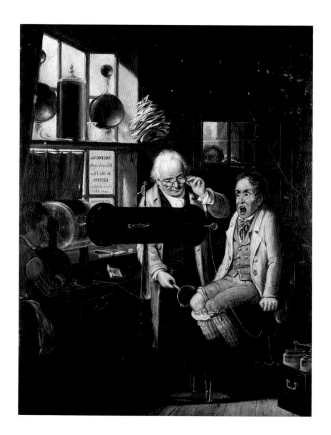

Above
In the era of physical therapies before the advent of psychoanalysis, electrotherapy became one of a number of fashionable treatments dispensed by nerve doctors for those suffering from hysteria and, later in the 19th century, neurasthenia. Painting by Edward Bristow, 1824.

Opposite
A patient suffering from shell-shock in the First World War. Some of the many mentally traumatized soldiers were helped by the talking cure.

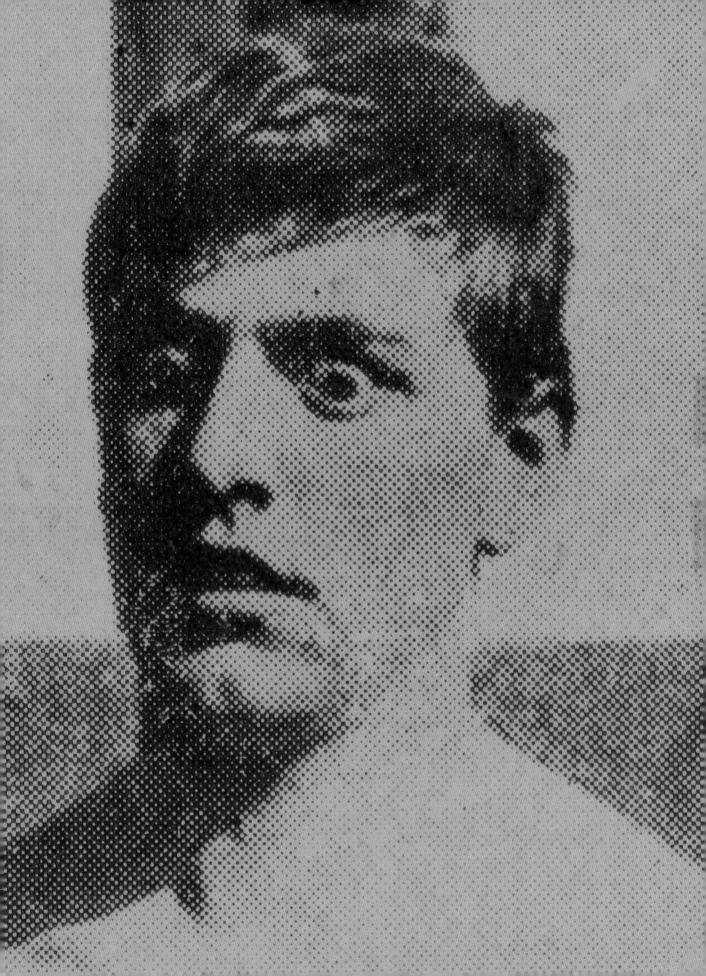

nerve doctors, so long as they could offer plausible explanations and suitable treatments for these mysterious pathologies.

Doctors had difficulty accepting therapies that did not operate through the body, and initially the treatments for these borderline disorders were of a demonstrably physical sort: various pills and patent remedies; hydrotherapy or water cures; diet; and electricity, in both static and galvanic forms. Many soon suspected, however, that these interventions worked as much through 'suggestion' as through any direct action on the patient's soma. Though controversial at first, increasingly some of those treating nervous invalids of various sorts began to experiment openly with what they came to call psychotherapy.

'MIND-HEALING CULTS'

The pressures to do so were amplified, particularly in North America, by the emergence of what physicians referred to disparagingly as 'mind-healing cults': groups such as the Christian Scientists encouraged by Mary Baker Eddy (1821–1910), or the Emmanuel Movement centred on an upper-class Boston church. The mesmeric trances of the discredited 18th-century Austrian physician, Franz Anton Mesmer (1734–1815), now rechristened as 'hypnosis' often formed part of the

new psychotherapeutic regimen, though suggestion and more directive forms of psychotherapy were also widely employed. Victims of psychological trauma – soldiers from the American Civil War, survivors of train crashes who developed mysterious symptoms – formed an important source of nervous patients, as did those who seemed burned out from too much ambition, stress and overwork. Though there was a temptation to attribute their disorders to physical trauma (war injuries or spinal concussion in train accidents), for many of their doctors these physical roots came to seem increasingly speculative and unlikely. Thus, the development of psychological treatments for mental disorders was often accompanied by psychological explanations of the causes of the disturbed thoughts and behaviours.

FREUD AND HIS RIVALS

Psychoanalysis, developed by Sigmund Freud (1856–1939), was to begin with just one of many such systems of psychological theorizing and treatments. The Swiss Paul Dubois (1848–1918) and the French Pierre Janet (1859–1947) – as well as Americans such as Morton Prince (1854–1929) and Boris Sidis (1867–1923) – advanced competing approaches to psychotherapy that for a time were at least equally as prominent, and some of Freud's inner circle, such as Carl Jung

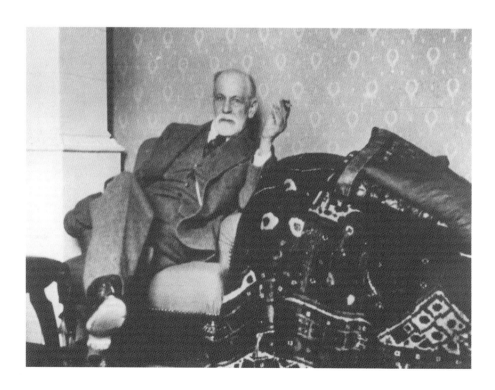

(1875–1961) and Alfred Adler (1870–1937), eventually broke with him and developed alternative systems.

Like many of his contemporary competitors among the nerve doctors, Freud had used hypnosis in treating his first hysterical patients in Vienna in the 1890s, and had come to regard repressed memories as the source of many of their difficulties. Having first assumed that abreaction (bringing repressed memories back into consciousness with the help of hypnosis) would suffice for a cure, Freud soon concluded otherwise. He also began to develop a far more elaborate account of the psychological roots of mental disorder, indeed of human psychology as a whole. Simultaneously, he abandoned hypnotism and began to experiment with what he called 'free association' – encouraging patients to lie on the proverbial couch and to speak whatever came into their minds, as well as to report their dreams. Such talk could, with the aid of skilled interpretation by an analyst, eventually lay bare the psychic roots of the mental symptoms, and ultimately lead to a cure.

Freud's talking cure ultimately surpassed and superseded its rivals. His visit to Clark University in Massachusetts in 1909 won him such prominent converts as the Harvard psychologist William James (1842–1910) and his neurological colleague James Jackson Putnam (1846–1918). Despite Freud's contempt for America and Americans, over time his ideas would establish their greatest beachhead in the United States. The massive epidemic of 'shell-shock' in the First World War (originally interpreted, as its name suggests, as the product of the concussive effects of high explosives on the human brain and nervous system, but gradually recognized by most as the product of psychic trauma), and the similarly widespread outbreaks of combat neurosis in the Second World War, did much to entrench psychoanalytic ideas and the talking therapy at the very pinnacle of American psychiatry, and to extend their influence into all quarters of its popular culture.

Elsewhere, psychoanalysis was never more than a minority taste, and it receded in the wake of the drugs revolution in psychiatry [48]. Psychotherapy in a very different form became the province of very distinct traditions with origins in academic psychology. The clinical branch of psychology, which developed within the university system in the immediate aftermath of the Second World War, most notably in North America, embraced short-term, experimentally based treatments of overt symptomatology. These interventions are usually collectively referred to as cognitive-behavioural therapy, or CBT, and underpin much of modern counselling.

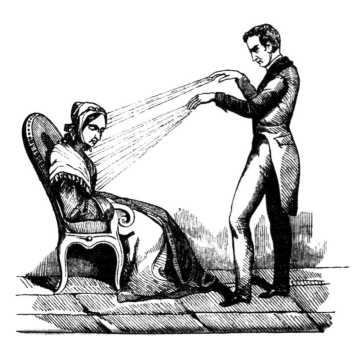

Opposite
Sigmund Freud, the founder of psychoanalysis, in his consulting room in Vienna, with his familiar cigar in hand and the famous couch on the right.

Left
A depiction, *c.* 1845, of the invisible rays of animal magnetism flowing from the fingertips of the practitioner of mesmerism to his seated patient. Mesmerism lost its respectability as the 19th century progressed, and many of its advocates were exposed as frauds. Transformed into hypnosis, the practice continued into the 20th century.

17. **HORMONES**
Chemical messengers

Robert Tattersall

*Agents which can determine whether an individual shall be a giant
or a dwarf, an idiot or a normally intelligent person, a 'sissy' or a real
male, a bearded lady or a woman; agents which are essential to normal
metabolism – indeed, whose destruction may lead promptly to death
– must evidently be respected.*
Walter B. Cannon, 1922

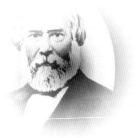

Charles-Édouard Brown-Séquard, who developed the idea of
internal secretion and the dubious (at least in his hands) practice
of organotherapy.

Hormones, or internal secretions, are chemical
messengers that are secreted by glands and coordinate
the functions of the body. Here we concentrate
on human hormones and related diseases, but all
multicellular organisms have hormones, including
plants (phytohormones).

FROM THE INTERNAL SECRETION THEORY TO ENDOCRINOLOGY

The originator of the internal secretion theory was
the physician and physiologist Charles-Édouard
Brown-Séquard (1817–93), who, in 1869, suggested
that all glands, with or without ducts, 'supplied to
the blood substances which are useful or essential
and the lack of which may produce physiological signs'.
In 1889, aged 72, he caused a sensation by describing
how he had rejuvenated himself with injections of
testicular extract from guinea pigs. He initiated the
movement called organotherapy, in which injections
of organ extracts were used therapeutically and
which was later blamed for the disrepute into which
this field of medicine descended over the following
30 years.

The first success of glandular treatment came in
1891, when George Murray (1865–1939) found that
injections of sheep thyroid extract cured mxyoedema
(thyroid failure). In 1902 the first direct proof of the
existence of hormones was produced by the London
physiologists William Bayliss (1860–1924) and Ernest
Starling (1866–1927), who found that production of
pancreatic juice in response to the arrival of acid in the
duodenum was not mediated by nerves as previously
believed but by a substance, secretin, carried in the
blood from the duodenum. In 1905 Starling invented
the term hormone from the Greek *ormao*, to 'stir up'.
Glands which discharged their secretion into the blood
became known as endocrine glands and the study of
their diseases became endocrinology. An American
society for the study of internal secretions was founded in
1916, with its journal *Endocrinology* appearing in 1917.

TOO LITTLE, TOO MUCH

Early progress in the field depended on removing
individual glands in animals to see what the effects
were and then looking for equivalent human
syndromes. Removal of the pituitary or adrenal glands

THE ENDOCRINE SYSTEM

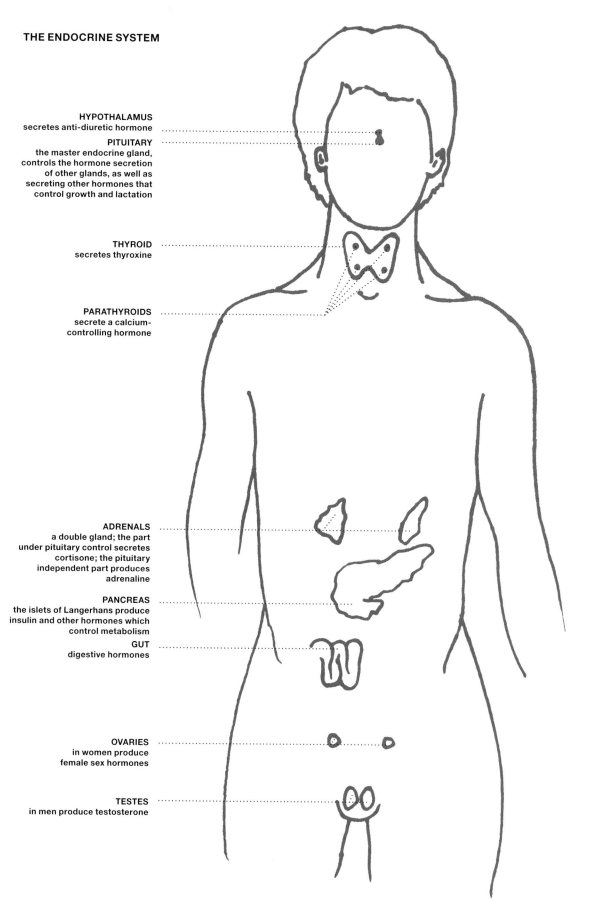

HYPOTHALAMUS
secretes anti-diuretic hormone

PITUITARY
the master endocrine gland,
controls the hormone secretion
of other glands, as well as
secreting other hormones that
control growth and lactation

THYROID
secretes thyroxine

PARATHYROIDS
secrete a calcium-
controlling hormone

ADRENALS
a double gland; the part
under pituitary control secretes
cortisone; the pituitary
independent part produces
adrenaline

PANCREAS
the islets of Langerhans produce
insulin and other hormones which
control metabolism

GUT
digestive hormones

OVARIES
in women produce
female sex hormones

TESTES
in men produce testosterone

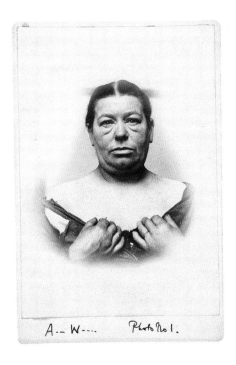 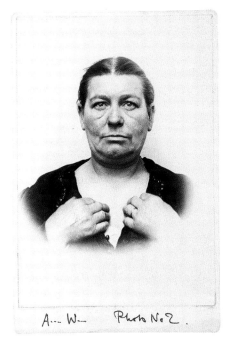

A--W----   Photo No 1.   A--W--   Photo No 2.

was fatal. Removal of the thyroid caused myxoedema and of the parathyroids, tetany (involuntary muscular spasms). Removal of the testes or ovaries affected secondary sexual characteristics. Removal of the pancreas caused severe diabetes.

It also became clear that some human diseases were due to overproduction of hormones, and were usually associated with enlargement or tumours of the relevant gland. Thus, a goitre was often accompanied by protruding eyes, anxiety, sweating and a fast pulse rate (thyrotoxicosis), symptoms which could be cured by removal of the gland. A disease involving bone cysts, kidney stones and abdominal pain was associated with parathyroid tumours (hyperparathyroidism). Gigantism and acromegaly (growth of the extremities) were associated with pituitary tumours, which produced growth hormone, first isolated in 1957. In 1932 another type of pituitary tumour was found to be associated with a distinctive clinical picture, Cushing's syndrome, which is the result of overproduction of cortisol, the hormone of the adrenal cortex that was isolated in 1948. During the 1930s it emerged that, in addition to growth hormone, the anterior pituitary

gland ('the conductor of the endocrine orchestra') produces hormones which control the thyroid (TSH), adrenal cortex (ACTH) and reproductive organs (FSH and LH); it also produces prolactin, which controls lactation. Anti-diuretic hormone, which is stored in the posterior pituitary, is produced by specialized nerve cells in the hypothalamus. One hormone which is not usually recognized as such is vitamin D, which is produced in the skin by sunlight and affects calcium absorption from the gut. Its chemical structure is similar to that of steroid hormones [64].

DEFECTIVE RECEPTORS

Hormones act on specific receptors and when these are defective it leads to diseases of end-organ resistance – the intended receptor organ fails to respond to the hormone. The first example of this was recognized in 1942 by Fuller Albright (1900–69) in a woman whose typical 'hypoparathyroidism' could not be cured by parathyroid hormone. Another example, which has caused problems in athletics, is androgen or male hormone insensitivity, which prevents masculinization of the fetus and leads to outwardly normal women

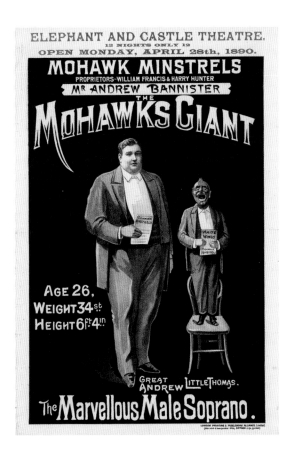

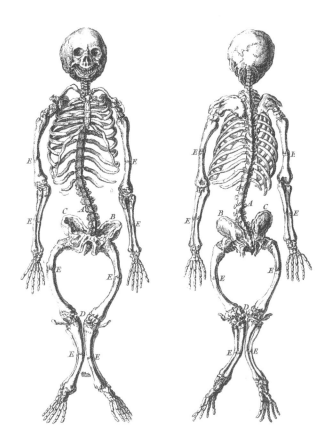

with XY chromosomes and intra-abdominal testes. Albright also recognized that some forms of kidney and lung cancer can produce hormones such as ACTH (adrenocorticotropic hormone) and parathormone (ectopic hormone production).

Until the 1960s diagnosis of endocrine diseases, whether resulting from under- or over-activity, depended on clinical acumen. Hormones are present in such small amounts in the blood that they were difficult to quantify using conventional biochemistry. This changed in 1960 when Solomon Berson (1918–72) and Rosalyn Yalow (1921–) invented the immunoassay, which could measure minute quantities of hormones even when, as in the blood, they were in a soup of thousands of other substances.

FURTHER COMPLEXITY

In addition to what might be called the 'classical' hormones, since the 1970s dozens of other hormones have been discovered in the gut and elsewhere. Many of these are involved in body weight maintenance. In 1994 leptin was found to be produced by fat cells and sensed by the hypothalamus. The very rare children with

leptin deficiency have insatiable appetites and become very fat; they can be cured by leptin, but unfortunately this is not the case with ordinary fat people. Ghrelin, produced in the stomach, stimulates appetite, while pancreatic polypeptide and peptide YY suppress it. It is tempting to think that manipulation of these hormones would be a magic bullet in treating obesity, but there is redundancy built into the system so that altering just one hormone has little effect.

Opposite
Photographs taken in 1895, before (left) and after (right) thyroid treatment for myxoedema (caused by an underactive thyroid gland) in a 55-year-old woman. The swelling of the skin and underlying tissues, part of the cluster of symptoms caused by this deficiency, has been reduced.

Above left
Not quite as vulgar as the earlier freak shows, the Mohawk minstrels advertised in this poster from c. 1890 may well have featured singers who were affected by hormonal growth disorders.

Above right
The skeleton of a child who suffered from rickets, caused by a deficiency of the hormone vitamin D, showing the characteristic bowed legs and spine.

18. **IMMUNOLOGY**
The body's defences

Gilberto Corbellini

*[Immunology] teaches us how to deal
with the complexity of organic functions.*
Frank Macfarlane Burnet, 1972

The modern discipline of immunology (the study of the immune system) emerged from bacteriology in the late 19th century [**14**]. In 1908 Simon Flexner, director of the Rockefeller Institute for Medical Research in New York, commented that, 'within just a few years, research into immunity had made unparalleled contributions to understanding disease causation and treatment'. The term 'immunology' first appeared in 1910 and the American Association of Immunologists (AAI) was founded in 1913. The *Journal of Immunology* was established in 1916, and in 1921 Eugenio Centanni published the first *Treatise on Immunology* in Italy – until then, only treatises 'on immunity' had appeared.

CELLULAR AND CHEMICAL IMMUNITY

The origin of the scientific approach to immunity was the idea, first suggested in 1884 by the Russian embryologist and zoologist Ilya Metchnikoff (1845–1916), that immune reactions are an organism's active and adaptive response designed to maintain its functional integrity against the threat of foreign substances. He emphasized the role of the white blood cells, called 'phagocytes' (literally, 'eating cells'). In 1890 Emil Behring (1854–1917) and Shibasaburo Kitasato (1852–1931) discovered that the blood serum of animals that had been immunized contains a substance called antitoxin, later known as 'antibody', which can neutralize a toxin (the 'antigen'), both in the living body and in the test tube, and thereby passively transfer protection. By 1910, the specific nature of immune reactions (agglutination, precipitation, complement fixation etc) was established. This in turn allowed the experimental study of the relationships between the species-specific nature of microorganisms, the clinical and aetiological specificity of infectious diseases, and the fact, empirically established for centuries, that immunization, whether active or

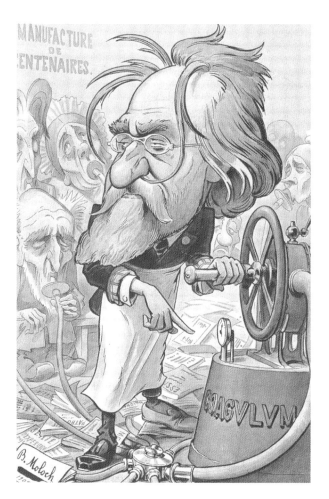

Above
Ilya Metchnikoff advocated the role of friendly gut bacteria, *Lactobacilli*, in helping to promote long life by maintaining a healthy body, which included a fully functioning immune system.

Opposite left
Metchnikoff's phagocytes or 'eating cells' are in action in this plate from his 1892 publication on the pathology of inflammation, ingesting the bacteria (red dots on the right) on the surface of the experimentally induced wound.

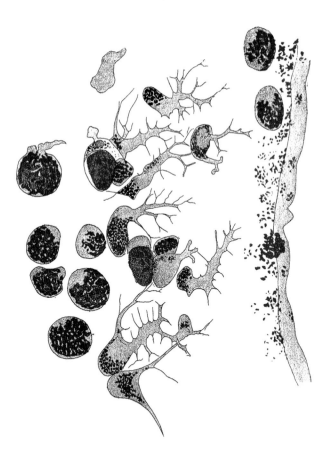

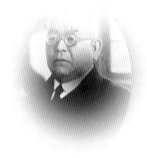

passive, against a specific infectious disease protects
only against that disease.

From the 1910s to the 1950s research focused on the
chemical and molecular aspects of immune responses,
and developments in immunology coincided with
the precise analysis of blood serum reactions. The
immunochemical approach demonstrated that immune
specificity is the result of a 'lock and key' molecular
relationship between antigen and antibody. It also
identified the chemical forces involved in antigen–
antibody interactions, and established that antibodies
are proteins. In the late 1950s, biochemical techniques
allowed Rodney Porter (1917–85) and Gerald Edelman
(1929–) to break the antibody molecule into pieces,
deducing its structure and sequencing its constituent
chains of amino acids.

SELF AND NON-SELF

The 1950s saw the return of a biological orientation to
the study of immune processes, alongside the chemical
approach. The adaptive nature of specific immunity
emerged again with the discovery of acquired immune
'tolerance' – the capacity of the immune system to learn
not to react against a foreign antigen that the organism
has encountered in its early development. Such a
function means that the immunological discrimination
between 'self' and 'non-self' depends on complex and
adaptive physiological mechanisms. The phenomenon
of immunological tolerance began to be studied at a
cellular level, and provided the scientific understanding
of why skin grafts and organ transplants were usually
rejected by the host organism; controlling the rejection
by powerful suppressant drugs has facilitated the
development of transplant surgery [60]. The 'chemical'
basis of the selectivity of immune responses was
redefined in terms of a Darwinian processing of
biological information, on a molecular and cellular
level, upon which antigen recognition and response
is dependent.

In this period, immunology became a fundamental
science, and the Australian immunologist and Nobel
Prize winner Frank Macfarlane Burnet (1899–1985),
renowned for his work on immune tolerance and the
theory of clonal selection, described immunology as
dealing with 'a microcosm that reflects vividly all the
essential features of the biological cosmos'.

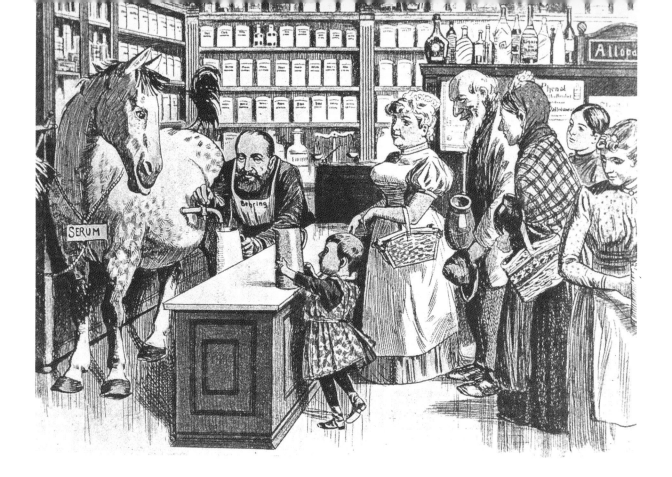

THE IMMUNE SYSTEM AND DISEASE

At the beginning of the 20th century serologists observed that the administration of the immune sera could sensitize the subject, and that such allergic reactions depended on the immune response. During the first half of the last century, clinical pathologists unveiled some of the complex immunological and inflammatory processes involved in allergic phenomena. The discovery of immunoproliferative disorders (such as the autoimmune diseases) and immunodeficiencies in the 1950s resulted in major methodological and therapeutic advances in medicine. Immunology received a boost from this clinical and experimental research that was as important as that previously created by the research into tolerance and secondary immune responses.

The study of congenital and acquired immunodeficiencies provided the medical and biological sciences with essential information about the normal and pathological functioning of the immune system – with its complex homeostatic mechanisms – and about the biological basis of immune responses. In addition, the concepts of medical genetics and the

emerging discipline of molecular pathology found fertile ground in the field of immunology, as the role of the histocompatibility molecule in regulating the processes of recognition and the control of molecular identity and of immune responses to foreign molecular structures gradually became apparent.

Immunological research has used sophisticated experiments to study the developmental processes of those cells of the immune system that are derived from the bone marrow (B lymphocyte, or B cell) and from the thymus (T lymphocyte, or T cell). Other investigations have led to diagnostic tools, treatments and animal models for autoimmune disorders and immunodeficiencies. In the process of the experimental approach to the understanding of the genetic basis of antibody production, techniques to create monoclonal antibodies were discovered. Monoclonal antibodies are the identical antibodies that arise when an antibody-producing cell is fused with a myeloma cell (a B-cell cancer). This discovery has yielded effective immunotherapies, such as for some cases of rheumatoid arthritis, and cancer-targeted therapies, as well as specific diagnostic tests.

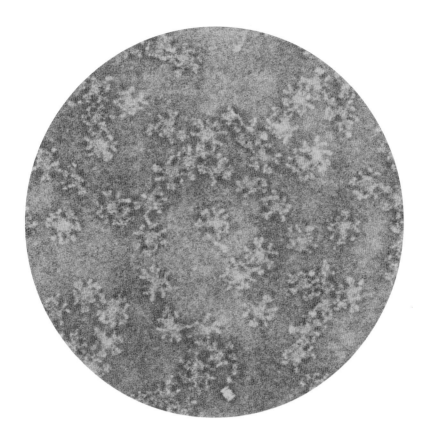

Recombinant DNA technology – combining two or more strands of DNA coming from different organisms – was first used to understand how antibodies are made. More recently recombinant DNA techniques have created libraries of millions of phages (viral particles that can infect other cells), each of which expresses a unique antibody on its surface and carries the antibody gene in its genome. The recombination of genes allows the creation of a repertoire of possible specific properties, from which antibodies can be selected for various therapeutic needs. The use of genetically modified mice – 'transgenic' and 'knock out' – has permitted the study of the role of different genes in the causal pathology of autoimmune diseases and immunodeficiencies.

Not only is the immune system accessible to such experimental research, but its cells (which are of different types and subtypes) can be isolated in a relatively pure form and the cell receptors can be biochemically identified and cloned. Immune cells can also be transferred to genetically similar hosts, within which specific markers make it possible to distinguish between host and donor cells and therefore to identify

the descendant cells and precursor cells that lead to clonal expansion (B and T cells can clonally proliferate as a consequence of a different kind of antigenic stimulation). At the frontier of research now is thus the study of the signalling mechanisms that control the complex changes in cell behaviour.

THE GENETIC REVOLUTION
From genes to genome

Angus Clarke

… just as no two individuals of a species are absolutely identical in bodily structure neither are their chemical processes carried out on exactly the same lines. Such minor chemical differences will obviously be far more subtle than those of form ….
A. E. Garrod, 1902

Right
The classic Mendelian inheritance of a recessive trait, in this case the colour white; red is dominant. Some diseases essentially follow this pattern. If two individuals both carry one copy of the affected gene, they will not be sick, but all their children will each have a 1 in 4 chance of having the disease.

Opposite
Chromosomes are pieces of DNA that contain genes. Various things can go wrong with the chromosomes, leading to disease. In Down syndrome there is an extra chromosome 21, visible here in the centre of the bottom row of a karyotype or chromosome set.

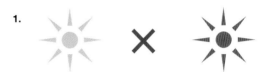

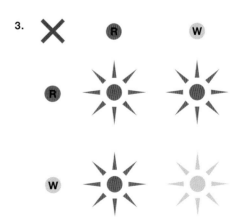

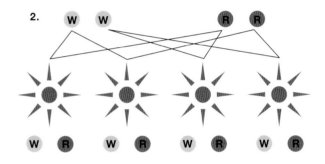

UNDERSTANDING HEREDITY

Before the famous work by Gregor Mendel (1822–84) with peas, it was often thought that heredity – how one generation influences the next – entailed a blending of both parents' contributions. Mendel showed instead that the hereditary factors causing offspring to resemble (and differ from) their parents were discrete, or 'particulate'. This insight was lost for some years, before being rediscovered in 1900. The behaviour of genes was then studied intensively, but without a knowledge of their material basis. Genes were dissected using inference, not a knife – their nature was elucidated by examining the progeny of careful breeding experiments in various organisms, including fruitflies, yeast and bacteria.

These experiments generated a detailed picture of what genes do. Together with the study of continuous variation or biometrics, promoted by Francis Galton (1822–1911), and the microscopic study of cells, they provided insights into the mechanism of heredity. It was necessary for these three approaches to merge before the modern science of genetics could develop, and subsequently tackle the 'Big Questions' of evolution, development and disease.

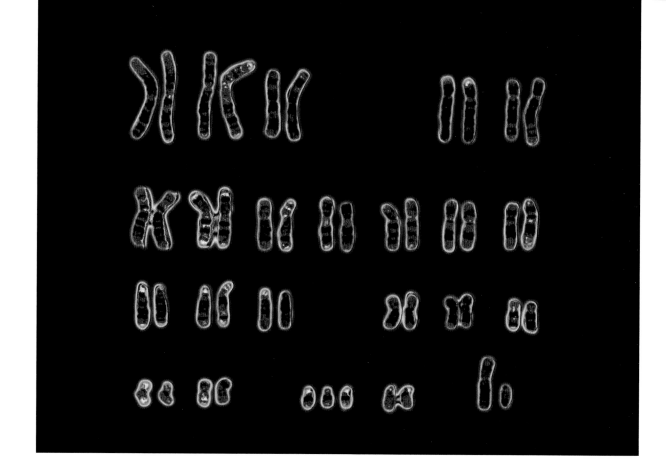

Biometrics and genetics were united in the 1920s with the recognition that many genes that have a small effect individually ('polygenes') together accounted for the influence of heredity on continuous traits such as body size, longevity and blood pressure. This 'modern synthesis' – the application of Mendelian (particulate) genetics to continuous variables – created the concept of evolution as a series of alterations in the relative frequencies of genetic variants as a result of natural selection and random drift.

For organisms that could be bred rapidly and easily, it was possible to create detailed maps of the linear order of genes on each chromosome. Their interaction with the organism's phenotype (appearance), including its development and behaviour, could then be charted, despite not knowing what a 'gene' actually was.

GENES, DNA AND DISEASE

While some diseases (e.g. cystic fibrosis) followed Mendel's laws, others that clustered in families more loosely, and with a less specific pattern of inheritance, were interpreted as the result of an unfavourable set of 'polygenes'. Where polygenic predisposition

was sufficiently high, even a minor environmental trigger might cause disease (or fetal malformation). This approach to gene–environment interaction has remained valid for many but not all diseases.

The material basis of genes was shown in 1910 by Thomas Hunt Morgan (1866–1945) to reside on chromosomes, but it was only in the 1960s that chromosome studies were applied clinically, when anomalies of chromosome number were recognized (e.g. Down syndrome, Turner syndrome). With improved resolution, cytogenetic techniques became progressively more useful, allowing small chromosomal deletions, duplications and rearrangements to be identified.

The recognition of deoxyribonucleic acid (DNA) as the chemical medium of heredity in 1944 by Oswald Avery (1877–1955), Colin MacLeod (1909–72) and Maclyn Macarty (1911–2005), and the elucidation of its structure in 1953 by Francis Crick (1916–2004) and James Watson (1928–) were of immense importance, leading directly to the development of molecular biology [10]. Its application to human disease took two tracks. One approach – as with sickle cell anaemia and

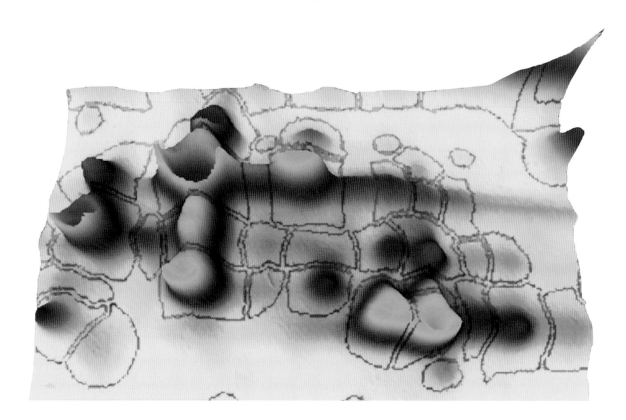

the thalassaemias – entailed the detailed molecular characterization of mutations that altered the level of gene expression or the structure of the protein produced (or both). This was possible because of the strong natural selection in favour of mutation at these loci as a defence against malaria in people carrying one such mutation. The condition of those affected by two altered genes brought their sufferers to medical attention.

The other approach was applied to those genes (almost all) whose chromosomal locations and corresponding proteins were unknown. A gene was mapped – its chromosomal location was found and its DNA isolated – by tracking sites of genetic variation (markers) through families affected by a disease. The effort entailed was enormous, often heroic, and brought together clinicians, laboratory scientists and those from affected families and their support associations.

GENE MAPPING AND THE GENOME

Gene mapping began in the 1980s and gathered pace in the 1990s. Immediate applications came in diagnosis, predictive testing for late-onset disease and prenatal genetic tests. It was against this background that the international Human Genome Project was conceived, and greatly assisted the subsequent identification of other gene loci.

Drafts of the human genome sequence were published from 2000, and the first nearly complete version appeared in 2003. Ready access to this information transformed biology. Subsequent knowledge and techniques have opened up the field of proteomics, the study of the structure and functions of the proteins expressed by the genes. The global pattern of gene expression can now be determined in different tissues, at different stages of development and in the face of different diseases, including tumours. There are already several categories of malignancy whose clinical management uses knowledge of the mutations present in the tumour.

Medical practice has incorporated knowledge about the major Mendelian genes, focusing preventive measures and surveillance for possible disease complications on those with rare disorders or the subset of those at very high lifetime risk of disease, typically around 5 per cent of those affected by the common, complex diseases. Insights into the 'polygenic' basis of other disorders, such as coronary artery disease, diabetes, breast cancer and schizophrenia, are helpful in research but not yet in practice. Genome-wide association studies indicate areas of the genome where genetic variants influence disease risk but have predominantly weak and indirect effects. Interestingly,

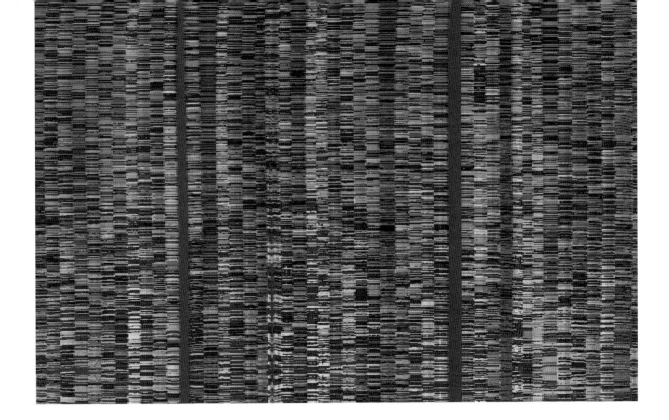

microarray studies of genomic DNA have shown that new mutations are making a bigger contribution to complex psychiatric disorders and malformations than had been appreciated.

FUTURE TRENDS

The price of a full genome sequence is expected to fall below the current cost of sequencing one or two large genes, making full genome sequence data available for research and clinical practice. It will take decades for clarification of the functional and pathogenic consequences of these DNA sequence variants, but the accumulating knowledge will result in improved therapeutics and disease prevention.

The same technologies are transforming developmental biology and generating vast quantities of data of great evolutionary significance. The evolutionary paths of different organisms and molecules are now much better charted. Although traditional skills remain important, in natural history as in laboratory techniques, biological research is progressively becoming ever more an exercise in information technology: the data are there, to be interrogated with sophistication.

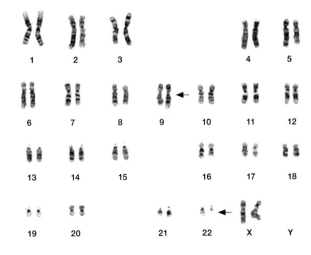

Opposite
After the genome came the proteome, exploring the proteins that an organism's genes produce. Proteomics is the study of all the proteins produced by the genome or of a smaller part, as seen here, that a cell produces. It is being used to explore familial motor neurone disease.

Top
The output of an automated DNA sequencing machine. Each vertical lane shows the base sequence in a stretch of DNA. Each of the four bases is differently coloured and their order analysed by computer. Here is just a tiny part of one chromosome.

Above
'The Philadelphia chromosome': parts of chromosomes 9 and 22 swap places (are translocated). The protein made by the fused chromosome causes uncontrolled cell proliferation of myeloid cells (in the bone marrow), which accumulate in the blood, producing the symptoms of chronic myelogenous leukaemia.

20. THE EVOLUTION OF CANCER
Hijacking the body

Mel Greaves

No man, even under torture, can say exactly what a tumour is.
J. Ewing, 1916

There's nothing new about cancer. It was well recorded by Galen, arguably the first oncologist, in 2nd-century AD Rome, and before him by Hippocrates (*c.* 460–*c.* 370 BC) and the ancient Greek physicians – who coined the insidious name after *carcinos* the crab, translated into Latin as cancer. All vertebrate classes of animal have cancers as do many invertebrate species, so we can safely assume the disease, in one form or another, has been an uninvited companion throughout all human history. But the question 'what is cancer?' remained a challenging mystery through 2,000 years of clinical observation, answers only being delivered, via technological innovation, in the past two or three decades. Galen, Hippocrates and their followers ascribed cancer to an excess of black bile or constitutive melancholy [04]. In the vacuum of understanding, unorthodox theories on causation have abounded, from neurotic personality to divine retribution or, in more current times, electromagnetic waves; or 'it's because you're old'. These lack credibility (or evidence) but play on public fears.

CELLS AND THEIR DNA
The biological nature or architecture of cancer was completely obscure until the invention of the microscope [23] and, later, the advent of cellular pathology in mid-19th century Germany [08]. This led to the recognition that cancer is a disorder of cells disrupting normal tissue structure, and that cancers develop, or evolve, via benign, localized tumours that invade within the tissue of origin and disseminate, via blood and the lymphatics, to form growths, or metastases, in other tissue sites such as the bones, liver or brain. It is the compromise, or hijack, of normal tissue function that is very damaging and ultimately lethal.

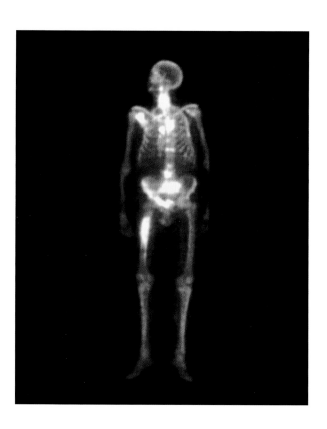

The hijack: a whole body image (gamma camera) of a patient whose skeletal bones have been invaded with prostate cancer. The white areas are cancer masses. The primary tumour was in the prostate and the invading cells in the bones are metastases.

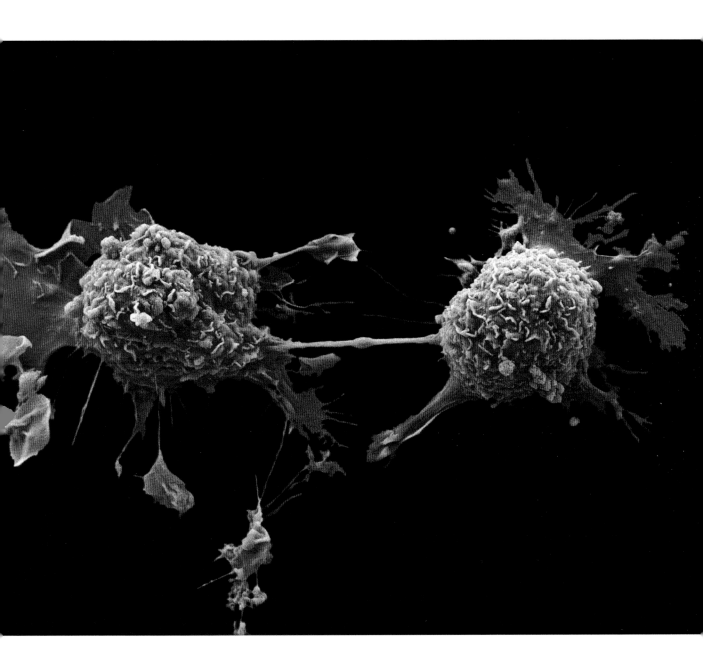

A lung cancer cell dividing into two daughter cells. Cancerous
cells harbour mutations in the genetic information that controls
their behaviour, but just as normal cells divide by cell division so do
their cancerous counterparts. In this image, produced by a scanning
electron microscope, the two daughter cells are only held together
by a very thin bridge of cytoplasm.

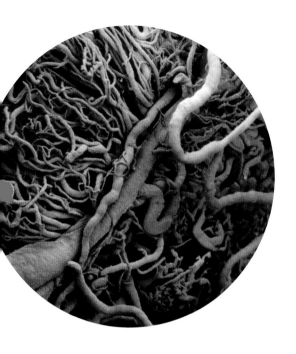

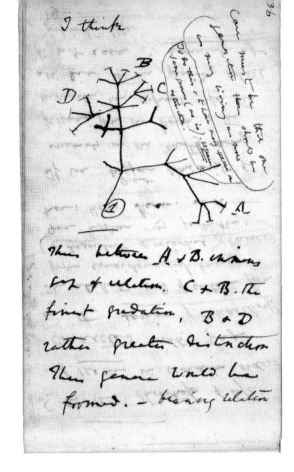

Very early in the 20th century, an insightful German embryologist, Theodor Boveri (1862–1915), speculated that abnormal chromosomes might provide the mechanistic drive or cause of cancer. This turned out to be prescient, though specific chromosomal abnormalities were not identified until the 1960s, and 'oncogenic' DNA mutations in cancer cells in the early 1980s. Today, it is widely recognized that although there are more than 100 varieties of cancer, what they all have in common is that they harbour acquired faults or mutations in the genetic information controlling cell behaviour. These abnormalities vary from gross copy number or structural changes in chromosomes [19], to very subtle modifications of the DNA sequence code; their mutational corruption results in changes to cell proliferation, cell death and cell migration.

CLONES AND NATURAL SELECTION

New technologies that can manipulate the genetic material, DNA, by amplifying small traces, clone individual genes (and assess their function) and, in the 21st century, scrutinize the whole genome sequence of individuals and their cancers have revolutionized our understanding of how the disease develops. And, extraordinarily, the picture that emerges of cancer cell evolution is remarkably similar to natural evolution in ecosystems, except that here we are dealing with the fast-track evolution of variant cells as 'pseudo-species', with our tissues acting as ecosystems. The principle involved is, as Darwin himself suggested, random genetic variation, competition, restraint and natural selection of the 'fittest' variant. In cancer, this translates to cells accidentally acquiring particular mutations – randomly or via so-called genotoxic insult (e.g. cigarette smoke) – and, usually, one single cell and its descendant, mutant clone escaping by bypassing the normal rules of restraint in tissues.

Such are the many evolved restraints that compel the normal social behaviour of cells, particularly in complex species such as ourselves, that a clone can only evolve to become seriously selfish, or cancerous, if it acquires sequentially, over time (usually years or decades) a series of mutations that collectively render the cell and all its clonal progeny blind to normal, physiological controls. The number of mutations per clone can vary from a handful to thousands.

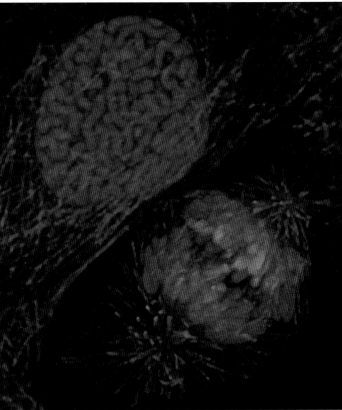

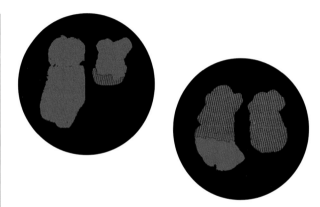

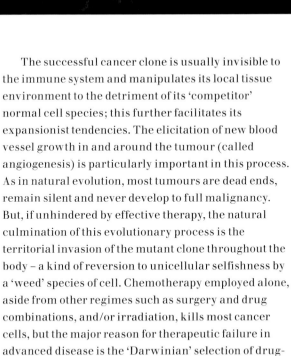

The successful cancer clone is usually invisible to the immune system and manipulates its local tissue environment to the detriment of its 'competitor' normal cell species; this further facilitates its expansionist tendencies. The elicitation of new blood vessel growth in and around the tumour (called angiogenesis) is particularly important in this process. As in natural evolution, most tumours are dead ends, remain silent and never develop to full malignancy. But, if unhindered by effective therapy, the natural culmination of this evolutionary process is the territorial invasion of the mutant clone throughout the body – a kind of reversion to unicellular selfishness by a 'weed' species of cell. Chemotherapy employed alone, aside from other regimes such as surgery and drug combinations, and/or irradiation, kills most cancer cells, but the major reason for therapeutic failure in advanced disease is the 'Darwinian' selection of drug-resistant mutants from within the cancerous clone.

THE FUTURE

The specific genetic changes or 'driver' mutations that have selective potency in cancer development are now – at least the majority of them – well recognized. This then spawns new diagnostic and predictive or prognostic markers and suggests novel, more sharply focused targets for therapy that are beginning to bear fruit.

Cancer, like any biological problem, is certainly very complex. But the smog has lifted. We now understand how it evolves as a cellular disorder. This, together with new insights into variable inherited susceptibility of individuals and predominant causal exposures (cigarettes, sunlight, some viruses), combined with a new armoury of biologically derived and molecularly based diagnostics and therapeutics, heralds a much brighter, if still challenging, future.

21. COMPLEMENTARY MEDICINE
Curing through nature

James Whorton

*Arrogant doctors are ready to take the place of nature, … and you
have to suffer the consequences, foot the bill – and fill the coffin.*
A. Erz, 1914

COMPLEMENTARY, ALTERNATIVE OR IRREGULAR?

The term 'complementary medicine' applies to
a number of approaches to healing lying outside
mainstream medicine, many dating back a century
or more. It is only during the past 20 years, however,
that these therapies have come to be thought of as
'complementary', that is, methods of treatment that
can be used as supplements to, or substitutes for,
conventional procedures. Before that time, such
systems were regarded by the medical establishment
as ineffective and sometimes dangerous, and dismissed
as 'irregular medicine' or 'sectarian medicine'. The
history of relations between the two sides is for the most
part one of bitter conflict.

Unorthodox systems of medical care began to
appear in Western society in the late 18th century.
Each constituted a 'system' by virtue of its practitioners
subscribing to the same set of therapies and supporting
theory, publishing books and journals proclaiming
their methods, forming professional associations
and operating educational institutions; all had a
professional structure, in short, that mirrored that
of conventional medicine.

Yet while each system formulated a unique theory
and employed unique therapies, all were guided by
a shared philosophy of healing: disease was to be
overcome only by procedures that supported the *vis
medicatrix naturae* – the healing power of nature
– innate in every person. Regular medicine, it was
maintained, used methods that operated contrary to
nature and thus inhibited recovery. Natural therapies
were to be discovered, furthermore, only through
experience, not by the abstract theorizing that, it was
charged, dominated orthodox practice. Finally, patients
were to be treated as suffering individuals, not as mere
cases of one or another disease.

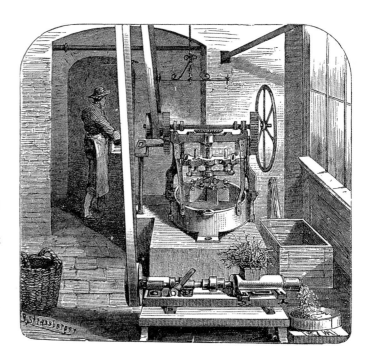

Above
In the early 19th century, Samuel Hahnemann's first experiments
with similars – drugs that produce the same symptoms as the
disease – were with Peruvian bark, the raw material of quinine [44].
He used many other botanicals in his treatments, preparing them
with his plant and herb press, as seen here.

Opposite
Despite their popularity, alternative healing schemes such as
homeopathy were often lampooned, as in this cartoon of 1850. Concern
about homeopathic drugs continues. Double-blind clinical trials
show no greater effect than a placebo, but patients worldwide
report positive experiences.

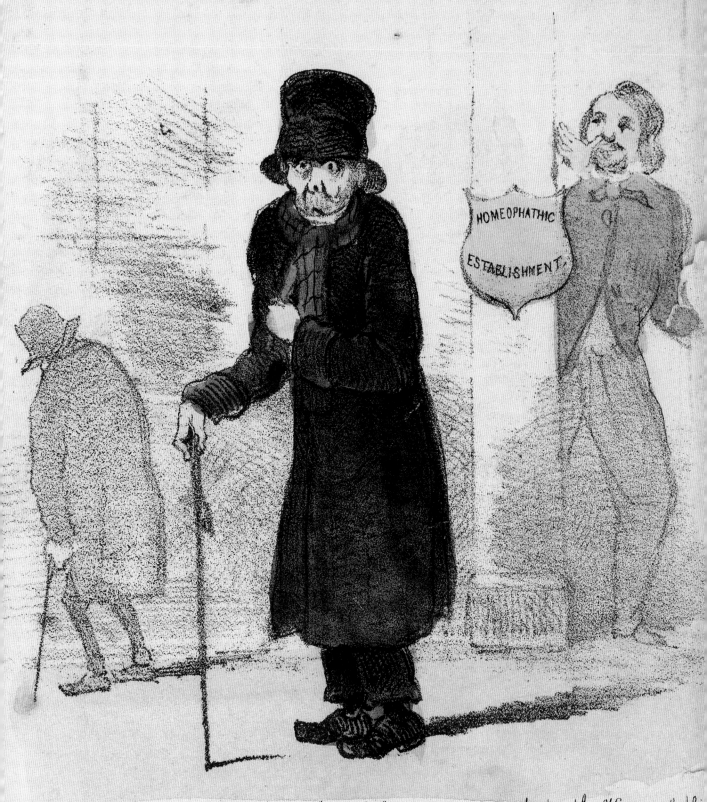

This is the appearance I presented when I became a convert to the Homœopathic theory, and placed myself under the care of Professor Hangthemann, who subjec— me to the globules or infinitesimal system.

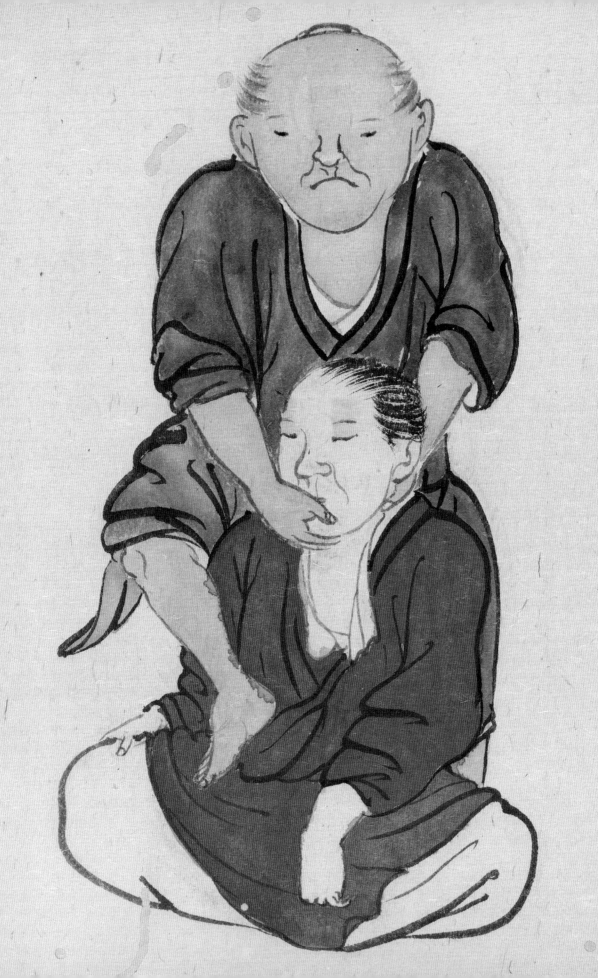

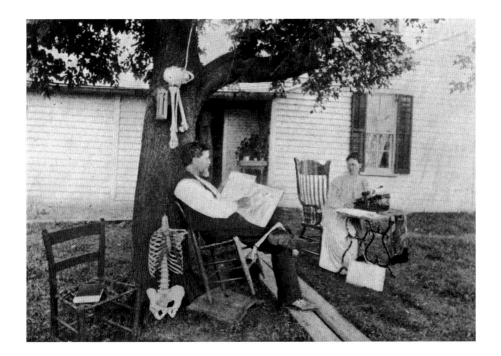

Opposite
While the healing systems of osteopathy and chiropractic were
developed in 19th-century North America, other cultures also
practised various forms of skeletal manipulation, as evidenced in this
19th-century Japanese watercolour.

Above
Andrew Taylor Still and his amanuensis, Miss Annie Morris, outside
her house, where Still conducted much of his research into osteopathy
with the help of his skeletal specimens.

HOMEOPATHY

A system of botanical healing called Thomsonianism
began in the 1790s, but did not last beyond the mid-19th
century. Another irregular system also introduced
in the 1790s, however, has survived and flourishes to
the present. Homeopathy was the creation of Samuel
Hahnemann (1775–1843), a German doctor who
became disillusioned with standard methods and
argued from the results of self-experimentation that
substances that produce certain symptoms in a healthy
subject will cure those same symptoms in a sick one.
To heal, the drug must be similar to the disease, hence
'homeopathy' (Greek *homoios pathos*). Since regular
physicians used drugs that counteracted symptoms,
Hahnemann coined the term allopathy ('other than the
disease') to characterize their work. Complementary
medical practitioners today still refer to conventional
practice as allopathic medicine.

Hahnemann also determined through experiment
that the power of any drug supposedly increased as
it was carried through a series of 100:1 dilutions,
reaching its most effective level when reduced to an
infinitesimal amount incorporated into tiny pills

of milk sugar. This principle of 'potentiation by
dilution' struck allopaths as absurd, of course, and
was mercilessly ridiculed. But despite opposition from
regular medicine, homeopathy spread throughout
Europe and North America during the early 1800s, and
was the most widely supported of all irregular systems
during the 19th century.

SKELETAL MANIPULATION

Another system that thrives still is osteopathic
medicine, developed in America in the 1870s by
Kansas doctor Andrew Taylor Still (1828–1917). Like
Hahnemann, Still grew disenchanted with orthodox
therapies and turned to intuitive trial-and-error
manipulations of the musculoskeletal system. When
these brought about recovery, he hypothesized that
all illness must be due to interference with the
flow of blood through arteries by pressure from
displaced bones; cure simply required the restoration
of skeletal integrity.

Initially, the practice of osteopathy (the name was
coined from Greek roots for bone and disease) involved
only manipulation; the drugs and surgical procedures

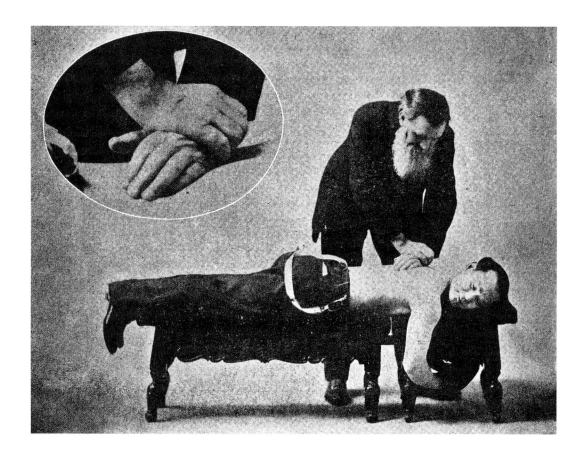

that formed the bulk of standard medical practice were denounced as unnatural and injurious. During the first third of the 20th century, however, first surgery and then drug therapy were gradually integrated into osteopathy. Towards the end of that century, most osteopaths would be virtually indistinguishable from allopaths in their methods, with manipulation playing a prominent role in the practice of only a minority.

In its early days, osteopathy was often confused with another system of musculoskeletal manipulation. Chiropractic was discovered in 1895 by Iowa lay healer D. D. Palmer (1845–1913) when he restored a deaf man's hearing by pushing a misplaced vertebra back into position. Postulating that all disease results from misaligned vertebrae impinging on adjacent nerves and thereby disrupting the flow of a mysterious 'Innate Intelligence', Palmer concluded that a cure could be effected by an 'adjustment' of the offending bone; the method soon became known as chiropractic, from the Greek for 'done by hand'.

As with osteopathy, chiropractic soon admitted the adoption of other therapeutic measures to support the 'adjustments', including items such as electrical

stimulation, heat and vibration. Not all practitioners welcomed these methods, however, and from the 1920s onwards there would be vigorous dissension between 'straight' chiropractors, who advocated manipulation only, and 'mixers'. There would be even greater animosity between chiropractors of both camps and osteopaths, each side accusing the other of stealing its therapeutic methods.

'Mixed chiropractic' was nevertheless modest in its assortment of therapies compared to naturopathy, a system that evolved from several 19th-century traditions, most notably herbal therapy and water-cure. Introduced in 1901 by Benedict Lust (1872–1945), a German immigrant to New York, naturopathy combined botanical remedies, water baths of various kinds, physical manipulations and massage, sunlight, electricity, and, indeed, any natural agent that might stimulate the body's natural recuperative powers.

FROM 'IRREGULAR' TO 'COMPLEMENTARY'
By 1920, then, there were four major rivals to conventional medicine in the Western world, all attracting enough patients to provoke efforts at

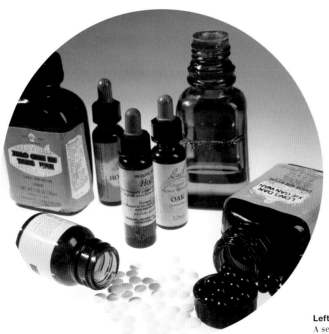

Left
A selection of alternative medicines, including Chinese, homeopathic and Bach flower remedies. Bach's 38 remedies are directed at specific characteristics; for instance, star of Bethlehem is advised for those in shock caused by grief or unexpected bad news.

Opposite
D. D. Palmer at work on a patient, from his *The Chiropractor's Adjuster: Text Book of the Science, Art and Philosophy of Chiropractic for Students and Practitioners* (1910).

suppression by allopaths. Orthodox practitioners loudly denounced alternative competitors as quacks, of course, but they went further politically by opposing attempts to legalize such practices and by having those who practised without a licence arrested and fined and even jailed. Chiropractors, in particular, often found themselves behind bars for offering their services.

In response, each system campaigned for legalization, and through the first half of the 20th century licensing protection was gained by all. Even so, intense hostility between orthodox and heretical practitioners continued into the 1970s. Since that time, however, relations have steadily improved, helped on the one hand by the development of much more rigorous scientific rationales and higher standards of education and practice among all the major unconventional systems, and on the other by alternative practitioners' acknowledgment of efficacy for allopathic medicine, particularly in handling trauma and acute infections.

Also vitally important has been the turn within mainstream medicine towards a more holistic orientation to illness and healing. Treating the whole person, mind and spirit as well as body, with gentler,

less invasive therapies, was, after all, the approach advocated by alternative systems from their inception. As the two sides moved on to this common ground, a spirit of acceptance and then cooperation came to prevail. Medicine's new openness to alternative healing traditions was perhaps most clearly demonstrated by allopathic physicians' interest in acupuncture, an ancient Chinese method [02], when it was introduced to the West in the 1970s. In America, the culmination of this transformation occurred with the 1991 establishment of an Office of Alternative Medicine within the National Institutes of Health; in 1998 the agency was upgraded to the National Center for Complementary and Alternative Medicine. Therapies that had once been despised as 'irregular' were now being welcomed as 'complementary'.

Tools OF
THE *Trade*

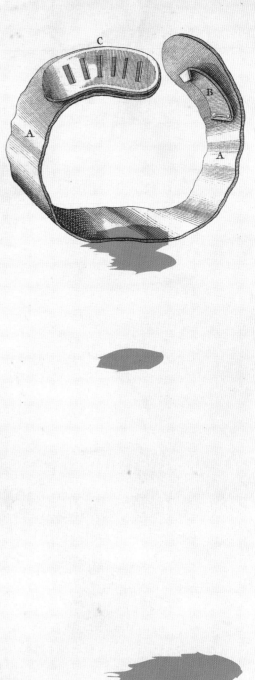

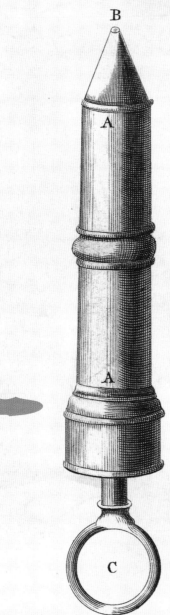

Nᵒ 3.

Modern medicine is surrounded by technology. Instruments and machines are everywhere to be seen in hospitals, health centres and even in the bags doctors carry. From the simple disposable syringe to the amazing MRI scan, instruments dictate what doctors can do and know.

In antiquity vaginal speculums could assist in diagnosing gynaecological problems, scalpels were used to let blood and therapeutic blisters were raised with special cups. However, the range of medical instruments was limited and remained relatively unchanged in the medieval and early modern periods. In medicine's long history before the 19th century, doctors used mostly their five senses, and their experience, to diagnose their patient's illness and to recommend a course of treatment. They felt the pulse, examined the tongue or urine, and listened to the patient's account of his or her affliction, all the while applying their clinical judgment.

During the 19th century doctors began to understand disease in specific rather than general terms. At the same time, they began to use a number of instruments to augment what they could discover about their patients. Thus, the stethoscope, thermometer, microscope, ophthalmoscope and other diagnostic aids came into use, especially when patients were treated in hospitals. By the end of the 19th century, medicine was much more closely allied with science and its emerging technology. Then, in the 1890s, the technology of medicine underwent a quantum leap, with the discovery of X-rays. Their clinical application was immediately recognized, and medicine entered the era of big technology, which is still with us.

Big meant expensive. X-ray machines were costly to build and run, and they required special technicians to operate them and properly trained doctors to interpret the images. A new pattern was set. It has been repeated in other diagnostic innovations featured here, including the new generation of endoscopes and imaging equipment – ultrasound, nuclear-magnetic imaging and PET scans. These and other instruments give the doctors of today a powerful ability to understand what is going on inside their patients' bodies. But there are also humbler technologies that provide vital information, such as the blood-pressure cuff (sphygmomanometer), and which patients can be taught to use themselves.

Diagnosis might dominate medical technology, but new tools have also aided medical and surgical treatments. Defibrillators, to shock the failing heart back into regular activity, can be found in most shopping malls in the US. Doctors use lasers to treat many disorders, especially of the eye. Incubators provide a special environment for premature or seriously ill babies. Medical robots augment the hand of even the most skilled surgeon. Surgical recovery rooms and intensive and coronary care suites are dominated by monitoring equipment, allowing doctors and nurses to keep a watchful eye on the moment-by-moment condition of the critically ill, and by the various machines that can keep us alive until our bodies recover.

All these tools of the trade have shaped medical diagnosis and treatment; they have also fuelled the spiralling costs of medical care, and, in many people's eyes, made modern medicine more impersonal and cold. No one has yet invented a sympathetic machine.

A selection of tools from an 18th-century surgical manual. Left to right: cubical scarificator used to make small incisions in the skin in preparation for cupping; syringe to introduce liquids into the urethra or vagina; leather strap to bind the arm during blood-letting.

22. THE STETHOSCOPE
Listening in

Malcolm Nicolson

*I have tried to place the internal organic lesions on the same
plane as the surgical diseases with respect to diagnosis.*
René Laennec, 1826

The stethoscope enables a medical examiner to hear sounds generated within the patient's body. The instrument was invented in 1816 by the French physician René Laennec (1781–1826), but its origins lie in the previous century. Leopold Auenbrugger (1722–1809), a Viennese physician, discovered that pathological alterations within the thorax could be revealed by tapping firmly on the patient's chest. He confirmed his observations by post-mortem dissection, conducting experiments in which he injected fluid into the lungs of cadavers. Auenbrugger published his results in 1761, but thoracic percussion, as it became known, did not gain in popularity until the early decades of the 19th century, with the work of the Paris School.

From the late 1790s onwards, in the large hospitals of the French capital, a systematic effort was made to correlate clinical signs and symptoms observed in the living patient with lesions revealed post-mortem [07]. This mode of investigation became known as the 'anatomico-clinical' method. One of its leading practitioners, Jean-Nicolas Corvisart (1755–1821), revived and refined Auenbrugger's innovation of thoracic percussion. Corvisart also encouraged his colleagues to employ auscultation – listening directly to the sounds that could be heard within the body cavities – which had been known to the Greeks but which had largely fallen into disuse.

Laennec, who had been a student of Corvisart, took a special interest in diseases of the chest. On one occasion, he was consulted by a young woman who seemed to be suffering from heart disease. She was plump and Laennec was unable to get her chest to resonate upon percussion and he felt inhibited from pressing his head firmly against the bosom of his female patient. Remembering a game he had seen played by children, he rolled several sheets of paper into a tube

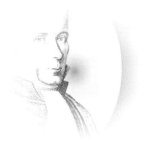

and placed one end against the woman's chest. Putting his ear to the other end, he was pleased to be able to hear the sounds of her heart quite distinctly. The stethoscope had been invented.

EXPERIMENTS AND DEVELOPMENTS
Laennec experimented with various materials and shapes for his new instrument, finally deciding on a simple hollow wooden cylinder, about 25 cm (10 in) long and 3.5 cm (just over 1 in) in diameter. With this tool, Laennec undertook a comprehensive investigation of the sounds to be heard emanating from the heart

Above
René Laennec, inventor of the stethoscope: he probably succumbed to tuberculosis of the lungs, one of the diseases that became easier to diagnose with a stethoscope.

Opposite above
The stethoscope was eminently transportable. In this late 19th-century illustration a doctor is depicted examining a gypsy child in a caravan on the roadside.

Opposite below
Four examples of the long form, or second type, of Laennec's stethoscopes. The one on the left has a slip joint, the other three have screw joints; both types allowed the rigid tube to be separated and put into the pocket, and all have removable earpieces. (See also p. 162.)

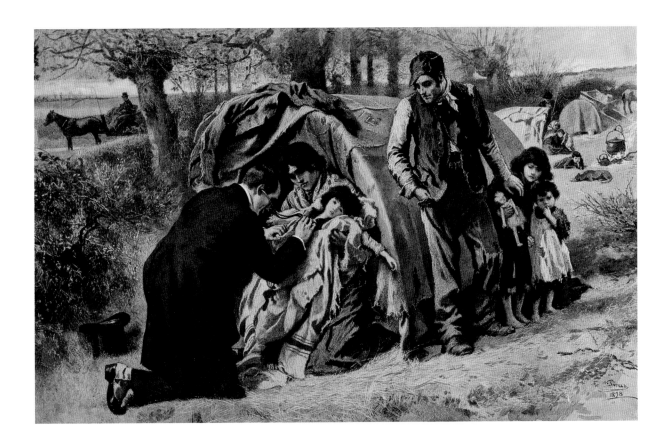

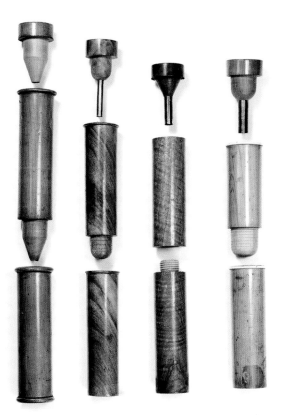

and lungs, comparing his findings, wherever possible, with pathological alterations observed on autopsy. His results were published in 1819 in his major work, *De l'auscultation médiate* (*On Mediate Auscultation*), which remains the basis of our modern understanding of the pathology of the lungs and, to an extent, also of the heart.

While there was a certain amount of opposition to the employment of the stethoscope from conservative doctors, who either felt the use of an instrumental aid would compromise their professional dignity or were unable to educate their ears sufficiently to apply the technique, Laennec's innovation came into general use quite quickly. The expansion of clinical teaching in hospitals that occurred in the 19th century provided students with the necessary supply of patients upon whom to practise and gain experience with the instrument. By the end of the century, the stethoscope had become an indispensable badge of office of the medical practitioner.

It should, however, be noted that, despite Laennec's claims to the contrary, the stethoscope possessed few acoustic advantages over the older technique of applying the ear directly to the patient's chest. In most

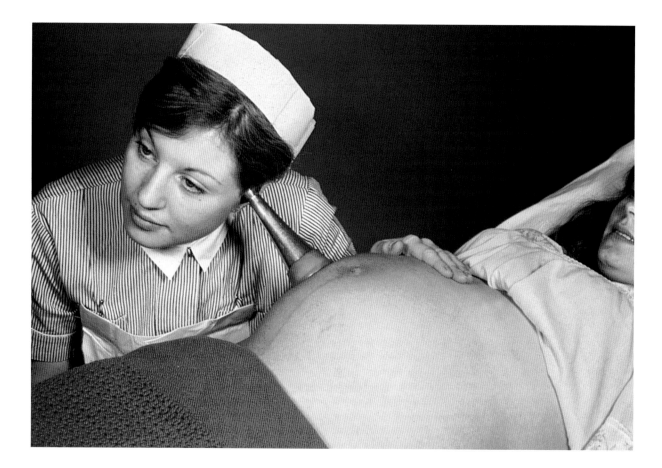

cases, the instrument did not enable the listener to hear the thoracic sounds any louder or clearer than with the naked ear. One exception is the detection of cavitation in the apex of the lung, an early sign of pulmonary tuberculosis, for which the doctor would have to insert an ear into the patient's armpit to investigate by direct auscultation. This circumstance notwithstanding, what was attractive about Laennec's invention was that it enabled the physician to examine the chest conveniently and hygienically, while preserving his personal and professional dignity and respecting the modesty of his patients, particularly female ones. The widespread adoption of the stethoscope accustomed lay people to being examined by the doctor and stimulated the development of other methods of physical diagnosis.

Considerations of professional convenience were to shape further developments of stethoscope design. In 1828 N. P. Comins, an Edinburgh physician, designed an instrument with a hinge between its two sections, which would enable the exploration of 'any part of the chest, in any position, and in any stage of disease, without pressure or inconvenience to the patient or to himself'. Numerous other modifications were

suggested to improve the acoustics or the ease of use of the instrument. C. J. B. Williams (1805–89) constructed a binaural stethoscope in 1843, but it was not until the introduction of flexible rubber tubes in the 1880s that employing both ears in auscultation became wholly practical. Another innovation was the provision of a bell-shaped end, often incorporating a diaphragm. Amplification of the heart and lung sounds was also experimented with.

A CONTINUED ROLE

Despite the invention of sophisticated imaging technologies, the stethoscope is still indispensable to the cardiologist and to the general practitioner. Numerous applications have been found beyond the thoracic region, such as in the measurement of blood pressure [27] and in the management of pregnancy. A variety of electronic digital stethoscopes, which can continuously monitor sound and provide recordings and visual displays, are now available. They have applications in cardiology and are also employed in teaching and telemedicine (electronic consultation at a distance).

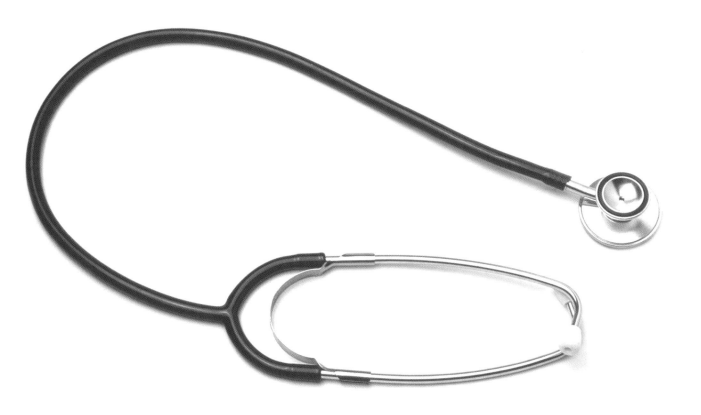

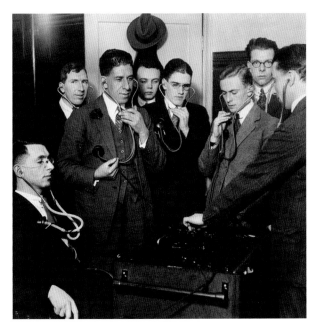

Opposite
Before the advent of electronic fetal monitoring, the fetal stethoscope trumpet enabled the midwife to listen to the unborn child's heartbeat.

Above
The introduction of the binaural stethoscope with rubber tubing, which could either be coiled into a pocket or, more frequently, hung around the neck, transformed the image of the doctor. It made examination easier and more dignified for both patient and doctor, with less intrusion into the former's personal space.

Left
Learning to listen and understand what was heard with a stethoscope were important skills for trainee doctors. What better way to begin than with a self-examination? Here a group of medical students from the 1920s listen to their own chests.

23. THE MICROSCOPE
Discovering new worlds

Ariane Dröscher

... by the help of Microscopes, there is nothing so small, as to escape our inquiry; hence there is a new visible World discovered to the understanding.
Robert Hooke, 1665

The first microscope was probably constructed in China. An ancient Chinese text describes how a tube with a lens at its bottom was filled with as much water as required to obtain different degrees of magnification; it seems the virtues of lenses were already known in antiquity. However, the broad diffusion of microscopy and its impact on natural philosophy began only in 17th-century Europe. Curiously, its invention initially created more puzzles than answers. Since the 19th century the microscope has become the symbol of biomedical research, linked to many great discoveries. Today, it is still indispensable for teaching and for clinical and forensic investigation.

THE FIRST INSTRUMENTS AND THEIR CHALLENGES

Throughout their history, microscopes were the product of the intimate collaboration between makers and users, aiming to overcome obstacles that were physical (resolution, magnification, aberrations); methodological (three-dimensionality, observation of living things, techniques); practical (manageability); and philosophical (interpretation of the image).

Light microscopes are actually straightforward constructions: simple microscopes consist of one lens (or magnifying glass drop); compound microscopes have two or more lenses assembled in a rigid tube. It might therefore be thought strange that the microscope's Western 'invention' occurred only in the early modern period. The reasons are multiple and show that more than technical skills were required; particular factors were the revival of atomism (the notion that things were made up of discrete particles), confidence in sensory experience, the spread of anatomical dissection, and the increasing market for spectacles. From the late 16th century onwards, convergent contributions were made by several

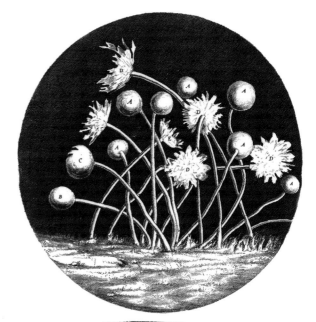

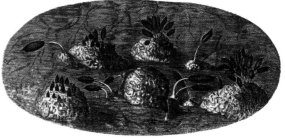

Above
Illustrations from Robert Hooke's masterpiece of microscopy, *Micrographia* (1665), showing, top, blue mould and, below, tiny 'plants' (fungi) growing on the blight spots on plant leaves.

Opposite
The frontispiece to Francesco Stelluti's *Melissographia* (1625), in which he presented the first anatomical details of the bee as seen with a microscope.

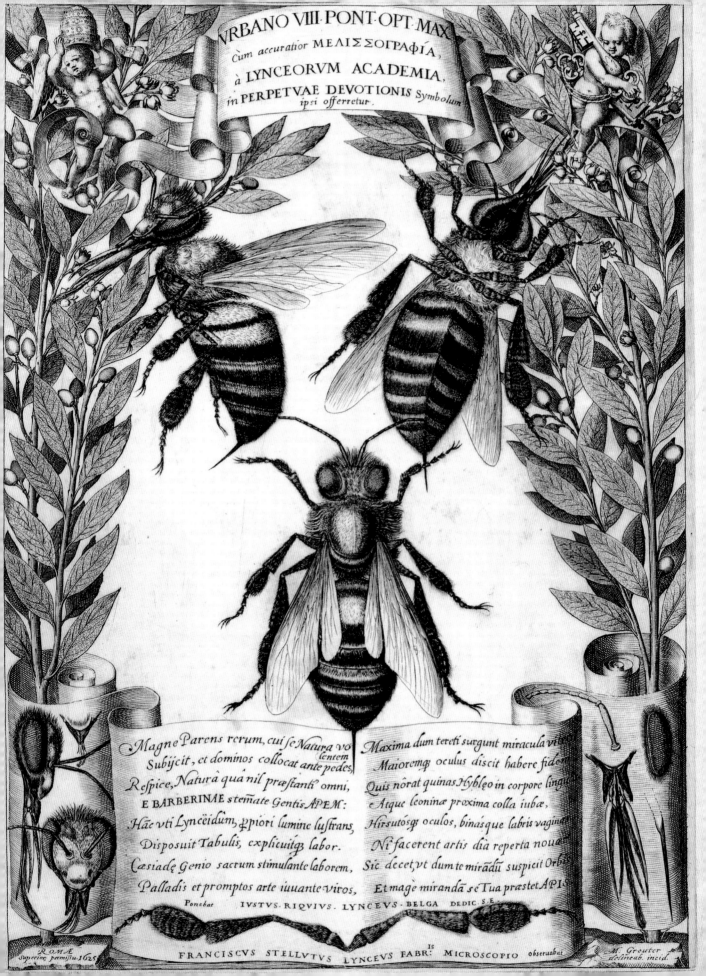

European scholars and craftsmen – Italian, Dutch and French in particular.

The first major promoters of microscopy were the scientific academies, namely the Accademia dei Lincei in Rome, and later the Royal Society of London. In 1612 Galileo Galilei (1564–1642) probably made the first scientific microscopic observation, of the eyes and hairy legs of a fly. His friend Giovanni Faber (1585–1630) coined the term 'microscopium' in 1625, and Francesco Stelluti (1577–1646) published the first micrograph (of a honey bee). Robert Hooke (1635–1703), curator of experiments at the Royal Society, greatly contributed to the technical improvement of compound microscopes and to their broad diffusion with his successful and splendidly illustrated *Micrographia* (1665).

However, even the important work of the Dutch draper and amateur lens grinder Antoni van Leeuwenhoek (1632–1723) and others failed to convince most physicians and natural philosophers of the veracity of the microscopic image and of the microscope's practical benefits. In the 18th century the microscope was mainly used by field botanists and for the study of microscopic organisms. Yet these *animalculi* or *infusoria* as they were called created great dilemmas for mechanistic natural philosophy. The most famous debate concerned the question of whether or not these microorganisms originated through spontaneous generation – an issue that became of great medical importance with the rise of microbiology and bacteriology in the 19th century [14]. Another advance made during the late 18th century was the increasing standardization of microscopes and of microscopic methodology.

THE GOLDEN AGE OF MICROSCOPY

The greatest technical breakthrough of the first decades of the 19th century was the development of achromatic lenses (that transmit light without separating it into its constituent colours), again due to several independent contributions, such as those of Giovanni Battista Amici (1786–1863), Jacques-Louis-Vincent Chevalier (1770–1841) and his son Charles Louis Chevalier (1804–59), and Joseph Jackson Lister (1786–1869).

Microscopy now entered its golden age, becoming indispensable for anatomical and pathological inquiry and underpinning the great discoveries of microbiology, cell biology [08] and neurology [09]. This in turn further stimulated advances in the construction of optical instruments and in microscopic techniques, especially in fixing, embedding, cutting and staining. Ernst Abbe (1840–1905) demonstrated mathematically the fundamentals of diffraction, aberration and optical resolution, and concluded that even the best microscope could not distinguish as separate entities two points less

The horizontal achromatic microscope of the French father and son team Jacques-Louis-Vincent Chevalier and Charles Louis Chevalier, manufacturers of microscopes and other optical instruments. This type was first made in 1834 and illustrated in Charles Chevalier's book on microscopes published in 1839. The eyepiece is on the left and the height-adjustable stage, where specimens were placed for study, is on the right.

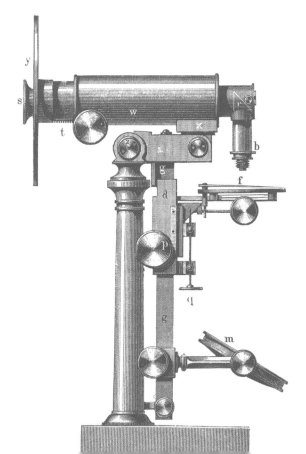

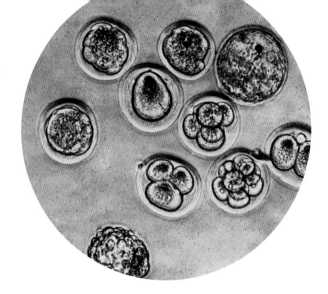

than 200 nanometres (20 millionth of a metre) apart. With Carl Zeiss (1816–88) he then established, a factory for the manufacture of high-quality microscopes.

NEW TYPES OF MICROSCOPES

Other light sources, mainly of shorter wavelengths, were captured by the dark field (1903) and the ultraviolet (1904) microscopes, which preceded the first fluorescence microscope (1911, Oskar Heimstädt). Today, there are also acoustic (using ultrasound) and thermal wave microscopes. Further improvements in contrast and in living-cell observation came, for instance, with the interference microscope (1931), the phase contrast microscope (1935, Frits Zernike) and the differential interference contrast microscope (1955, Georges Nomarski), while confocal microscopes (1957, Marvin Minsky) were developed for thick specimens.

A qualitative jump was made with the invention of electron microscopy, which does not diffract light but uses magnetic lenses and beams of electrons. The first 'supermicroscope' was constructed in 1928 by Ernst Ruska (1906–88); it soon exceeded the maximum power of resolution of light microscopes, reaching the level of 30 nanometres (300 millionth of a metre) in 1940, and able to see the tobacco mosaic virus (TMV). In the 1950s the development of specific techniques for the electron microscope opened the door to ultrastructure research

in biology. The scanning tunnelling microscope (1981, Gerd Binnig and Heinrich Rohrer) provides three-dimensional images of objects down to the atomic level and has been applied to examining viruses.

Today, theoretical and technical improvements continue. New tools such as digital microscopes and stimulation emission depletion microscopy, and microscopes that can localize single molecules offer still new entrance points to unveil the intimate structure of matter. The potential benefits of such developments for medicine would no doubt astound the microscope's earliest practitioners.

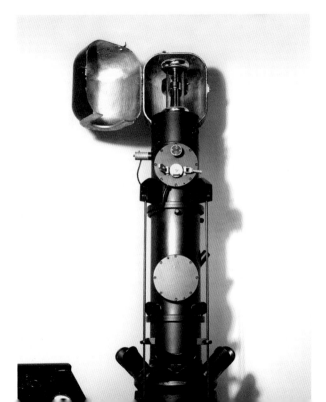

Above
A collection of early human embryos at different stages of development. The embryos are visualized using Nomarski Interference Contrast, developed by the Polish optical physicist Georges (Jerzy) Nomarski. This technique uses a special kind of prism and polarized light, enhancing the contrast in unstained, living biological samples and giving excellent results in these delicate structures.

Left
This Metropolitan Vickers EM2 electron microscope of 1946 was part of a new way of seeing microscopically, using electron beams and magnetic lenses rather than diffracted light. Each of its two lenses has a maximum magnification of 100, giving a combined magnification of 10,000, which could increase to 50,000 times magnification if the plates were enlarged photographically.

24. THE HYPODERMIC SYRINGE
Getting under the skin

Robert Tattersall

Sherlock Holmes took his bottle from the corner of the mantelpiece, and his hypodermic syringe from its neat morocco case. With his long, white, nervous fingers he adjusted the delicate needle, and rolled back his left shirt-cuff. For some little time his eyes rested thoughtfully upon the sinewy forearm and wrist all dotted and scarred with innumerable puncture-marks. Finally he thrust the sharp point home, pressed down the tiny piston, and sank back into the velvet-lined arm-chair with a long sigh of satisfaction.
Sir Arthur Conan Doyle, 1890

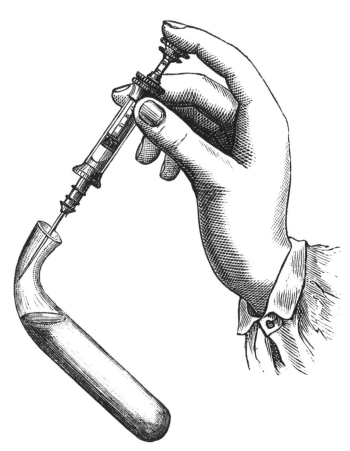

In 1657 the architect Christopher Wren injected various drugs intravenously into animals, which were 'immediatly purg'd, vomited, intoxicated, kill'd, or reviv'd'. The method was used sporadically on patients but gradually fell into disuse. During the 18th century metal or wood syringes were used for vaginal and rectal administration, but attempts were not made to puncture the skin until the mid-19th century. In 1844 Francis Rynd (1811–61) of Dublin used a gravity-fed device to introduce morphine along the course of a nerve to treat neuralgia. The Frenchman Charles-Gabriel Pravaz (1791–1853) made a metal syringe with a screw plunger and hollow needle to inject a coagulant into the arteries of horses, hoping that this could be used to treat aneurysms in humans.

The first hypodermic injection was done by a Scot, Alexander Wood (1817–84), who used what we would recognize as a syringe to inject morphine along the course of a nerve. He was aiming for local analgesia but noted that his patients became sleepy, which implied that morphine must have reached the brain. Wood's 1854 paper in an Edinburgh journal attracted little attention, but following one in the *British Medical*

A glass Pravaz syringe: here the vaccine is being returned to the tube after initial filling to avoid the risk of air bubbles. Tiny air bubbles will be absorbed, but larger bubbles are potentially dangerous, causing an obstruction or air embolism if introduced into a blood vessel during an injection.

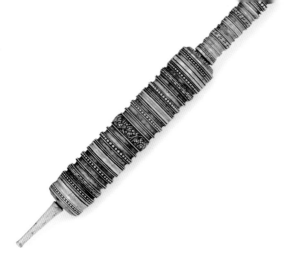

Journal in 1858, he was deluged with letters asking where syringes could be bought. A young London surgeon, Charles Hunter (1834/5–78), pointed out that painkilling injections did not have to be given around nerves but worked when injected into any area of the body. He used the term hypodermic as opposed to Wood's subcutaneous (both meaning 'under the skin'), and they conducted a long and acrimonious correspondence in the *Medical Times and Gazette* about priority for recognizing the remote effects following injection.

Opiates were freely available in Victorian Britain and soon many middle- and upper-class women had become addicted and often used injections of morphine to get to sleep [43], while Sherlock Holmes used cocaine to stimulate his powers of deduction. Self-injection was helped by such devices as mini-syringes, which could be attached to key chains, and 'automatic injectors'. By the 1920s metal syringes with leather plungers had been replaced by all glass syringes.

The use of syringes was greatly increased by the introduction of insulin in 1922–23 [65]; in the 1930s 60 per cent of all injections were to diabetics. The business of injecting insulin was cumbersome, however – syringes were supposed to be boiled before each injection, which led to breakages, and needles had to be resharpened with a stone. The first (plastic) insulin syringe with a permanently attached needle was marketed in 1969, and in 1981 John Ireland (1933–88) invented Penject, which combined the vial of insulin and syringe in a single unit in which the required dose could be dialled. The idea was taken on board by the Novo company of Copenhagen, who in 1985 launched NovoPen, the precursor of the modern insulin injectors that will soon make the insulin syringe obsolete.

Until the 1950s blood for (relatively infrequent) laboratory tests was taken with ground glass syringes, which had to be sterilized after each use. In 1947 the American firm Becton Dickinson developed the vacuum tube system for withdrawing blood, and in 1961 produced the first disposable plastic syringe for venepuncture.

Above
A highly decorative 16th-century Sri Lankan ivory syringe (for the delivery of enemas), said to have been a gift from King Kirthisin Rajasinghe to his royal physicians.

Below
A French syringe and accessory kit used for blood transfusion during the Second World War.

Below right
This fine-needled injection 'pen' enables diabetics to self-regulate their blood glucose level and thus actively manage their condition. The correct amount of insulin is calibrated against the number scale on the end.

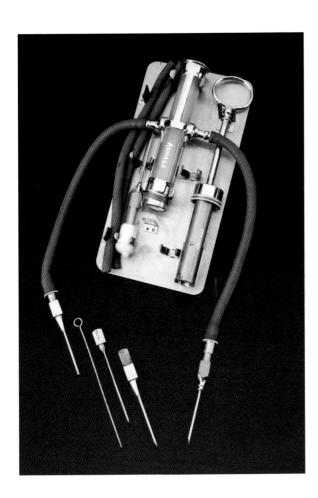

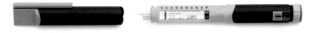

25. THE THERMOMETER
'Measure is medicine'

John Ford

*A knowledge of the course of temperature in disease
is indispensable to medical practitioners.*
Carl Wunderlich, 1871

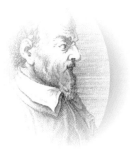

The heat of patients suffering from fever has been
noted since antiquity. Hippocrates (*c.* 460–*c.* 370 BC)
used his hand to measure it, but the Italian Santorio
Sanctorius (1561–1636) is credited with inventing the
first thermometer used in clinical practice. At about
the same time, Galileo Galilei (1564–1642) described
an instrument using the expansion of air over water
to measure temperature, but he did not investigate the
significance of temperature changes in disease. Other
experimenters used the expansion of such substances
as water, wine, oil of aniseed and mercury, but it
was difficult to produce a standard against which to
graduate the different instruments.

To overcome this problem, the German physicist
Gabriel Fahrenheit (1686–1763) proposed three fixed
points: zero was the freezing point of a mixture of ice,
water and sea salt; 32° the freezing point of water; and
96° the external body temperature measured by his
instrument. The scale devised by Swedish astronomer
Anders Celsius (1701–44) took the freezing point of
water as 0°, while 100° was the point at which it boiled.
Clinically useful thermometers could be produced
with improved glass-blowing techniques and the

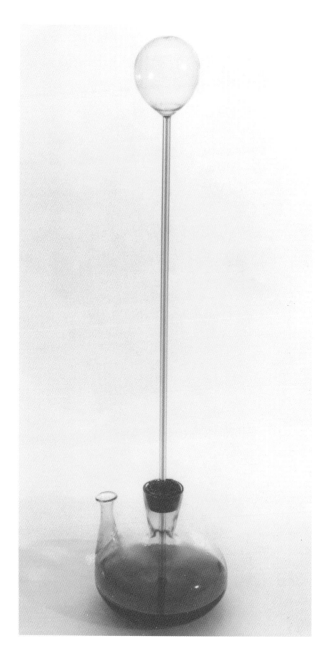

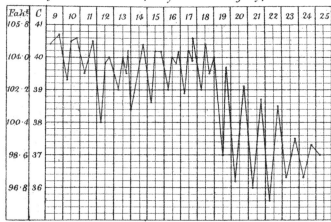

Fig 3. Intense, rapidly recovering Typhoid.

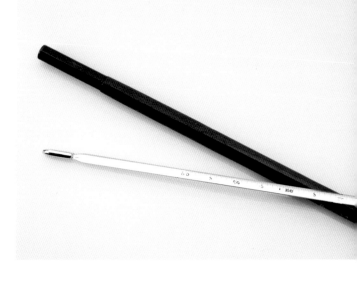

introduction of hydrocyanic acid to etch the glass with gradations of scale.

Several clinicians tried to correlate temperature with disease. In Vienna Anton de Haen (1704–76) took regular measurements from febrile patients, and thought that recovery occurred when the temperature returned to normal. Standards for the variation of temperature with disease were produced by Gabriel Andral (1797–1876) at the university of Paris. James Currie (1756–1805) is credited with the first systematic record in English of clinical observations with the thermometer. The importance of measuring a patient's temperature regularly was emphasized by the work of Carl Wunderlich (1815–77) in Germany. He reported having taken the temperatures of about 25,000 patients and correlated the patterns of the readings – which he showed graphically with the introduction of the temperature chart – with different diseases.

The accumulation of this mass of statistics demonstrating the importance of thermometry in regular clinical practice was a remarkable achievement, especially as Wunderlich's thermometer was 30 cm (1 ft) long and took 20 minutes to register.

Importantly, he showed that it was not necessary for the doctor to take the temperature, but that the task could be delegated to a trained nurse or member of the family. In Britain Clifford Allbutt (1836–1925) introduced a thermometer that was only around 15 cm (6 in) long and which took five minutes to register. This advance meant that, by the late 1860s, taking the temperature was a normal part of the clinical assessment of a patient.

Traditionally the temperature has been taken with the thermometer in the mouth, but this can be difficult with unconscious or uncooperative patients. Alternative sites used have been the armpit, the vagina and the rectum – the last being for many years the preferred site for babies. The difficulty of re-setting a glass mercury thermometer after use by vigorous shaking and the dangers associated with breakage led to the development of safer devices. Electronic digital instruments are now in common use, often taking the temperature in the ear, and strips applied to the forehead using thermal imaging technology are frequently used by the parents of sick children.

26. X-RAYS & RADIOTHERAPY
Invisible light illuminates the body

Michael Jackson

The surgical imagination can pleasurably lose itself in devising endless applications of this wonderful process. If it becomes possible to drive these mysterious rays through the entire body as clearly as they now penetrate the hand, the realm of utility will be practically boundless.
Dr Henry Cattell, 1896

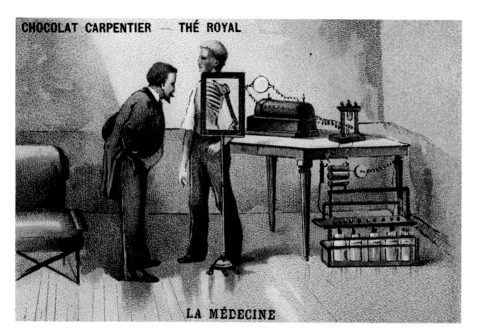

CHOCOLAT CARPENTIER — THÉ ROYAL

LA MÉDECINE

Left
X-rays were quickly taken up in popular culture. An advertising card for the French company Chocolat Carpentier from around 1896/1900 shows a doctor looking into an X-ray screen placed in front of a man's body and seeing the ribs and the bones of the arm.

Opposite
The iconic X-ray image of the bones of Mrs Röntgen's hand, with a ring on one finger, taken by her husband in 1895.

The origin of both radiology and radiotherapy can be traced back to Friday, 8 November 1895. Working in his laboratory, Wilhelm Conrad Röntgen (1845–1923), Professor of Physics at the University of Würzburg in Germany, noted unexpected glowing from some paper coated in barium platinocyanide solution. He had been passing current through a coil inside an evacuated glass tube – a method known at the time to generate cathode rays. Röntgen knew such rays could cause fluorescence in platinocyanide screens, but he had wrapped the tube in black cardboard – impervious to cathode rays – and he realized the cause of the glowing green light from the paper must be 'a new kind of ray'.

Aware of the significance of his finding, Röntgen spent the following month meticulously investigating what he labelled X-rays. He revealed them to penetrate not only card but also books, wood, rubber and a variety of thin metal sheets. Placing his wife's hand between the coil and a photographic plate produced the first radiographic image of the human body – the bones of the hand seen clearly, with skin and flesh rendered translucent. Röntgen presented his work to the Würzburg Physico-Medical Society on 28 December 1895.

News of the discovery spread with remarkable speed around the globe, generating excitement among the scientific community and public alike. The clinical

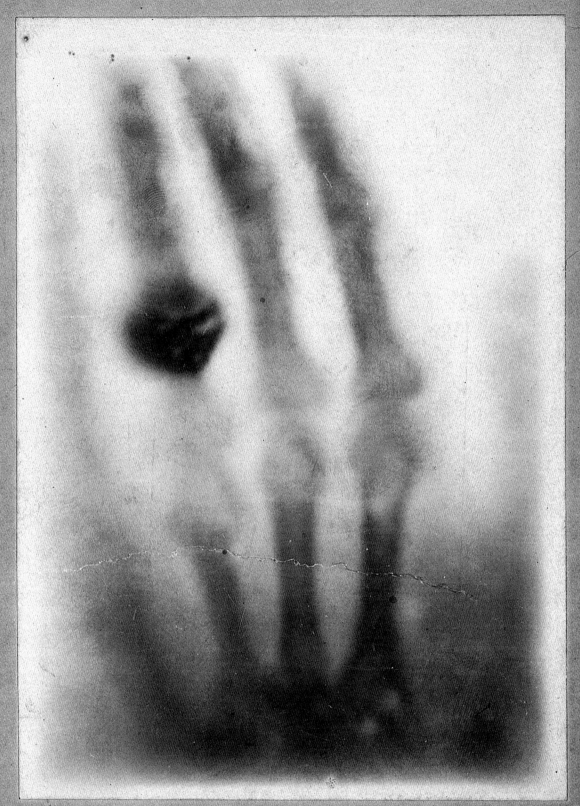

utility of X-rays was recognized instantly, and the first radiograph for medical purposes was taken within a month of Röntgen's announcement. Early images were largely of broken bones, bony tumours and gunshot or bullets embedded within soft tissue – structures of high density that could be demonstrated with (relatively) short exposure times. Images of the chest and abdomen were initially of poor quality, requiring exposure times of longer than 30 minutes [31].

RADIOTHERAPY

Harmful effects of X-rays were seen at an early stage. Röntgen himself noted skin ulceration and hair loss following prolonged exposures, and radiation dermatitis became increasingly common in those operating X-ray equipment. A Chicago medical student, Emil Grubbe (1875–1960), realized that X-rays also had therapeutic potential and used them to treat a woman with breast cancer in early 1896. This was soon followed by treatment of stomach cancer in France, skin tumours in Vienna, and apparent cures of head and neck cancers in Sweden, establishing radiotherapy as a promising new treatment for a variety of cancers.

Partly inspired by Röntgen's work, Henri Becquerel (1852–1908), working in Paris, discovered spontaneous radioactivity in uranium in 1896. Two years later, Becquerel accidentally left some radium in his chest pocket for a number of hours, leading to ulceration of the underlying skin for several weeks. The realization that radioactive elements could produce similar physiological effects to X-rays led to the technique of brachytherapy – treating cancerous tumours by placing a radioactive source in direct contact with them.

Increased understanding of the nature of X-rays and radioactivity, together with biological models to explain their effects, led to safer, more effective radiotherapy throughout the 20th century. Fractionated radiotherapy, in which several smaller doses of radiation are administered separated by intervals, reduced side effects to healthy tissue compared to one big dose while retaining the equivalent potency to the target tumour. Increased power of X-ray tubes allowed the type of radiation to be tailored to the tumour being treated.

DEVELOPMENTS IN MEDICINE AND BEYOND

More powerful tubes also reduced exposure times for radiographs, enabling good-quality images of the chest and abdomen. Tumours, infection and evidence of heart disease became readily apparent on chest radiographs,

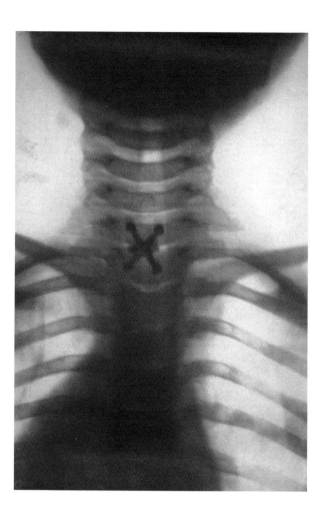

Above
A typical early diagnostic X-ray image, *c.* 1906, in which a metal toy is clearly visible. The metal (like bone) shows up so well because of its high density – blocking the X-rays and preventing them from exposing the photographic plate.

Opposite above
The control panel in the deep X-ray therapy department at the Marie Curie Hospital for Cancer and Allied Diseases, 1934. The hospital building was bought after a fund-raising appeal and staffed by women doctors. Marie Curie, who discovered radioactive polonium and radium, endorsed the hospital's work.

Opposite below
A Jackson X-ray tube from 1896. On the right is a cup-shaped cathode that focuses the cathode rays on to the target (to the left in the central bulb), a platinum anode. When the rays hit the anode, their energy is changed into invisible X-rays, which pass through the glass.

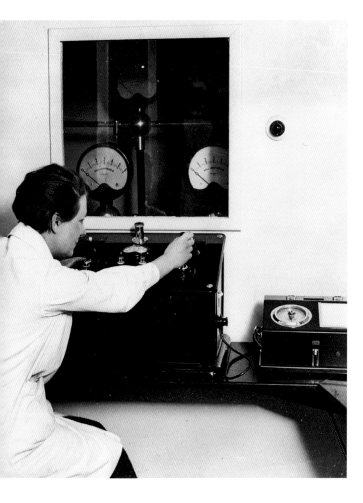

which rapidly became one of the most common medical investigations in the world. The use of barium, which is opaque to X-rays, whether swallowed or administered as an enema, provided new insights into the gastrointestinal tract and its diseases. Intravenous contrast agents were to follow, allowing visualization of blood vessels and the renal tract.

A succession of technical improvements in combination with a growing appreciation of how valuable radiodiagnosis and radiotherapy were becoming to patient care led to massive uptake of equipment and personnel in hospitals in the first half of the 20th century. This was accompanied by the development of training structures and professional bodies for radiographers and radiologists.

By the end of the Second World War both radiology and radiotherapy were firmly established within the practice of modern medicine. Yet it was only with the concluding acts of the war – the bombings of Hiroshima and Nagasaki in 1945 – that radiation safety was finally to become embedded within the specialties. Survivors of the atomic bombs provided sobering proof of the danger of radiation, both in the form of severe sickness soon after the bombings, and in cancers occurring in the years and decades that followed. These individuals not only provided the impetus to prioritize radiation safety within medicine, but also, in the form of follow-up studies correlating radiation dose with disease, provided the data with which this could be achieved.

Beyond the clinical arena, Röntgen's discovery would lead to profound insights into the physical nature of the universe, from the intergalactic to the subatomic scale. The award of the first Nobel Prize in Physics to Röntgen in 1901 heralded a new era of discovery within this field. X-ray crystallography would furthermore provide the tool for discovering the structure of DNA [10]. Within popular culture X-rays and their (often fictional) applications have likewise had a major impact, beloved of superheroes and voyeurs alike. Yet had the discovery of X-rays (or Röntgen rays as they are known by way of tribute in North America) led only to plain radiographs and X-ray beam radiotherapy, this would still remain a remarkable legacy.

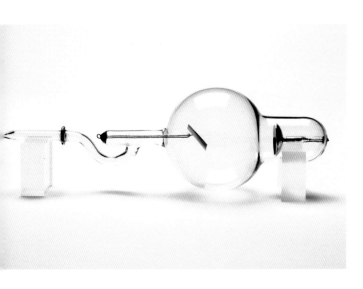

THE SPHYGMOMANOMETER
Feeling the pressure

Carsten Timmermann

Since arterial pressure is easily and quickly measured, high blood pressure has become one of the conditions most frequently diagnosed by the doctor and dreaded by the patient.
George White Pickering, 1955

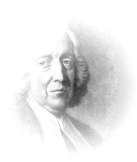

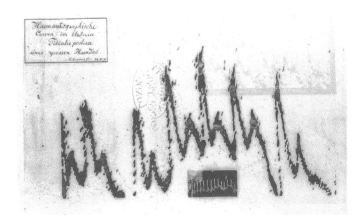

The sphygmomanometer is a piece of 19th-century physiological laboratory equipment that has become part of routine medical practice. The instrument, connected to the inflatable blood pressure cuff, is one of the most basic and common diagnostic tools in modern medicine. Its ease of use made blood pressure an ideal parameter for large-scale epidemiological studies aiming to identify risk factors for heart disease in the post-Second World War era.

EXPERIMENTAL MEASUREMENTS

The first documented experimental blood pressure measurements were performed on animals, notably horses and dogs, by the English naturalist Stephen Hales (1677–1761) in the early 18th century. Interested in the mechanics of circulation [11], Hales measured the pressure of the blood by severing a major blood vessel of a horse and inserting a brass tube connected to a long, upright glass tube, enabling him to observe the height of the blood column. In early 19th-century Paris, Jean Louis Marie Poiseuille (1799–1869) replaced Hales's long glass tube with one that was shorter and filled with mercury to build his haemodynamometer. In his 1828

medical school thesis he was the first to use the unit mm Hg (millimetres of mercury). The German physiologist Carl Ludwig (1816–95) combined Poiseuille's setup with a recording cylinder to create his kymograph (Greek for 'wave writer'). Depending on which blood vessel was severed, these experiments often resulted in the subjects' deaths. Clearly, such invasive approaches were not suitable for clinical routine.

Clinical interest in blood pressure measurement grew out of the traditional practice of taking the pulse and 19th-century attempts to identify its tension. Pulse-taking was a qualitative practice, relying on the touch and judgment of a learned physician. A variety of sphygmographs (*sphygmo* is Greek for pulse) were developed in the late 19th century. These instruments recorded pulse waves non-invasively and allowed the move from animals to human subjects. Sphygmographs turned the pulse of an experimental subject into a graphical trace that could be stored, studied, reproduced and compared. They did not, however, produce standardizable, numerical blood pressure readings. Most clinicians, moreover, ignored the new instruments, preferring traditional pulse taking.

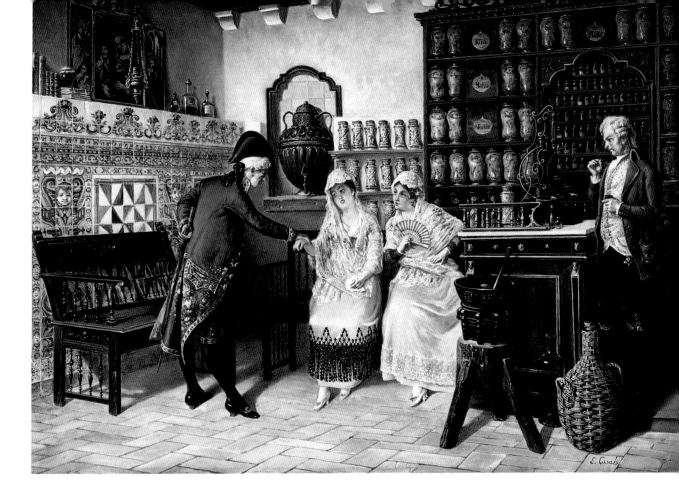

THE MODERN SPHYGMOMANOMETER

Modern sphygmomanometers do not measure the strength of the arterial pulse directly, but rather the pressure that needs to be applied to the arm in order to obliterate it. The first of these instruments was invented and presented in 1881 by the Austrian pathologist and physiologist Samuel von Basch (1837–1905). The man credited with the invention of the modern sphygmomanometer and the inflatable cuff around the arm was an Italian physician, Scipione Riva-Rocci (1863–1937). Riva-Rocci was one of several research-minded doctors who adapted von Basch's instrument and developed it further.

However, Riva-Rocci did not work in any of the major centres of 19th-century medicine and he published in obscure places. The success of his sphygmomanometer was owed to the enthusiastic embrace of the instrument by reform-minded medical teachers in the United States, such as Harvey Cushing (1869–1939; see also [56]), George Crile (1864–1943) and Theodore C. Janeway (1872–1917). This was a reflection of a move of the centre of gravity in academic medicine across the Atlantic.

Cushing observed the use of a Riva-Rocci sphygmomanometer during a visit to Italy in 1901 and took one of the instruments back to Baltimore, encouraging its use at Johns Hopkins University Hospital. It was also thanks to American supporters that the auscultation method proposed in 1905 by an equally obscure Russian military physician, Nikolai Korotkoff (1874–1920) was widely adopted. This comprised the use of a stethoscope in combination with Riva-Rocci's inflatable cuff and, while deflating the cuff, recording a systolic pressure reading when the sound reappeared, and a diastolic one when it disappeared again.

Opposite left
Stephen Hales: as part of his experiments into the mechanics of circulation in the early 18th century he measured the blood pressure of a horse.

Opposite right
Tracing of the pulse of a dog recorded on a kymograph (1873).

Above
In a pharmacy an elegant medical practitioner feels the pulse of his young female patient while her mother or chaperone looks on. The subjective quality and quantity of the pulse would be transformed in Western medicine by the sphygmomanometer. Oil painting by Emili Casals i Camps, c. 1882.

Below

The complex apparatus designed by Samuel von Basch in 1881: rather than using the familiar inflatable cuff, the arterial pulse was obliterated by the bulb pressing down on the radial artery and read off an attached kymograph (not shown).

Right

The aneroid barometer and attached bulb, which would be pressed down on to the artery as in the illustration below. The barometer replaced the kymograph as Samuel von Basch refined his instrument.

Opposite

The inflatable cuff (left) and u-tube recording device of Scipione Riva-Rocci's sphygmomanometer (1896) – these highly practical adaptations made this apparatus portable and therefore of use anywhere.

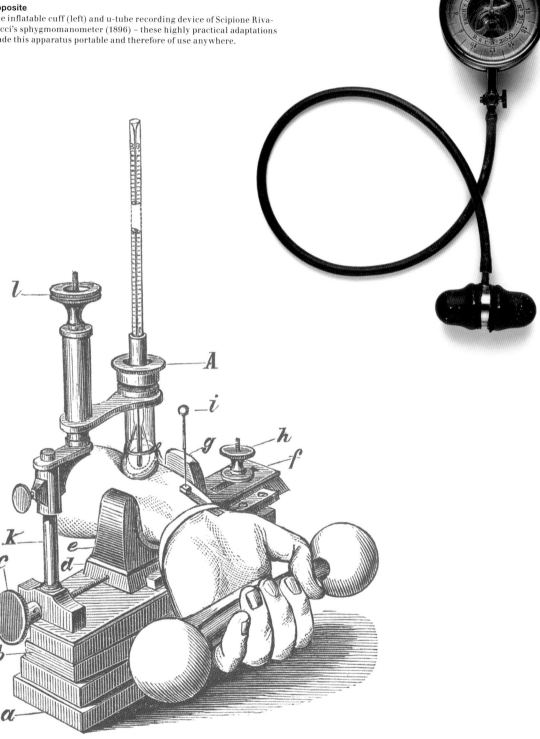

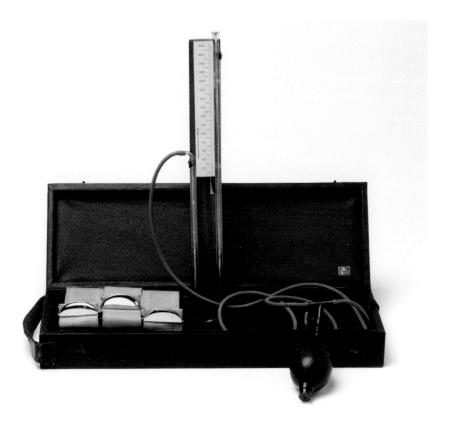

BLOOD PRESSURE AND CLINICAL ROUTINE

Despite the enthusiasm of Cushing, Janeway, Crile and others, many physicians continued to doubt the usefulness of blood pressure measurements. It took until well after the Second World War for consensus to be reached about what abnormal blood pressure readings signified. Some assumed that a rise in blood pressure was a necessary physiological response to ageing. Others demonstrated that very high blood pressure was linked to observable pathological changes, coining the term malignant hypertension. A controversy over the nature of essential hypertension unfolded in the 1950s between the eminent British clinicians Robert Platt (1900–78), who believed that hypertension was a distinct disease entity with genetic causes, and George White Pickering (1904–80), who argued that it was simply the upper extreme of a normal distribution of blood pressure in the population. There was no simple answer.

Physicians employed by American life assurance firms used blood pressure measurements as a key to predicting an applicant's risk of premature death soon after Cushing introduced the sphygmomanometer to America. They compiled blood pressure data from thousands of policy holders, and some of their observations were taken up by the organizers of epidemiological studies on the causes of what many believed to be an epidemic of heart disease. These studies, the best known of which is the Framingham Heart Study (see also p. 212), revealed associations between high blood pressure and premature deaths from strokes and heart attacks. Framingham researchers coined the term 'cardiovascular risk factor' for physiological markers such as blood pressure or blood cholesterol level.

High blood pressure became treatable in routine practice in the late 1950s, when drugs with relatively mild side effects were developed – the thiazide diuretics. Earlier drugs such as the ganglion blockers demanded close monitoring and because of their serious side effects were used almost exclusively in the treatment of malignant hypertension. Experiences with these and more recent drugs [50] led to the issuing of successive guidelines recommending treatment for ever lower blood pressure readings.

28. **DEFIBRILLATORS**
Rescuing the dying

Douglas Chamberlain

Anyone, anywhere, can now initiate cardiac resuscitative procedures.
W. B. Kouwenhoven, J. R. Jude & G. G. Knickerbocker, 1960

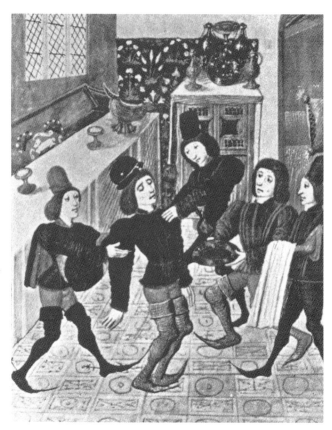

In Froissart's *Chronicles* (written in the 14th century), Gaston de Froix is said to have died after suffering heart oppression and great pain.

Cardiac arrest – the cessation of an effective heart beat – most commonly starts with the uncoordinated activity of the heart's myriad muscle components such that it would be seen to quiver rather than contract. No blood can be pumped, and if not rapidly reversed then death is inevitable. This is called ventricular fibrillation. But it *can* be reversed by applying a shock of a suitable nature and strength that restores coordinated action. This is called defibrillation.

The first plausible defibrillation occurred in 1775 when a Danish vet, Peter Christian Abildgaard, used electricity from Leyden jars to render hens senseless and showed that a subsequent shock could prevent otherwise certain death. He even foresaw that fatalities from lightning might be reversed. Two Swiss physiologists, Jean-Louis Prévost and Frédéric Battelli, conducted similar experiments with dogs over 100 years later. The first well-organized research, begun in 1930 by Donald Hooker, William B. Kouwenhoven and Orthello R. Langworthy in the USA, was interrupted by the Second World War.

Claude S. Beck (1894–1971), a cardiac surgeon, was the first to use an alternating current defibrillator on the exposed heart: he successfully treated a 14-year-old boy during surgery in 1947. It was Paul Zoll (1911–99), an expert in pacing (the electrical control of the timing of the heart beat), who then produced the first defibrillator for use through the intact chest in 1955. The age of clinical defibrillation had arrived. It advanced rapidly from 1960, after external chest compression combined with artificial ventilation made resuscitation possible both within and outside the hospital.

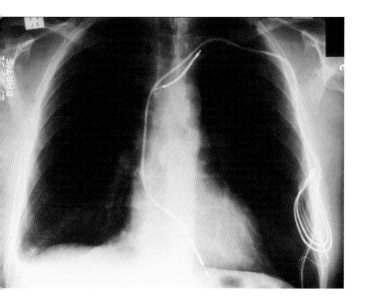

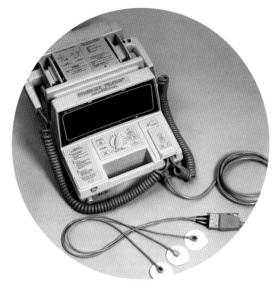

An X-ray showing an implanted cardioverter defibrillator (ICD). It is placed under the skin outside the ribcage and the wires introduced into the heart through a vein.

A defibrillator with paddles (on the side of the machine attached by the spiral wires) and sensing equipment to provide an ECG (electrocardiogram) of the patient's heartbeat.

The early defibrillators had limited application. They were large and heavy, and the alternating current required a transformer to step up the voltage to around 1,000 volts. In 1962 Bernard Lown (1921–) produced a direct current defibrillator using a capacitor to deliver a unidirectional single shock ('monophasic'); much lighter than a transformer, this solved the portability problem. The timing of the shock in relation to an electrocardiogram (ECG) could also be controlled to avoid worsening the heart rhythm if used to terminate non-malignant but abnormal heart rhythms.

Bidirectional ('biphasic') shocks are, however, more effective. William B. Kouwenhoven (1886–1975) produced the 'Mine' biphasic portable defibrillator in 1963. Its advantages were not well appreciated at the time, and it was soon forgotten after being described only in an engineering journal. A portable defibrillator designed by John Anderson specifically for use outside hospitals was made popular by Frank Pantridge (1916–2004); the first was installed in a Belfast ambulance in 1965. Biphasic defibrillators have been available commercially in the Western world since 1996, though they were in use from 1967 in the USSR.

Thus far, defibrillation was a matter only for health care professionals, but this changed with the introduction of automated external defibrillators (AEDs) in 1980; these are capable not only of delivering a shock to terminate fibrillation, but can also analyse the heart rhythm. They will not deliver a shock unless fibrillation is present and so are safe for lay use. Although manual defibrillators need to be used with an oscilloscope (to show the ECG), this is not essential for an AED. The rescuer follows simple verbal instructions; training is advisable but not strictly necessary.

Miniaturization has proceeded apace, with some devices now weighing less than 500 g (18 oz). Such small devices have a role, but in many situations easy visibility is important. Miniaturization has, however, been crucial for defibrillators that are implanted subcutaneously in patients known to be susceptible to malignant arrhythmias. These must have reliable automatic function and are generally combined with a pacing facility. The major development stage is over. Progress now will depend more on the more widespread use of defibrillators in various contexts. Their life-saving potential has not yet been fully realized.

29. LASERS
Light amplification by stimulated emission of radiation

Helen Bynum

Blasted with excess of light.
Thomas Gray, 1757

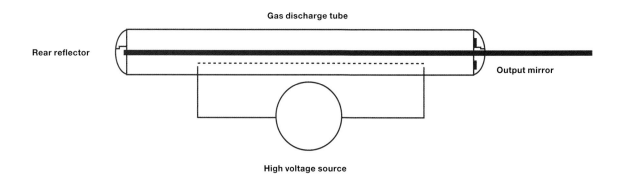

Gas discharge tube

Rear reflector

Output mirror

High voltage source

Lasers produce special light beams – intense, very pure and of the same wavelength. Different materials (solids, liquids and gases) are used to produce different wavelengths in the visible and invisible (infrared/ultraviolet) spectrum. All lasers harness a basic principle in physics: atoms and molecules occur at differing energy levels and those at lower levels can be induced or stimulated (S) by various means to reach higher energy levels. As these excited atoms return to their natural state they emit electromagnetic radiation independently and in different wavelengths. Lasers manipulate this emission (E) phenomenon. At the moment of excitation, if a source of light (L) is applied to the target atoms, the radiation (R) they emit will be in step with this source, amplifying (A) it. Suitably multiplied and controlled, the result is a tremendously powerful focused light beam, continuous or pulsed.

Following Einstein's suggestion of the concept in 1917, researchers investigated 'stimulated emission', and in 1960 the American Theodore H. Maiman (1927–2007) produced the first visible laser beam using a synthetic ruby crystal. Despite initial difficulties in handling the beam (it was a short pulse not a continuous wave), medical interest was keen. Light from a xenon arc lamp was already employed as a photocoagulator

Above
Components of a laser.

Below
A publicity shot of Theodore H. Maiman at the Hughes Research Laboratories in 1960 with his ruby crystal (the cube inside the tube) laser, with which he produced the first laser beam in the visible light spectrum.

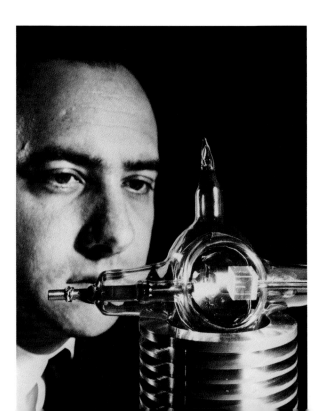

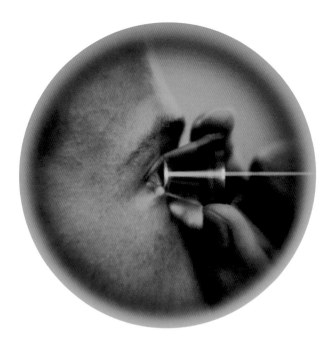

Above
Shining an intense beam of light into the eye might seem counterintuitive, but it has a wide range of uses in surgery, from restoring detached retinas to the correction of visual impairments.

Below
Richly coloured light shows are probably the most familiar use of lasers. The same ability to produce and control a narrow beam that medicine employs allows finely detailed images for entertainment.

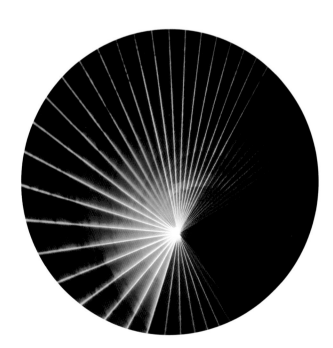

(changing blood and tissue from a fluid to a clotted state using the heat of an intense beam of light) to weld detached retinas back in place and remove intraocular tumours. The laser would take over in both these situations. In 1961 ophthalmologist Charles J. Campbell (1926–2007) and physicist Charles J. Koester used a ruby laser to destroy such a tumour. In 1964 the development of the argon gas laser greatly expanded the scope of retinal surgery thanks to its greater controllability and haemoglobin's high absorption of its beam. Lasers are now used in the repair of detached and torn retinas, in ameliorating the retinal complications of diabetes [65], and assisting in glaucoma treatment and certain types of age-related macular degeneration.

Just as the argon gas laser augmented eye surgery, the carbon dioxide (CO_2) laser, also developed in 1964 at the Bell laboratories, opened up new possibilities elsewhere in the body. The continuous wave, infrared beam of the CO_2 laser is well absorbed by water, a major constituent of soft tissue, which allows it to act as a light scalpel. Causing negligible bleeding, such lasers create a clean operating environment. The Hungarian-born surgeon Geza Jako pioneered the use of CO_2 lasers in laryngeal cancer. Other applications – ablation of pre-cancerous cells on the cervix and laparoscopic (keyhole) surgery [62] in the abdomen – followed in the 1980s.

The pulsing dye lasers of the later 1980s introduced selective thermolysis. This discriminatory destruction of abnormal or unwanted tissue (without damaging the surrounding area) was used in the removal of disfiguring birth marks. Q switches – another development in pulse control – made unwanted tattoos, body hair and thread veins treatable. Combined with scanners allowing precise computer control of the laser, resurfacing of the skin in plastic and cosmetic surgery became much safer.

Currently the most common laser procedure is the correction of some visual impairments (myopia, astigmatism and hyperopia). The Excimer laser emits a cold, non-thermal beam, which neither burns nor cuts. Instead it adds energy and breaks the carbon-carbon bonds between molecules, disintegrating the tissue and reshaping the cornea. First LASIK (laser assisted in-situ keratomileusis) and subsequently LASEK (laser subepithelia keratectomy) surgery have rendered glasses and contact lenses redundant for millions of people.

30. THE ENDOSCOPE
Seeing round corners

Rodney Taylor

You go not, till I set you up a glass
Where you may see the inmost part of you.
William Shakespeare, *Hamlet*, Act 3, Scene 4

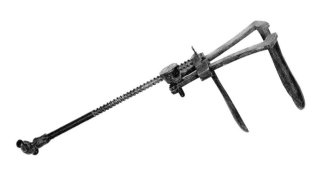

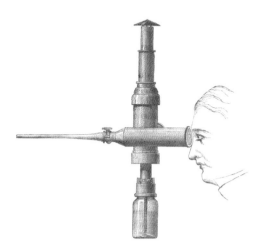

Hippocrates (*c.* 460–*c.* 370 BC) first described attempts to look within the body using a rectal speculum in the treatise *On Haemorrhoids.* A three-bladed vaginal speculum, dating from *c.* AD 70, was found in the ruins of the Roman city of Pompeii. Avicenna (Ibn Sina, 980–1037; see also [05]) describes using reflected sunlight and mirrors to provide better illumination to make an observation within the body. Despite scientific advances in the Renaissance, however, two fundamental problems remained. Most of the inner parts of the body are not straight; and it is dark inside. An instrument was needed that could pass round corners and had a suitable light source.

In 1805 Philip Bozzini (1773–1809), a German doctor, devised a light-conducting system, which he called the *Lichtleiter*; this carried light and allowed the observer to see into the body's inner cavities. A more refined instrument for examination of the bladder was described by Pierre Segalas (1792–1875) in Paris in 1827. Antoine Jean Desormeaux (1815–82) used a much improved version in 1853 for urological cases, which he called an 'endoscope'. The light source was a lamp flame focused by mirrors and lenses, risking burns

to the patient. The invention by Thomas Edison of the incandescent lamp in 1878 solved the light problem. Maximilian Nitze (1848–1906) used this for urological procedures. Adaptations of such instruments were made to examine the rectum, vagina and pharynx.

The first examination of the stomach was undertaken on a sword-swallower by Adolph Kussmaul (1822–1902) in 1868 in Germany, using a 47-cm (18-in) long metal tube. But the first practical rigid gastroscope was devised by Johann von Mikulicz-Radecki (1850–1905) in 1881. Only in 1932 did Rudolph Schindler (1888–1968) and Georg Wolf (1873–1938) design a flexible gastroscope that allowed fuller examination of the stomach by being able to bend the final third of the instrument. The optical problem of looking round corners was overcome partially by using a succession of convex lenses throughout a rubber tube. Gastrocameras were developed in the 1950s to take pictures blind using a miniature camera at the instrument's tip.

FIBRE OPTICS
But it was with the development of fibre optics in the early 1950s by the British physicist Harold Hopkins

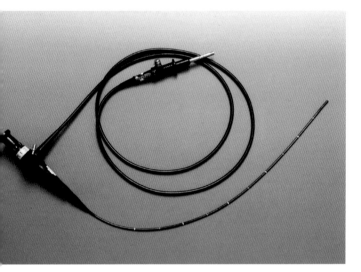

(1918–94) that the real breakthrough came in seeing round corners. Light is transmitted by total internal reflection through a flexible glass fibre; a coherent bundle of fibres can transmit light or an image even when the instrument is bent. The fibre-optic gastroscope was developed in 1957 by Basil Hirschowitz (1925–). Image-quality constraints of fibre optics were subsequently overcome by using a microchip that can produce a digital colour image on a television screen, which was developed in 1969 and incorporated into endoscopes ten years later. Endoscopes can also carry an ultrasound probe.

Instrument control systems now allow much greater flexibility and better access, while instrument channels enable access for diagnostic procedures, such as biopsies, as well as therapeutic uses such as polyp removal in the colon or tying off veins in the oesophagus. Endoscopes are now employed throughout the gastrointestinal tract, though as the small intestine is more difficult to see, specialized versions called enteroscopes and now capsule endoscopes that can be swallowed have been developed (see also [33]). Specific endoscopes make possible full examination of the upper and lower respiratory system, the urinary tract, the gynaecological system and other inner spaces. Laparoscopes inserted through the abdominal wall have been important diagnostically and for complex intra-abdominal surgery [62].

In endoscopy, the partnership between clinician and scientist has enabled considerable technological, diagnostic and therapeutic advances in the previously less accessible parts of the body.

Opposite left
A bronze three-bladed vaginal speculum dating to *c.* AD 70, found at Pompeii, where a rectal speculum was also preserved.

Opposite right
The Desormeaux 'endoscope' (1853) was used for urological visualization. An improved design, it still required a burning flame as the light source, which was hazardous.

Above
A fibre-optic endoscope. Fibre optics provided the looked-for flexibility in the light source for endoscopes and greatly improved the patient's experience of an essentially unpleasant procedure.

Right
Not a fishing trip at all, but the Nitze-Leiter cystoscope of 1879 (for looking into the bladder), packed for easy transport.

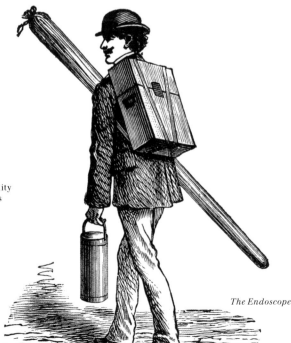

IMAGING THE BODY
Beyond the X-ray

Malcolm Nicolson

I must say I like doing obstetrics this way and removing as much of the traditional guesswork from our subject as possible.
Ian Donald, 1967

Right
'The scan' is part of the excitement for prospective parents. It is immeasurably useful when all does not go according to plan; happily, this is a normal 24-week-old fetus.

Opposite
False-coloured CT brain scan showing the effects of a bleed, which led to a stroke. The dark area (top left quadrant) is damaged brain tissue. In a scan of a normal brain the coloration would be symmetrical.

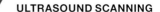

Throughout the 19th century, as pathological anatomy [07] became more dominant within medicine, doctors often expressed the wish to see what was going on inside the bodies of their living patient, without having to resort to exploratory surgery. The discovery of X-rays [26] in 1895 made this dream come true. But X-ray images have many limitations. Soft tissue is less successfully imaged than bone, and certain clinically significant structures – gall bladder stones for instance – may not be revealed at all.

During the Second World War, the United States and Britain invested heavily in instruments for communication and computation, as well as in the echolocation technologies of radar and sonar. In peacetime, engineers and clinicians sought to find civilian applications for their newly acquired expertise and their sophisticated electronic equipment. One of the fields that benefited from the 'electronic revolution' was diagnostic imaging of the human body.

ULTRASOUND SCANNING

The first of the new imaging technologies to achieve clinical utility was ultrasonic scanning. Ultrasound is sound of a frequency too high to be detected by the human ear. In modern medical equipment, ultrasound is produced by the piezoelectric effect: a rapidly alternating electric charge produces physical oscillation in a ceramic element, thus propagating high-frequency sound waves. Most ultrasound instruments work by echolocation: a pulsed beam of high-frequency sound is directed towards the object that the investigator is interested in and the echoes reflected by the target are detected. This information is then displayed, generally in two-dimensions and in real-time, on a screen.

Shortly after the Second World War, several investigators realized the diagnostic potential of ultrasound. By the early 1950s there were two major programmes of research under way in the US, one led by Douglass Howry (1920–69) in Denver, and the other by John Wild (1914–2009) in Minneapolis. Collaborating with several engineers, Howry produced

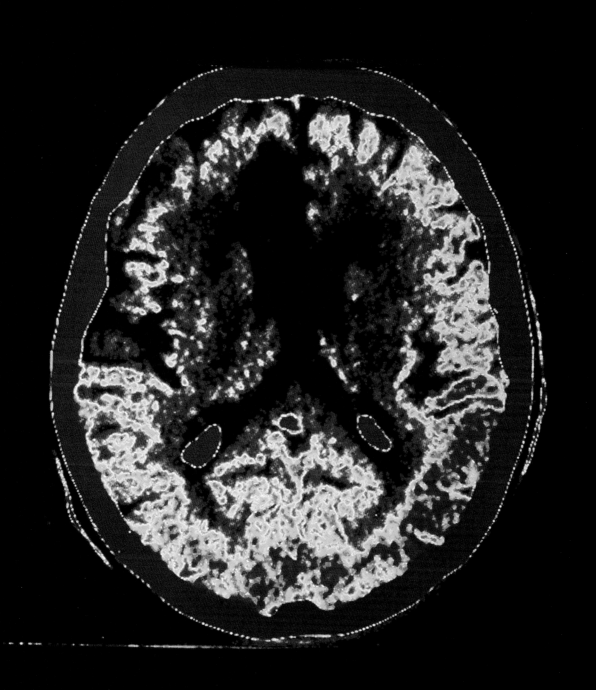

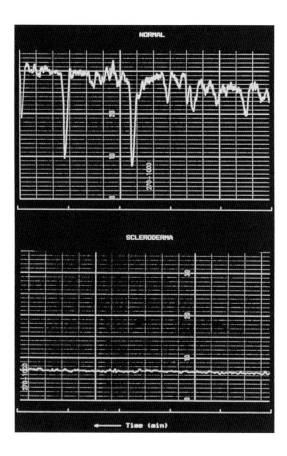

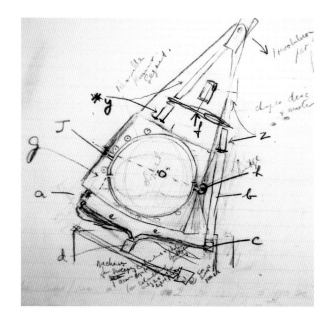

detailed images of the soft tissue of the neck. However, his instrument, which required the scanned subject to sit in a water bath for long periods of time, was not clinically applicable. Wild designed a smaller, hand-held scanner, and had considerable success in the detection of breast cysts, but again the complexities of his technique discouraged its general adoption.

The first team to produce unequivocally useful results with ultrasound was that based at the University of Glasgow and led by Ian Donald (1910–97), an obstetrician and gynaecologist, and Tom Brown, an engineer. Brown greatly increased the clinical utility of the method by designing a scanner that did not need to be contained in a water bath but could be placed directly on the patient's abdomen. He improved the scanning procedure and devised a means of two-dimensional, cross-sectional display, which made optimal use of the information gathered by the probe. It was also fortuitous that the fetus, a solid structure surrounded by fluid, turned out to be a very suitable target for ultrasound examination, being rather 'like a submarine', as Wild put it. Donald and Brown published their first images of the pregnant uterus in 1958.

Using increasingly sophisticated equipment, in the 1960s and early 1970s Donald and his colleagues transformed our understanding of the early stages of pregnancy and greatly improved the management of complications, such as placenta praevia, occurring in the third trimester. Roughly simultaneously, Inge Edler (1911–69) and Hellmuth Hertz (1920–90) in Sweden developed a system to examine the heart.

While most ultrasound images are produced using the pulse-echo technique, the Doppler scanner operates by a different principle. Using a continuous beam of ultrasound, Doppler instruments can detect whether a fluid (usually blood) is moving towards or away from the probe, and also determine its velocity. Thus the speed and direction of flow can be visualized. This is useful, for instance, in monitoring fetal wellbeing during labour, and in detecting abnormal patterns of blood flow.

COMPUTERIZED TOMOGRAPHIC (CT) SCANNING

Conventional X-ray equipment has several limitations. The image is produced by the shadows cast on a photographic plate as the X-radiation passes through the

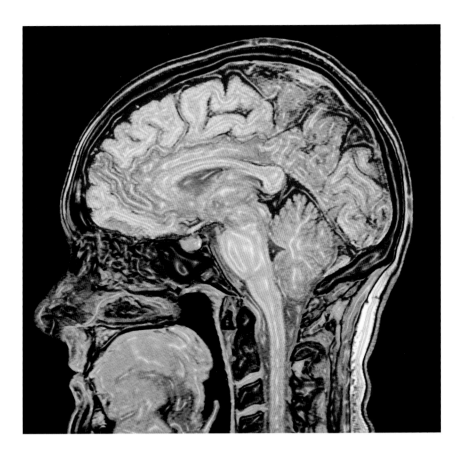

body and is absorbed more strongly by some tissues than by others. This process produces a two-dimensional projection of a three-dimensional target and can be difficult to interpret as structures at different depths within the body are visualized together on the one flat surface. The obvious solution was to find some way of displaying the same information as a tomograph, a cross-sectional 'slice' across the body, which would show the various structures in their correct anatomical orientation to one another. Several attempts were made to achieve this throughout the 20th century, but it was not until the development of powerful computers in the 1950s and 1960s that the technique became feasible.

The first practical tomographic scanner, designed by Godfrey Hounsfield (1919–2004), working for EMI in the UK, came into clinical use in 1972. In modern instruments, the patient lies within a ring of detectors, while an X-ray source rotates around the body. When sufficient data have been gathered, a computer program constructs the tomographic image according to an algorithm designed to maximize its specific clinical utility. One of the great advantages of this procedure is that it enables small differences between the density of

Opposite left
Doppler ultrasound scanning can measure the rate of blood flow over time. Here it is possible to compare results of scans in a normal person (above) and a patient with a case of scleroderma (below), an autoimmune disease in which the blood flow is restricted, evidenced here by the almost flat line.

Opposite right
The electrical engineer Godfrey Hounsfield shared the 1979 Nobel Prize for Physiology or Medicine with South African born physicist Allan Cormark for their independent work that led to the CT scanner. Hounsfield made this preliminary sketch in his notebook.

Above
Digitally enhanced MRI scan of the head. The brain and spinal cord are shown in orange and yellow, the other tissues in blue and pink – all in exquisite detail.

the various tissues to be detected, allowing muscle to be distinguished from fat, for instance.

MAGNETIC RESONANCE IMAGING (MRI)

Tomographic techniques do not, however, remove all the shortcomings associated with X-ray imaging. The strongly absorbent characteristics of bone can create distortions in the visualization of adjacent tissue. Inevitably, also, the patient receives a dose of ionizing radiation. Magnetic resonance scanning does not have these disadvantages and is capable of very high image resolution.

In an MR scanner, the patient is placed within a strong magnetic field. Incoming pulses of electromagnetic radiation excite the nuclei of the body's hydrogen atoms, which subsequently release back the energy, and this is detected by radiofrequency receivers. The data are processed by a computer program, as in CT, to produce a two-dimensional tomographic image. Whereas all the earlier imaging modalities (Doppler excepted) produce only anatomical information, MRI can detect the biochemical properties of tissues and can thus provide a snapshot of physiological processes, such as blood flow and muscle contraction.

Magnetic resonance techniques were developed to study the molecular structure of chemical compounds by Felix Bloch (1905–83) at Stanford and Edward Purcell (1912–97) at Harvard in the 1940s. In 1971, Raymond Damadian showed that cancerous tumours had distinctive MR characteristics. By 1974, two British groups, one in Aberdeen led by John Mallard, and another in Nottingham led by Peter Mansfield, were at work building prototype scanners. Damadian and his colleagues published the first cross-sectional image of a living animal, a mouse, in 1976. MRI machines were in commercial production by 1981.

While most of the MR images used diagnostically are static cross-sections, it is possible, by scanning very quickly at low resolution, to produce sequences of images virtually in real-time. Functional MRI, as it is called, has applications in physiological research and in the pre-operative assessment of brain tumour patients.

POSITRON EMISSION TOMOGRAPHY (PET)

The achievement of the computational capacity necessary to produce cross-sectional images for the CT scanner also inspired the development of Positron Emission Tomography. In this technique, radioisotopes with a short half-life are injected into the body. As they decay, the gamma rays they emit are detected by arrays of scintillation counters. PET scanners were first deployed in the late 1970s. They produce very detailed images, which visualize the movement of the isotopes through specific parts of the body. The pictures can be refreshed very quickly, providing information about physiological processes as they occur. Some of the most remarkable PET images display the brain responding to different cognitive and emotional challenges. PET scanners are expensive, however, and thus are largely confined to research, rather than clinical contexts.

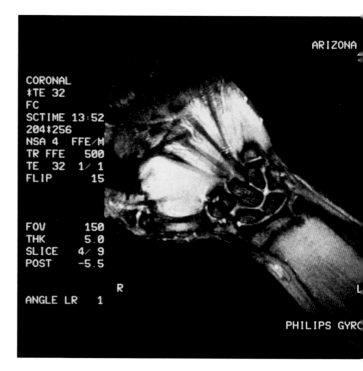

A magnetic resonance imaging or MRI scan of the blood vessels of the wrist, which appear to stand out in dramatic relief in this image.

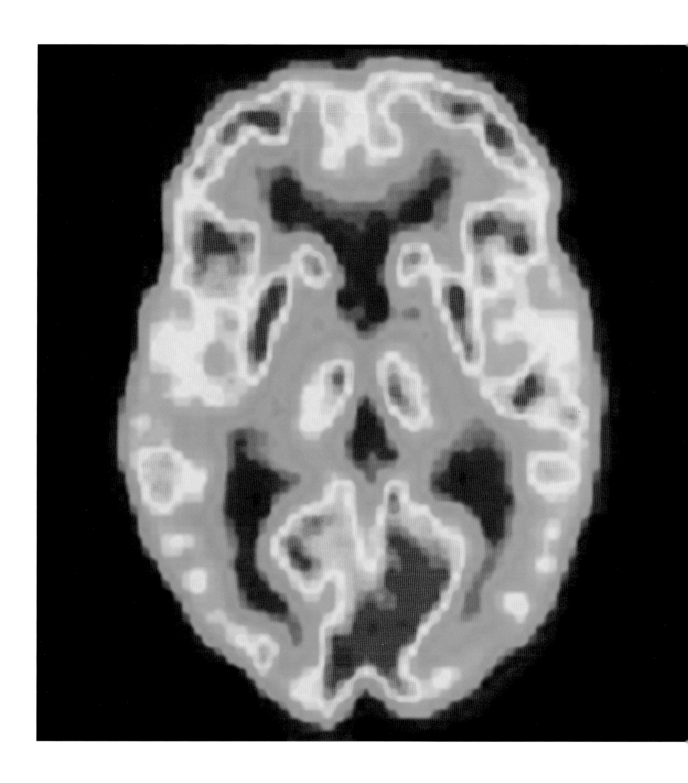

A positron emission tomograph (PET) of the healthy brain of a 20-year-old. PET neuroimaging relies upon the assumption that areas where the introduced radioisotopes are highest are those associated with active areas of the brain. What is indirectly measured is the flow of blood to different parts of the brain.

32. THE INCUBATOR
Re-inventing the womb

Jeffrey Baker

*First, save the infant, the essential point; second, save it in such a way
that when it leaves the hospital it does so with a mother able to suckle it.*
Dr Pierre Budin, 1900

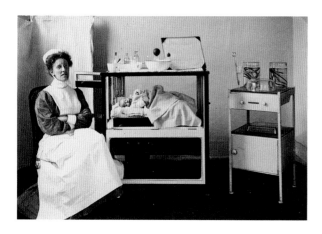

The incubator reaches England: a nurse watches as her tiny charge lies
in an incubator at the General Lying-In Hospital, York Road, Lambeth,
London, *c.* 1906. The glass walls encouraged the carer to interact with
the baby.

Premature birth was one of the leading contributors
to the extraordinary infant mortality rates (15–20
per cent) afflicting 19th-century European and
North American cities. While the smallest of such
infants had little chance of survival until the rise
of neonatal intensive care in the 1960s, many more
were born only one to two months early. Lacking
the 'brown fat' that enabled full-term infants to
maintain their temperature, many of these babies
succumbed to a downward spiral of hypothermia,
lethargy and starvation. Their fate was entirely in
the hands of mothers, who had few options other
than breast-feeding and the use of hot-water bottles
for warmth.

In Britain and the United States social Darwinist
and eugenic assumptions long discouraged physicians
from treating these so-called 'weaklings'. French
obstetricians, however, took a more favourable view.
Their nation's embarrassing defeat in the Franco-
Prussian War of 1870–71 had prompted politicians and
doctors alike to re-frame high infant mortality not as a
law of nature but rather as a social problem robbing the
country of its future workers and soldiers.

Troubled by the high mortality of the premature
infants on the cold wards of the largest lying-in hospital
in Paris, the Maternité, obstetrician Stéphane Tarnier
(1828–1927) found a solution during a visit to the
chicken incubator display at the Paris zoo. A similar
device for infants was promptly installed on the hospital
ward, with impressive results: mortality of infants born
weighing under 2,000 g (70 oz) fell from 66 per cent to 38
per cent – a decrease of nearly half.

MACHINES AND MOTHERS
Propelled by this success, incubators spread rapidly
from France to the rest of Europe and the United States.
As they did so, popular attention increasingly shifted
to the technology itself. Tarnier's early collaborators
favoured simple incubators heated by hot-water bottles
that could be kept next to the mother, who breast-fed the
infant and acted as nurse. Later innovators developed
ever more complex models equipped with amenities
such as thermostats, weighing scales and ventilation
systems. These formidable devices, as tall as the mother
and striving to embody many of her functions as a
mechanical 'womb', greatly excited the public.

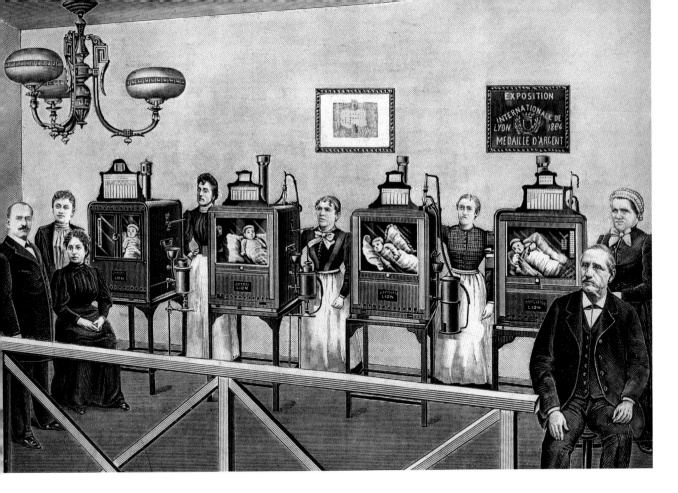

Most remarkably, 'incubator baby' shows featuring live infants sprang up in storefront institutes and world fairs. These exhibits, whose popularity peaked at the turn of the 20th century, resembled not so much side shows as today's medical dramas celebrating the power of technology. Americans were particularly enraptured by the promise of highly complex incubators in rescuing babies small enough to fit in the hand.

PROFESSIONAL CARE

Despite all this excitement, incubators entered routine medical practice far more slowly. Incubator-based premature nurseries did not become widespread until well into the 20th century, as hospitalized birth became routine and economic resources made possible the rise of specialized nursing. Incubators remained the central therapeutic technology directed at premature infants until finally supplanted by mechanical ventilators and neonatal intensive care in the 1960s. They embodied a conservative style in the treatment of premature infants, dominated by nurses rather than physicians, and emphasizing meticulous feeding and minimal handling of the fragile infant.

Simple by today's standards, incubators none the less were one of the first therapeutic 'machines' to attract widespread public attention. They played a critical role in expanding the authority of medicine into the domain of the newborn infant. At the same time, they functioned as a lightning rod for broader anxieties regarding the limits and ends of that project.

The Maternité Lion incubator exhibit at the Exposition universelle et coloniale de Lyon, in 1894. Exhibits such as these were extremely popular wherever they appeared in the early years of the incubator, attracting large crowds and inspiring articles in the lay press. They frequently featured large and complex incubators equipped with thermostats and separate ventilation systems, as seen here.

33. **MEDICAL ROBOTS**
A helping hand

Andrew Robinson

Many mini- and micro-robots have biologically inspired designs which emulate the crawling and wriggling motion of worms and insects, or the swimming motion of bacteria. We turned to biological inspiration because worms have locomotion systems suited to unstructured, slippery environments and are ideally suited for use in the human body.
Dr Arianna Menciassi, 2009

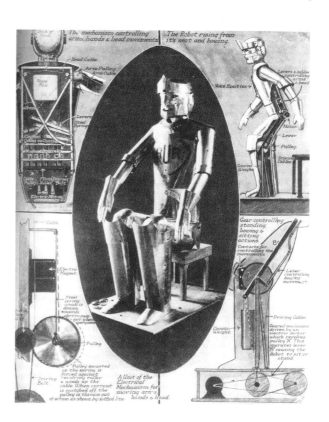

The word 'robot' was invented in 1920 by the Czech writer Karel Čapek in his play *R.U.R.* (*Rossum's Universal Robots*). In 1941 the scientist and science-fiction writer Isaac Asimov coined 'robotics', which became famous as a result of his fiction *I, Robot*, published in 1950. During the 1960s, robots began to be used in manufacturing processes, space exploration and bomb disposal, to perform tasks deemed too tedious, dangerous or precise for humans. In 1966 Asimov published a novel, *Fantastic Voyage*, in which he imagined a team of doctors miniaturized and injected into a patient, in order to eliminate a life-threatening blood clot in his brain. While miniaturizing human beings remains an 'Alice in Wonderland' fantasy, medical robots may soon be small enough to realize Asimov's vision.

In 1985, the first real medical robot, the PUMA 560, was used, under CT guidance, to place a needle for a brain biopsy. Robot-assisted medicine increased in scope during the 1990s. By 2010 a wireless 'digital plaster' was in prototype – a disposable device worn by the patient in hospital or at home for monitoring and transmitting temperature, heart rate, respiration

An illustration from an English edition of Karel Čapek's play *R.U.R.*, showing the workings of a robot, a machine programmed to perform human functions and often made to resemble a person.

Below
Intuitive Surgical Inc.'s Da Vinci Surgical System includes
'EndoWrists', which mimic but enhance human dexterity, precision
and control. A variety of specialized tips – forceps, needle drivers,
scissors, electrocautery instruments and scalpels – allow various
procedures through a tiny incision.

Bottom
The future of nanomachines is not likely to look like this miniature
robot grappling with a red blood cell; instead, they will be molecules
pre-engineered to undertake specific tasks.

rate and other data to a computer database. If the vital signs fall outside predefined ranges considered safe, the patient, doctor or carer is alerted. Also in prototype are mini-robots, only 10–15 mm in diameter – for example, a remote-controlled camera pill for endoscopy of the gastrointestinal tract, with hooked legs to grip gently on to the intestinal wall so that surgeons can guide it to points of interest, somewhat like a rover on the surface of Mars. At the same time, the possibility of injecting still smaller micro-robots, less than 1 mm across, into the bloodstream is an active area of research. Although robots are still newcomers in medicine, during the early decades of the 21st century they seem set to become familiar not just to surgeons but also to every medical practitioner.

Among the best-known operational medical robots is the Da Vinci Surgical System, a so-called master–slave robot introduced in the 1990s for minimally invasive surgery [62]. In 1998 it was used to perform the first robot-assisted heart bypass operation under the control of Dr Friedrich-Wilhelm Mohr at the Leipzig Heart Centre in Germany. Da Vinci comprises three components: a surgeon's console; a patient-side robotic cart with four arms that can be manipulated by the surgeon – one arm to control the camera, the other three to control the surgical instruments; and a high-definition 3D vision system. The robot senses the movements of the surgeon's hands and translates these into scaled-down micro-movements, while at the same time detecting and filtering out any tremors in the hand movements. The Da Vinci system is now routinely used for surgical procedures such as hysterectomy, mitral valve repair and the removal of prostate cancer.

The chief function of medical robots is to improve existing diagnostic and operating techniques for the benefit of patients. The aims of robotic surgery are decreased blood loss, reduced pain and faster healing. Such medical robots will probably not be designed as independent or autonomous – like the robot servants in Woody Allen's futuristic comic fantasy *Sleeper* – but kept under direct, precise, human control. Robots should permit smaller incisions with greater accuracy; the decisions, however, will continue to be made by human beings.

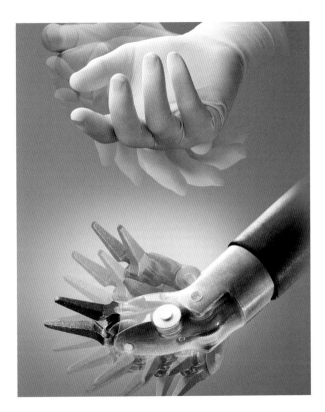

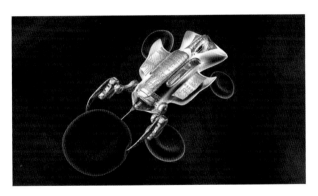

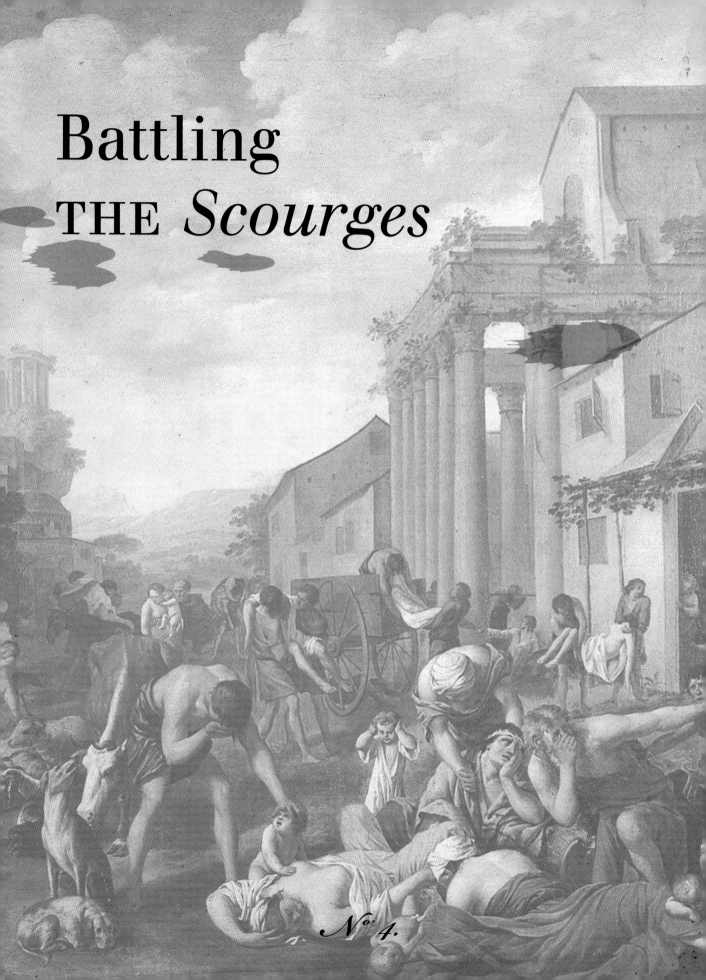

Battling
THE *Scourges*

Nº 4.

Half a century ago, people in the West assumed that infectious diseases had more or less been conquered. A combination of public health, vaccinations, antibiotics and improved medical care had rendered the old enemies a thing of the past. This has all changed. The rise of fast international travel has created the global village. The causative agents of infectious diseases have shown themselves capable of developing their own defences against antibiotics and other modern therapeutic agents. New strains of the influenza virus seem constantly about to jump from their normal reservoirs in pigs, domestic fowls and other animals, and to acquire the capacity to spread from human to human. New infectious agents, of which the Human Immunodeficiency Virus (HIV) is only one, threaten to provide fresh challenges to our efforts to prevent and to treat. Infectious diseases constituted a dying medical specialty in the 1950s; now they are a growth industry.

In this section we examine some of the major scourges of the past, their impact on human history and the counter-measures they have stimulated. It offers sober reading. The eradication of smallpox is a human triumph, though the disease still presents a worry as a potential weapon for terrorists. Polio, the 'summer plague', has retreated and might also be eradicated. Childbed fever, too, is now rare in the West, and only one of several causes of maternal mortality around the world.

The report card on the other scourges examined here is mixed. Bubonic plague – the 'Black Death' of the 14th century and the Great Plague of London in the 17th century – created a serious worldwide epidemic in the late 19th century, when its causative organism was identified, and is still around (there are sporadic cases in the USA today). Fortunately, the plague bacillus can be treated with antibiotics. Typhus, the traditional disease of overcrowding and insanitary conditions, can also be managed by modern medicine, even if conditions favouring its spread are all too common in the world today, and in places where expert medical care is in short supply. The same applies to cholera, one of the most feared diseases of 19th-century Europe, though it can actually be managed with low-technology therapy consisting of a simple solution of clean water, sugar and salt, administered orally.

Tuberculosis is another disease that commentators a couple of generations ago liked to speak of in historical terms. But the disease never went away in developing countries, and was still present in the West. It is a threat once again, with the rise of drug-resistant strains and a vulnerable population whose bodily defences have been compromised by AIDS. It is treatable, but the patient has to complete a sustained course of drugs, otherwise they risk their health and endanger others through the rise of drug resistance. Who ever said health care was easy?

HIV has contributed to the tuberculosis issue, but it is of course a worrying concern in its own right. A symbol of the increasing pace of life today, the disease has evolved from a rare acute disorder to a widespread chronic one in little over a generation. It also invites us to think about other aspects of health: gender, sexuality, poverty and lifestyle, and to remember that Nature may still have unpleasant surprises in store for us.

In the Old Testament a plague afflicted the Philistines at Ashdod in retribution for their theft of the Ark of the Covenant. This was not necessarily bubonic plague, but epidemic disease arriving to decimate a community has a long history and is still with us. Oil painting by Pieter van Halen, 1661.

PLAGUE
Death on the grand scale

Dorothy Crawford

Ring-a-ring o'roses
A pocket full of posies
Atishoo, atishoo,
We all fall down.

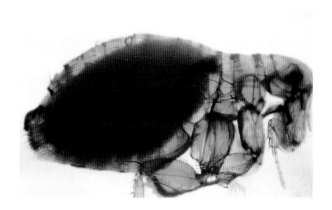

Above
An oriental rat flea infected with the plague bacillus. After three days the bacteria are evident as the dark finger-like projection in the blood-engorged stomach. When the flea bites a person, regurgitated blood containing the live bacilli passes into the bite site.

Below
The black rat's colloquial names – ship rat, roof rat, house rat, Alexandrine rat, old English rat – indicate its place in history and human lives. Originally a tropical Asian native, it spread through the Near East during the Roman period, reaching Europe by the 6th century.

Throughout our history, plague has been one of the most feared diseases, and among the most lethal. It has caused cyclical epidemics that spread inexorably from one household to another and condemned up to 50 per cent of those infected to an excruciatingly painful, though mercifully rapid, death. Typified by 'bubos' – hugely swollen lymph glands (hence the term 'bubonic' plague) – the symptoms were graphically described by Michael of Piazza, a Franciscan monk who witnessed early cases of the Black Death in Sicily in 1347:

> … boils developed in different parts of the body: in the sex organs, in others on the thigh, or on the arm, and in others on the neck. At first these were of the size of a hazelnut and the patient was seized by violent shivering fits, which soon rendered him so weak that he could no longer stand upright, but was forced to lie on his bed, consumed by a violent fever and overcome by great tribulation. Soon the boils grew to the size of a walnut, then to that of a hen's egg or a goose's egg, and they were exceedingly painful, and irritated the body, causing it to vomit blood by vitiating the juices. The blood rose from the affected lungs to the throat,

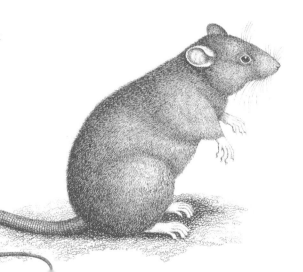

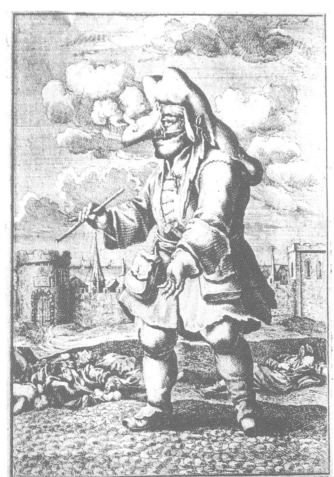

Abriß und Vorstellung derer Herrn Doctorum Medicinæ zu Marseille, alß welche währender Pest-Zeit in Cordyan leder gekleidet, mit einem die Pest verscheuchende Rauchwerck angefüllten Nasen-Futer und mit einem kleinem Stecklein in der hand den Krancken den Pulß damit zu fühlen, versehen gewesen.

Portrait Véritable d'un Medecin à Marseille, étant revetu du marroquin et d'un etui de nez, rempli des parfums contre la peste, de même que portant à la main un petit baton pour en tater le pouls, aux malades.

Above
The Great Plague of Marseille (1720–22), the most significant in 18th-century Europe, arrived on a ship from the Levant and killed around 100,000 people in the city and its hinterland. This Marseillan plague doctor is smoking as a protection against miasma (foul smells) in the air, then believed to cause the disease.

producing a putrefying and ultimately decomposing effect on the whole body. The sickness lasted three days, and on the fourth, at the latest, the patient succumbed.

There have been three pandemics of plague in the last 2,000 years: the first was the Justinian plague in AD 542; the second began with the legendary Black Death in 1346; and the third originated in China in the 1860s. The first two each lasted for at least 200 years and the third is still ongoing today. The pandemics spread along trade routes, virtually engulfing the whole of the Old World, with the third reaching the New World via international shipping.

GERMS, FLEAS AND RODENTS: CLOSING THE LOOP

The beginning of the third pandemic coincided with the general acceptance of the germ theory [14] and the 'golden age of bacteriology'. Isolation of disease-causing microbes was a recognized practice when plague hit Hong Kong in 1894 and Alexandre Yersin (1863–1943) travelled from the Pasteur Institute in Paris to investigate. He rapidly isolated the causative bacterium, now called *Yersinia (Y.) pestis* in his honour. Three years later, Paul-Louis Simond (1858–1947), also from the Pasteur Institute, working in plague-infested India, unravelled the microbe's complex life cycle [15].

Y. pestis naturally infects burrowing rodents, spread among them by their fleas. Most of these animals, including gerbils, marmots and ground squirrels, show no ill effects from the infection, and the microbe circulates continuously in their underground cities. There are several infected colonies, called plague foci, around the world. The foci in the Himalayas, Eurasia and Central Africa are ancient, whereas the others, including those in the Americas and South Africa, were only established during the third pandemic.

Plague threatens humans only if they come into contact with infected rodents, especially black (house) rats (*Rattus rattus*), as these animals are particularly susceptible to *Y. pestis*. Classically the chain of infection passes from wild rodents to black rats, which then die rapidly. Their fleas promptly desert the corpse in search of their next meal and, since until quite recently each human household hosted its own black rat colony, the hungry fleas generally fed on human blood, passing on a dose of *Y. pestis* in the process. Victims of classic bubonic plague are not directly infectious to others and each new human infection must start

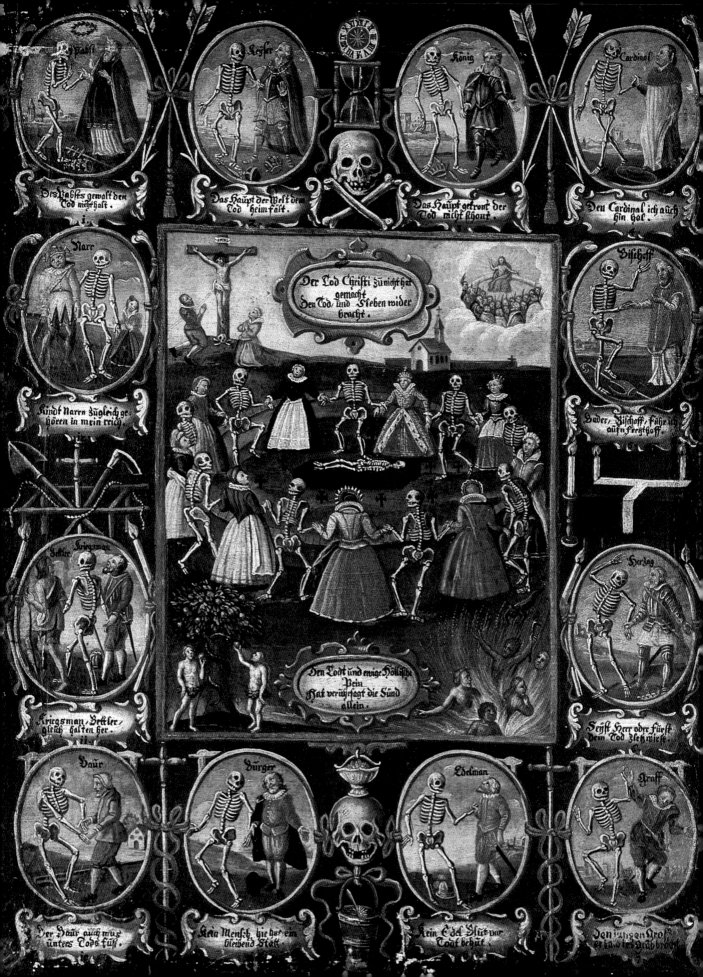

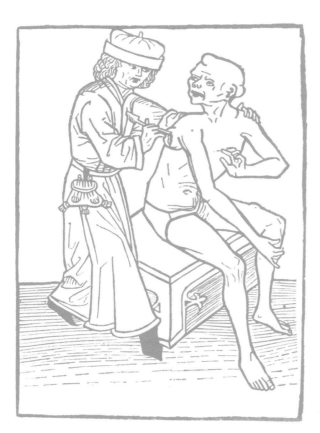

with a bite from a rat flea. This is contrary to beliefs during the Black Death, when plague doctors donned elaborate protective clothing and quarantine laws were introduced for the first time to prevent further spread. Just occasionally, however, bacteria travel through the blood to a victim's lungs, producing pneumonic plague and allowing direct spread to other people via coughing.

DEATH AND DISRUPTION

In each pandemic the death tolls were immense, with far-reaching consequences felt for several generations. The Justinian plague, for example, struck Constantinople in the 6th century AD, just as Emperor Justinian was striving to reunite the old eastern and western Roman empires. It caused recurring epidemics for the next 200 years, with an estimated death toll of 100 million. The severe lack of manpower left the Byzantine empire's borders unguarded, and invasion ultimately led to its long-term decline.

Similarly, the Black Death caused the most dramatic fall in the population of Europe ever recorded, with numbers only recovering after 300 years. There were 1.4 million deaths in England alone, accounting for around a third of the population. As no one had any idea where the visitation came from, or how to avoid or treat it, panic ensued. Charlatans and quacks fully exploited people's terror, but although lancing bubos gave some relief, there was no effective treatment.

The third pandemic saw a huge epidemic in India, China and parts of Africa. It is still ongoing and causes over 5,000 cases worldwide every year. The bacterium arrived in San Francisco in the late 1890s, causing a small outbreak, infecting ground squirrels and establishing a plague focus in California. This enlarging focus now stretches from Canada to Mexico and halfway across the US, causing around 10–20 cases in the US annually. But, unlike in previous episodes of infection, we now have antibiotics to combat the bacterium, taking the sting out of its tail for those who can gain access to treatment.

35. TYPHUS
Preying on the weak

Mark Harrison

Typhus is not dead. It will live on for centuries, and it will continue to break into the open whenever human stupidity and brutality give it a chance.
Hans Zinsser, 1935

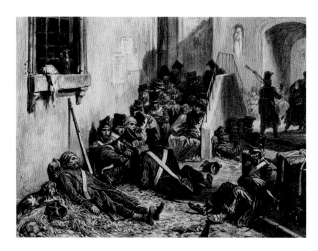

Above
Typhus has had many colloquial names, including camp fever. An epidemic could easily devastate an army's ability to fight, or could prey upon those already weakened by a long campaign as depicted here. As Napoleon withdrew his defeated army in 1814, his troops, suffering from camp fever, littered the streets of Mainz in Germany.

Opposite
In his *Inquiry into the sanitary condition of the labouring population of Great Britain* (1842) Edwin Chadwick mapped out in meticulous detail the social evils of overcrowding and inadequate sanitary facilities, along with the incidence of various diseases, including typhus. It made for grim reading.

Typhus is an infectious disease characterized by sudden fever, skin rash and headache, with the potential to cause epidemics and multiple deaths. The long-time companion of war and social upheaval, it is associated with some of the most turbulent periods in human history. Often widespread among armies and displaced persons, typhus also added regularly to the misfortunes of agriculturalists in times of dearth. Indeed, the association between typhus and food shortage was so close that it was often dubbed 'famine fever'. Typhus was also, notoriously, a disease of overcrowding. Among the many other names given to typhus in the course of its biological history, the appellations 'jail fever', 'ship fever' and 'camp fever' are among the most common.

It was the intimate association between typhus, prisons and armed forces that led to the first important efforts to control the disease. As standing armies and navies were formed from the late 17th century, more attention was paid to preserving their health. Jails, ships and other confined spaces began to be cleansed and disinfected, in the belief that this would neutralize the putrid odours then thought to produce the disease. By the end of the 18th century, such methods were beginning to reduce the incidence of contagious fevers on naval vessels, but such illnesses were becoming increasingly common in the slums of rapidly expanding industrial cities. Sanitary reformers such as Edwin Chadwick (1800–90) identified these diseases as social evils and believed they could be prevented by the removal of filth and overcrowding.

RICKETTSIA AND THEIR VECTORS
Typhus undoubtedly loomed large among these dreaded fevers, but at that stage it could not be easily differentiated. It was not until 1849 that the London physician William Jenner (1815–98) distinguished

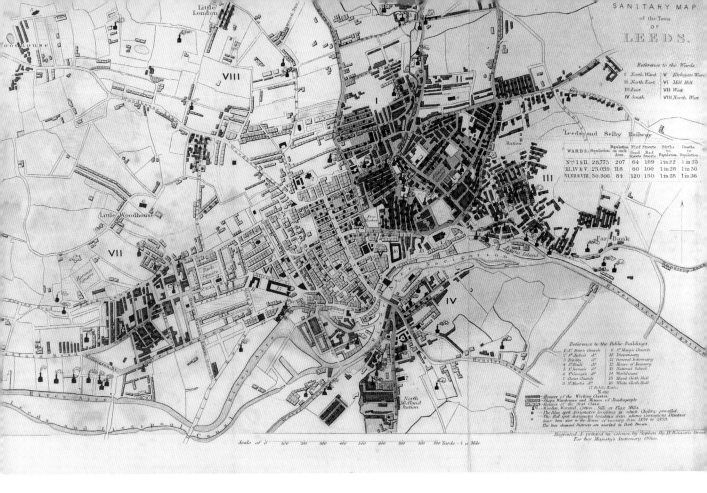

typhus clinically from the disease we now call typhoid, for example, and up to that point there was still much debate about whether typhus was a separate disease at all. But clinical descriptions of 'typhus' were becoming progressively more detailed and by the late 19th century, medical works were describing typhus with some accuracy. Moreover, by the beginning of the 20th century, the discoveries of Pasteur and Koch [14] had induced others to search for what they assumed to be the infective agent of typhus.

The discovery of the first of several diseases in the typhus 'family' occurred in 1909, when Howard Taylor Ricketts (1871–1910) identified the organism causing Rocky Mountain spotted fever. Noting the similarity between the symptoms of this disease and typhus, Ricketts proceeded to Mexico City in 1910, where the latter was epidemic. After isolating the organism, Ricketts tragically died from the disease, but his work was continued by others during the First World War. The Austrian bacteriologist and zoologist Stanislaus von Prowazek (1875–1915) confirmed that the typhus then raging in Serbia was caused by the organism identified by Ricketts. He, too, died from the disease

when investigating an outbreak in a prisoner-of-war camp, but his assistant, Henrique da Rocha-Lima (1879–1956), managed to isolate the causal microorganism and named it *Rickettsia prowazekii* in honour of both men. After the war, other eminent bacteriologists, including the author of an acclaimed book on typhus, Hans Zinsser (1878–1940), identified other forms of typhus and their causal organisms.

It is now known that there are numerous rickettsial diseases, with different clinical manifestations, the most fatal being that identified by Ricketts himself and the mildest being 'rickettsial pox', caused by *Rickettsia askari*. These forms of 'typhus' are spread by different insect or arthropod vectors, the identification of which began at much the same time as of the causal organism of the disease itself. The original insight into its method of transmission is generally attributed to the French Nobel laureate Charles Nicolle (1866–1936) who, in 1909, determined that typhus fever was transmitted by the human body louse [15]. This made possible a clear distinction between louse-borne and so-called 'murine' typhus, transmitted by the rat flea. But while Nicolle's discovery took priority, two American researchers,

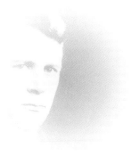

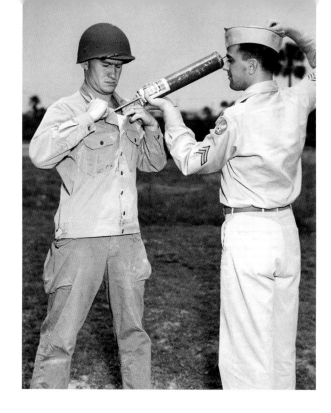

John Anderson and Joseph Goldberger, independently
demonstrated the louse-borne transmission of typhus
a few months later. Subsequently, the transmission of
other rickettsial diseases was elucidated, and it thus
became apparent that some could be transmitted by
ticks and mites.

CONTROL AND TREATMENT

The prevention and cure of these related diseases
made great strides in the course of the 20th century.
In the early 1930s the Polish biologist Rudolf Weigl
(1883–1957) developed the first effective inoculation
against epidemic typhus, which was soon used in the
field by Belgian missionaries in China. During the
Second World War, the vaccine became widely available
to troops, but the main problem remained the incidence
of typhus among displaced civilians and the inmates of
prison camps.

During the First World War, steam and chemical
disinfection had been widely used to prevent louse-
borne diseases and this helped to control typhus in
Western Europe and the Middle East. But the insecticide
DDT, developed prior to the Second World War, offered

a more powerful weapon. In the winter of 1943–44 it
rapidly brought an epidemic in Naples to a halt and was
used to good effect on active service in Burma, where it
was employed against the vector of scrub typhus. And
yet, the high mortality rate from louse-borne typhus
meant that it continued to arouse great fear. This did
not abate until the development of antibiotics such as
the tetracyclines after the war, which proved to be very
effective against a range of rickettsial diseases [46].

Today, typhus is rare by comparison with the mid-
20th century, although various forms of rickettsial
disease are widely distributed, and in some cases
are spreading, possibly due to climate change and
encroachment upon wild environments. Although
typhus poses less of a threat today than when Zinsser
wrote about it in 1935, we should perhaps continue
to heed his warning.

КРАСНАЯ АРМИЯ РАЗДАВИЛА БЕЛОГВАРДЕЙСКИХ ПАРАЗИТОВ — ЮДЕНИЧА, ДЕНИКИНА, КОЛЧАКА.

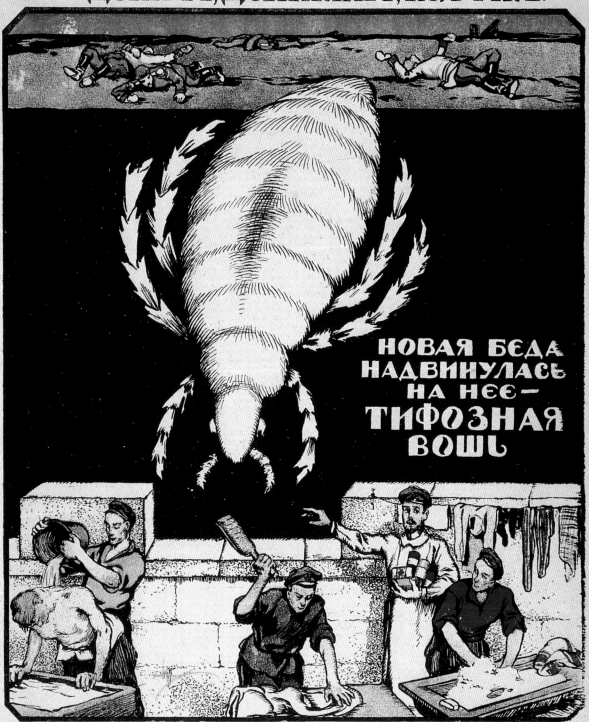

НОВАЯ БЕДА НАДВИНУЛАСЬ НА НЕЕ — ТИФОЗНАЯ ВОШЬ

ТОВАРИЩИ! БОРИТЕСЬ С ЗАРАЗОЙ! УНИЧТОЖАЙТЕ ВОШЬ!

№ 67.

Christopher Hamlin

Anyone who has seen the disease of cholera realizes its
fearsome power as an instrument for societal fear and change.
Richard L. Guerrant, Benedito A. Carneiro-Filho & Rebecca A. Dillingham, 2003

John Snow believed cholera was water-borne, but he could not identify what exactly was carried into people's bodies as they drank. The microscopic life in the New River Company's supply reminds us that drinking water teemed with life.

The early history of the disease we call cholera is obscure. Among ancient chronicles of mass outbreaks of deadly diseases are some which report severe and protracted diarrhoea and vomiting, spasms and coldness of limbs. Awareness of such a disease spreading relentlessly from place to place arose only in the early 1820s, however, as it became clear that a deadly epidemic with such symptoms had begun advancing to the east and northwest from Bengal in 1817. That disease would come to be understood as an Asian, Indian and particularly a Bengali form of cholera. The term itself came from classical Greek medicine, where it referred to a usually self-limiting disorder associated with the expulsion of excess bile.

During the heyday of European imperialism, cholera repeatedly spread over the world: new technologies of rapid transportation by rail and steamship aided its spread, but it also moved along ancient corridors of trade and pilgrimage. By 1930 it had largely been confined to Asia, yet in the early 1990s, cholera crossed over much of Latin America and more recently has become endemic in parts of Africa. Modern cholera is often a disaster disease, emerging when war or some other crisis brings large numbers of people together in unsanitary conditions.

A 19TH-CENTURY EPIDEMIC

For most of the 19th century, what exactly cholera was and how it spread were matters of controversy. Whether it was a distinct disease, whether it required the arrival of a person carrying its contagion or represented the resurgence of some pathological entity in the environment were unclear. After 1854, following groundbreaking epidemiological work by London physician John Snow (1813–58), it was recognized that the consumption of contaminated water was at least one important cholera-transmitting factor. Already cholera had come to be associated with poor sanitation and poverty. Snow hypothesized there was a specific contaminant in water, though he could not identify it. Robert Koch's isolation in 1883 of the so-called 'comma

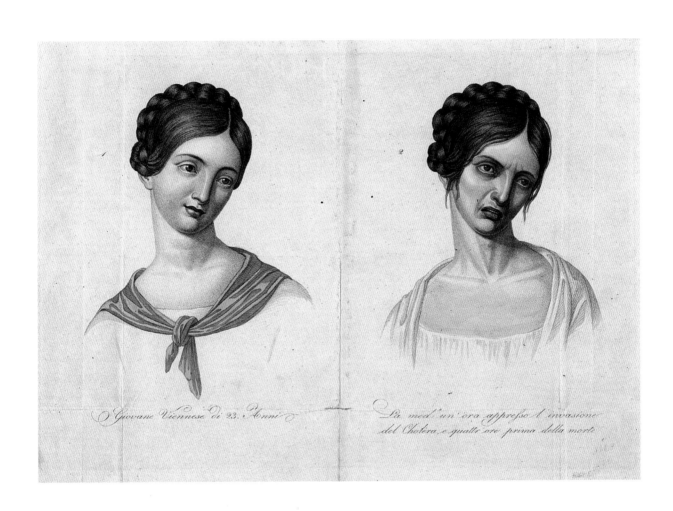

Giovane Viennese di 23. Anni

La med. un'ora apprefso l'invasione del Cholera, e quattr ore prima della morte

Before and after. This demure 23-year-old Venetian woman was rendered into a shrivelled, blue-lipped, near-corpse as the cholera toxin in her intestines caused the water to be drawn out of her bloodstream and tissues into the guts, to be vomited or passed out as the characteristic rice-water stools of cholera. Some victims of the disease would die in just a few hours.

vibrio' (later called *Vibrio cholerae*; see p. 72) brought an era of great confidence in cholera control, yet it would prove challenging to distinguish the few strains that caused dangerous disease from the many which did not. Almost immediately after Koch's discovery attempts were made to produce a vaccine, but the immunity provided by cholera vaccines has usually been partial and short-lived [63].

Cholera's stay in any place was typically brief but extremely deadly: to many physicians a death rate of only half those stricken was a mark of success. Higher cure rates were lies or misdiagnoses, they claimed. In part, differences in cure rates probably depended on definitions: in some places mild cases were called something else, such as 'choleraic diarrhoea'. Modern authorities note that most cholera cases are mild. Often they go undiagnosed.

HOW TO CURE?

To pre-19th-century physicians this was a disease that could be managed – by helping the body expel poisons, treating the coldness and spasms, and restoring strength. Pressed on by a public in panic, 19th-century doctors often took a 'nothing to lose' approach. Some reasoned that a disease producing such radical changes in the body must require equally radical therapies. Cholera involved almost every part of the body save the mind; with its pathology so uncertain, there was ample rationale for innumerable bizarre, painful and even dangerous therapies. Cholera also proved a great opportunity for quacks to market infallible cures.

Given the prominence of fluid loss in cholera, it might have been expected that doctors would try to replace them. Earlier cholera management had often included restorative fluids; the problem was getting them to stay down. As early as the 1830s there had been attempts to restore fluids (and salts) by injection. Improvement was often dramatic, but usually temporary; most experimenters gave up when the technique showed no benefit over other therapies.

At the beginning of the 20th century, Leonard Rogers (1868–1962), working in Calcutta, was able to reduce mortality to about 4 per cent, following studies of changes to blood composition in cholera. Better anticipation of complications that often proved fatal in the disease allowed further improvements. Growing success brought confidence that hospital- and laboratory-based therapeutics were usually

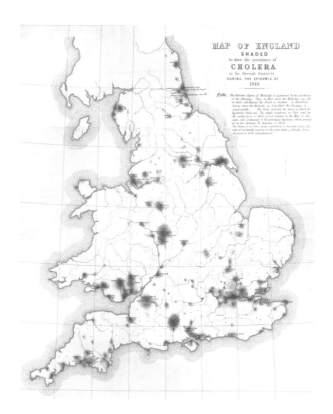

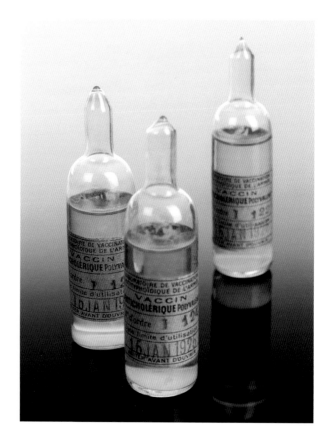

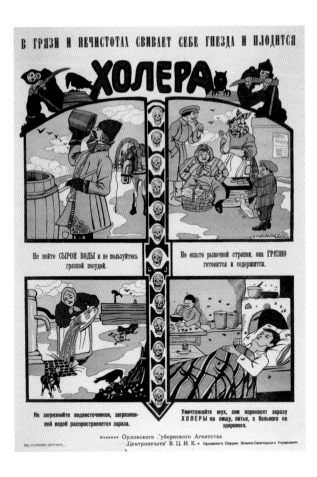

unnecessary; in the early 1970s it was recognized that oral restoration of fluids with a simple solution of sugars and salts was usually sufficient. And not only for cholera, but also for most other forms of gastrointestinal diseases that produced severe dehydration. The discovery that sodium and glucose in the oral rehydration solution are transported together across the small intestine, promoting the absorption of water, has been described as 'potentially the most important medical advance of the 20th century'.

MODERN CHOLERA

Our picture of cholera has changed radically in recent decades. *Vibrio cholerae* has proved to be widely distributed, particularly in warm brackish seas, and to be genetically unstable. How much cholera still exists is not clear. Most modern authorities believe it to be significantly under-reported, partly from the persistence of a cholera stigma. For practical purposes there is usually little incentive to distinguish it from other diarrhoeas – all can be prevented by public and private hygiene (with, perhaps, some help from vaccines) and generally cured by oral rehydration. Still, there remains the possibility of renewed spread. A century ago cholera terrified populations; it still puts governments and authorities into crisis mode – as evident in a Haitian outbreak in November 2010.

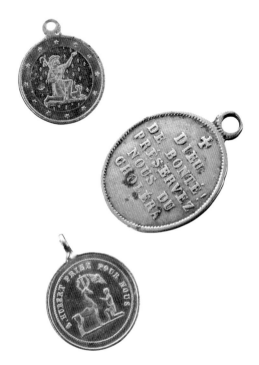

Opposite above
In the aftermath of the cholera epidemic that reached Britain in 1848 its effects were mapped. The relative degree of mortality is expressed in the darkness of the shading.

Opposite below
Ampoules of cholera vaccine produced by the French 'Army Laboratory for Anti-Typhoid Vaccination'. The use by date is prominently displayed.

Above
'Don't do the following, if you want to stay clear of cholera': a Russian public health poster from *c.* 1920 reminds its audience how to avoid contracting the disease.

Left
French or Belgian pendants from the 19th century used as a protection against cholera by invoking the guardianship of St Roch. In the Middle Ages this saint had served a similar service in preventing plague.

Cholera **155**

PUERPERAL FEVER
Killer of mothers

Christine Hallett

It is a disagreeable declaration for me to mention, that I myself
was the means of carrying the infection to a great number of women.
Alexander Gordon, 1795

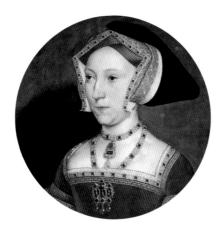

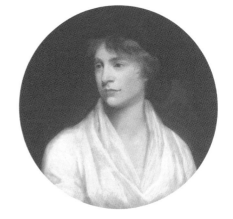

A DEVASTATING DISEASE

Childbed fever – also known as puerperal fever or puerperal sepsis – is one of the most famous iatrogenic diseases (those caused by doctors) of modern times, and was common until the early 20th century. It is the result of the inadvertent introduction of an infective agent into a woman's uterus from the hands of the birth attendant during labour. The infection may originate in the practitioner's nose and throat, or may be transmitted directly from a previously infected patient. The most common causative organism is a particular type of *Streptococcus*, the virulent beta-haemolytic (group A), though other bacteria may also be involved [14].

The disease has an acute onset, beginning, usually on the third day after delivery, with classic symptoms of bacterial infection: high temperature, severe headache, raised pulse and debility. Severe abdominal pain becomes worse over the course of the disease, and is accompanied by abdominal distension, vomiting and diarrhoea. Death is caused by the infection's spread, often culminating in peritonitis and septicaemia. Famous victims include Jane Seymour, Henry VIII's third wife, the cookery-writer Isabella Beeton, and

author Mary Wollstonecraft, who died days after giving birth to her daughter, Mary Shelley.

NEW HOSPITALS AND NEW SCIENCE

The first epidemic probably occurred in Paris in the mid-17th century, but the incidence of the disease increased rapidly in the mid-18th century, the era of the rise of the great public hospitals and the growth of a more 'scientific' and 'empirical' approach to medicine. The new 'lying-in hospitals' admitted the poor and destitute. In return for care, food and shelter, patients became teaching objects and were subject to frequent examinations by doctors and medical students. Here, the 'epidemic form' of puerperal fever usually occurred. Its case fatality rate could exceed 30 per cent.

A new group of medical men emerged in the 18th century: the men-midwives or 'accoucheurs', belonging to a specialist branch of surgery whose practitioners focused on obstetric practice. Many men-midwives studied puerperal fever. They drew on theories of 'contagion' and 'infection' extant since ancient times, but viewed these as a sideline to the more important business of finding out how the disease developed

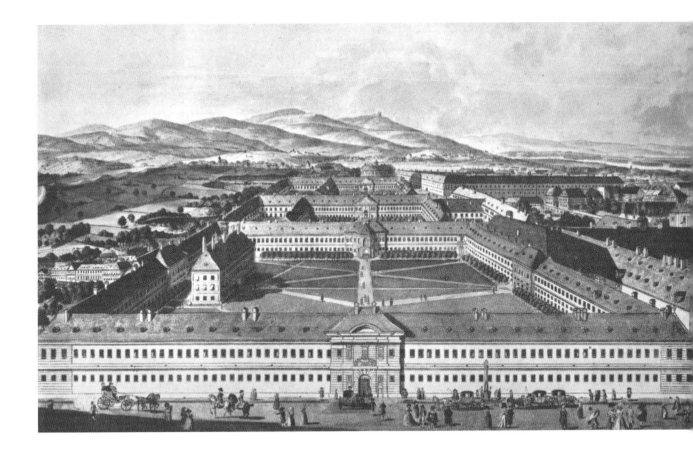

within the human body, a study increasingly dependent on anatomical dissection to discover the 'lesion's' organic location [07].

The great hospital epidemics were undoubtedly the result of the common practice of doctors and medical students moving directly from the hospital's dissecting room, where they worked on the infected bodies of the dead, to the delivery ward without washing their hands or changing clothes, thus transferring the infective microorganism from the dead to the living. The tragedy of childbed fever was that the more time doctors spent in the anatomy dissection theatres struggling to discover the sources of the disease, the greater the chance that they would infect their unfortunate patients.

DAWNING REALIZATION

The first medical writer seriously to consider that puerperal fever could be transmitted to an otherwise healthy woman from the hands or clothes of her birth attendant was Alexander Gordon (1752–99). His private practice as a man-midwife in Aberdeen enabled him to observe large numbers of cases, and he came to realize that a woman's survival apparently depended on who had delivered her. His *Treatise on the Epidemic Puerperal Fever of Aberdeen* (1795) caused uproar: he named those doctors and midwives who appeared to be transmitting the infection.

In 1843, the American physician Oliver Wendell Holmes (1809–94) published 'The Contagiousness of Puerperal Fever' in the *New England Quarterly Journal of Medicine and Surgery*, recommending birth attendants wash their hands and change their clothes between patients, and avoid attending autopsies on days they delivered parturient women.

Opposite left
Jane Seymour (1508–37), third wife of Henry VIII of England, died of puerperal fever contracted during the birth of Edward, Prince of Wales; detail of a portrait by Hans Holbein the Younger.

Opposite right
Mary Wollstonecraft (1759–97) was an advocate of the equality of men and women (she was the author of *A Vindication of the Rights of Woman*, 1792), so it is particularly poignant that she should die of this essentially female affliction.

Above
The Vienna General Hospital, where Ignaz Semmelweis linked together deaths in the obstetrical clinic with attendance by medical students who came there from the dissecting room without washing their hands properly.

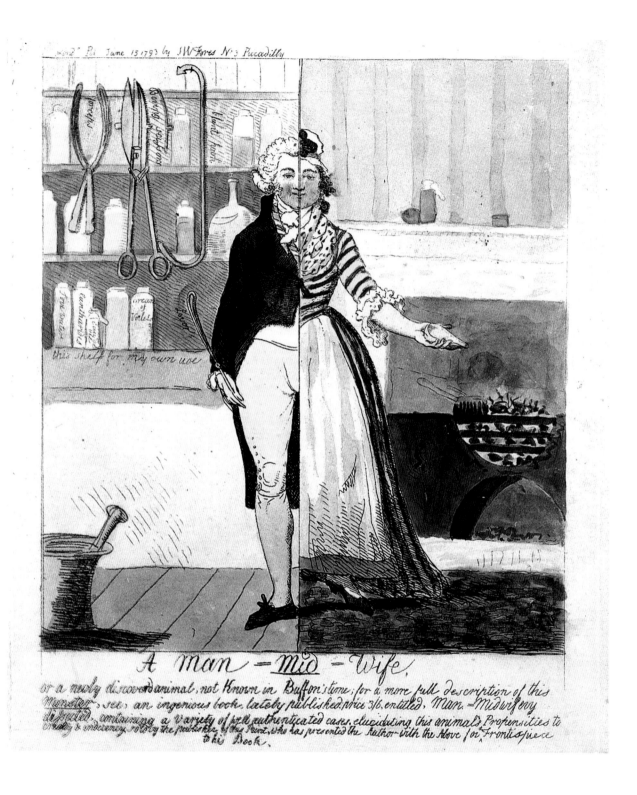

Published June 15 1793 by SW Fores No 3 Piccadilly

A man — mid — wife.

or a newly discovered animal, not known in Buffon's time; for a more full description of this Monster; see, an ingenious book, lately published, price 3/6, entitled, Man—Midwifery dissected, containing a variety of well authenticated cases, elucidating this animal's Propensities to cruelty & indecency, sold by the publisher of this Print, who has presented the Author with the above for Frontispiece to his Book.

Above
A late 18th-century caricature of the 'new' man-midwife, by Isaac Cruikshank. Male professional encroachment on the female sphere of childbirth sadly increased the risk of puerperal sepsis for some women.

Opposite below
A tube of Prontosil tablets – the first sulphonamide antimicrobial drug – developed at the Bayer laboratories in Germany by Gerhard Domagk. He was awarded the 1939 Nobel Prize in Medicine, but was prevented from accepting it by the Nazis.

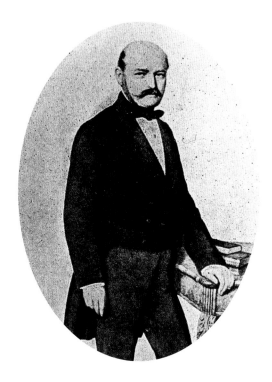

The name most inextricably linked with the discovery of the infectious nature of puerperal fever is that of Hungarian man-midwife, Ignaz Semmelweis (1818–65). The tragedy of his own life mirrors that of the disease itself. Appointed assistant to the First Obstetrical Clinic of the Vienna General Hospital in 1846, he noticed that the mortality rate from puerperal fever was much higher in his clinic, where medical students were trained, than in the Second Clinic, where midwifery students (who were not allowed to attend dissections) received their instruction.

When a colleague, Jakob Kolletschka, died of septicaemia after accidentally cutting his hand during an autopsy, Semmelweis realized it was matter (which he named 'cadaverous particles') carried on the hands of doctors and students that caused puerperal fever. In 1847 he ordered all staff and students to wash their hands in chloride of lime solution before entering his ward; its mortality rates fell dramatically, but his ideas were ridiculed and his three-year contract not renewed. He was forced to leave Vienna in 1849 and only published his ideas in a book, *The Aetiology, Concept and Prophylaxis of Childbed Fever*, in 1860. In 1865 he became mentally ill and was confined to an asylum, where he died of an infected injury aged 47.

BREAKTHROUGHS OF THE 20TH CENTURY

After Louis Pasteur's discovery of the *Streptococcus* organisms in the 1870s (see [14]) Semmelweis's ideas began to be taken seriously. Rebecca Lancefield (1895–1981) classified the *Streptococci* in the 1920s, enabling Leonard Colebrook (1883–1967), assisted by his sister Dora (1884–1965), to establish that the most common causative agent of puerperal fever was a haemolytic streptococcus. In 1935 Leonard Colebrook discovered the first effective treatment: the active ingredient, sulphanilamide, in the dye Prontosil. With the advent of aseptic procedures and antibiotics [46], childbed fever was almost completely eradicated. By the middle of the 20th century, treatment of the disease had been transformed from a medical failure into one of the great achievements of medical science.

Above
Ignaz Semmelweis had a difficult time convincing his colleagues of their complicity in the spread of puerperal sepsis; like Alexander Gordon in the 18th century, his ideas brought him extreme unpopularity rather than praise.

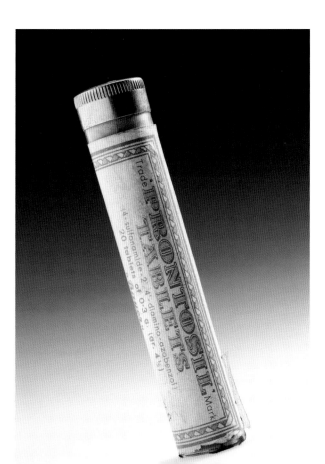

38. TUBERCULOSIS
Spitting blood

Helen Bynum

*The captain of all these men of death that came against
him to take him away, was the consumption; for it was
that that brought him down to the grave.*
John Bunyan, 1680

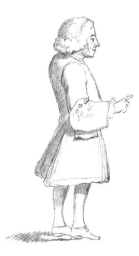

Left
The hunchbacked Alexander Pope probably suffered from Pott's
disease. The causal bacteria spread in the bloodstream (often from
the lungs) to the thoracic vertebrae and discs in between, which are
gradually destroyed, just as the lung tissue is.

Opposite above
The causative microorganism of tuberculosis, a *Mycobacterium
tuberculosis* bacillus, seen here inside a macrophage, the white blood
cells that engulf and consume such invaders as part of the body's
immune response.

Opposite below
A gold touch-piece from the reign of James I of England (1566–1625).
The monarchs of France and England 'touched' those suffering
from scrofula (tuberculosis of the lymphatic glands): being divinely
appointed, they were regarded as God's intermediaries.

Tuberculosis is one of the greatest killers of all time.
In the early 19th century it accounted for 17 to 20 per
cent of all deaths, making it the commonest cause. Most
widespread as pulmonary tuberculosis, it is transmitted
by contact with sputum infected with *Mycobacterium
tuberculosis* – the most ubiquitous of the tuberculosis-
causing mycobacteria. A third of the world's population
is currently infected, and of these 10 per cent will go on
to develop the active disease.

Tuberculosis is also one of the oldest human
diseases. *Mycobacterium tuberculosis* has long been
part of our evolutionary history. DNA sequencing
techniques indicate its presence in 9,000-year-old
skeletons. Ancient texts from India, China, the Middle
East and classical Greece describe tuberculous
symptoms, while mummified human remains reveal
its ravages. Humans share tuberculosis germs with
animals, importantly with cows; *Mycobacterium bovis*
causes tuberculosis in both. Veterinary and public
health measures can safeguard milk supplies and
prevent animal to human spread.

TUBERCLE TO GERM
Once inside the body, tuberculosis can lead to
widespread tissue damage. The collapsed spine of the
poet Alexander Pope (1688–1744) was tuberculous, as
were the swollen lymphatic glands on the necks of those
suffering from scrofula, or the 'king's evil', treated by
the royal touch of monarchs of France and England
from the medieval period until the 18th century.
Queen Anne touched the lexicographer Dr Samuel
Johnson (1709–84) as a scrofulous baby. He wore the
commemorative coin for the rest of his life. Frenchman
René Laennec (1781–1826), inventor of the stethoscope
[22] unified these and other apparently disparate
conditions. He realized that tubercles, found in the
lungs at autopsy and long associated with cases
of phthisis or consumption, were also found in the
spine, intestines and lymph glands, for instance – the
same disease process occurred throughout the body.

Laennec himself died of tuberculosis not long after
publishing his seminal research in 1819, one of the
disease's many wealthy, talented victims. Some even
perceived a link between tuberculosis, genius and
heightened sensibility. It fuelled the Romantic obsession

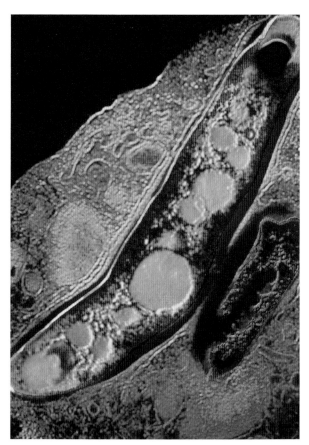

years for everyone to be convinced. Koch won the Nobel Prize in 1905.

BED-REST AND BEYOND

Knowing what caused the disease was vital, but brought no immediate therapeutic advances. Koch's own tuberculin treatment was a sad failure. Instead, the new bacteriology demonized sufferers, who were now perceived as dangerous to their family and neighbours. Sanatoria offered rest, a restorative diet and kept the sick away from the healthy, but it was a grim and isolating existence: the monotony of the all-year round open-air treatment broken perhaps by artificially collapsing an infected lung to 'rest' it. Conditions might be more pleasant for the better off on Thomas Mann's *Magic Mountain* (1924), or in Dr Edward Trudeau's sanatorium beside Saranac Lake in the Adirondacks, but unless the body halted the progress of the disease there wasn't much hope.

That arrived in 1943, when Selman Waksman (1888–1973) and Albert Schatz (1922–95) produced streptomycin, the first antibiotic against tuberculosis [46]. Waksman earnt tuberculosis's second Nobel Prize in 1952. Streptomycin treatment was unpleasant, requiring intramuscular injections. It quickly became

of being, as the poet John Keats wrote, 'half in love with easeful death', as if dying from tuberculosis was beautiful. It was not. Exhausted sufferers coughed, spat out blood, saw their flesh waste as they could neither swallow food over a diseased larynx nor stop their diarrhoea, and felt the sweat soak the bedclothes during their nightly fevers. For every case in a comfortable household there were many more among the malnourished poor. The tuberculosis epidemic followed urbanization and industrialization around the globe, decimating those in the prime of their working and childbearing lives from the age of 18 to 30.

Rich or poor, tuberculosis seemed to strike some families hard. Think of the Brontës: five of the six children, including the writers Emily, Anne and Branwell, had the disease. Their father was probably scrofulous (although he outlived them all). Was it infectious or hereditary? In 1882 the German doctor and proponent of the germ theory of disease [14], Robert Koch (1843–1910), announced his discovery of the tubercle bacillus (hence the subsequent abbreviation TB), bringing a new certainty to tuberculosis's aetiology, although it still took a few

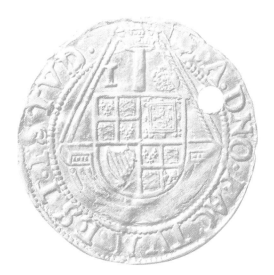

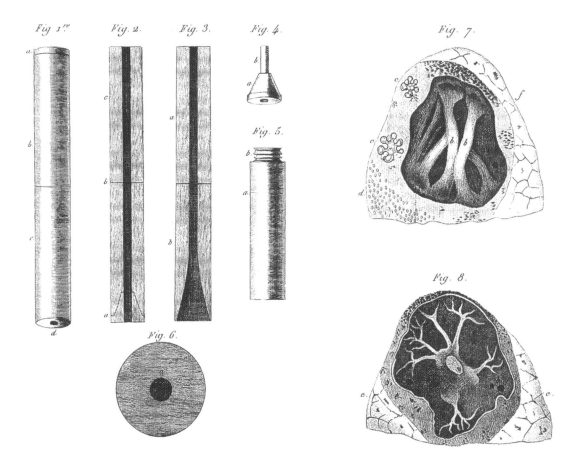

apparent that a combination of streptomycin, isoniazid and para-aminosalicylic acid was both more efficacious and helped to prevent the development of antibiotic resistance. Subsequently, rifampicin tablets replaced injected streptomycin.

Ironically, by the time this drug triad was available the incidence of tuberculosis was already waning. In the developed world improving living standards had turned the tide and there was some benefit from BCG (Bacillus Calmette-Guérin) vaccination, introduced in 1921 [63]. With mass X-ray campaigns to identify early, pre-symptomatic cases, medication mopped up the end of the epidemic, but the disease's apparent disappearance was illusory. In the developing world there was still plenty of it, if people bothered to look.

In the last two decades of the 20th century, with the rise of AIDS/HIV [42] and the growth of a new urban underclass in the developed world, tuberculosis re-emerged with a new force. In the developing world and in the deteriorating social conditions in the former communist countries the problems were more acute and public health infrastructures poor. Various degrees of drug-resistant bacteria led to new protocols of drug delivery. DOTS (directly observed treatment, short course) aims to ensure that patients (and those they have been in contact with) take their medication for the full six-month course. Extensively drug-resistant tuberculosis presents a significant future challenge to the ingenuity of pharmaceutical research, while we can hope that improved living standards and a reduction in other infections might once more lead the way.

Above
Engravings of Laennec's original stethoscope (left) and sections through a tuberculous lung (right) from *De l'auscultation mediate* (*On Mediate Auscultation*; 1819), in which he announced his unitary theory of tubercles – wherever these lesions appeared in the body, the same disease process was at work.

Opposite
Fresh air and sunshine were thought to help prevent tuberculosis in the pre-antibiotic era. Children of tuberculous parents could enjoy summer camps run by anti-tuberculosis charities. The sale of stamps, as advertised in this French poster of 1917, helped to fund such activities.

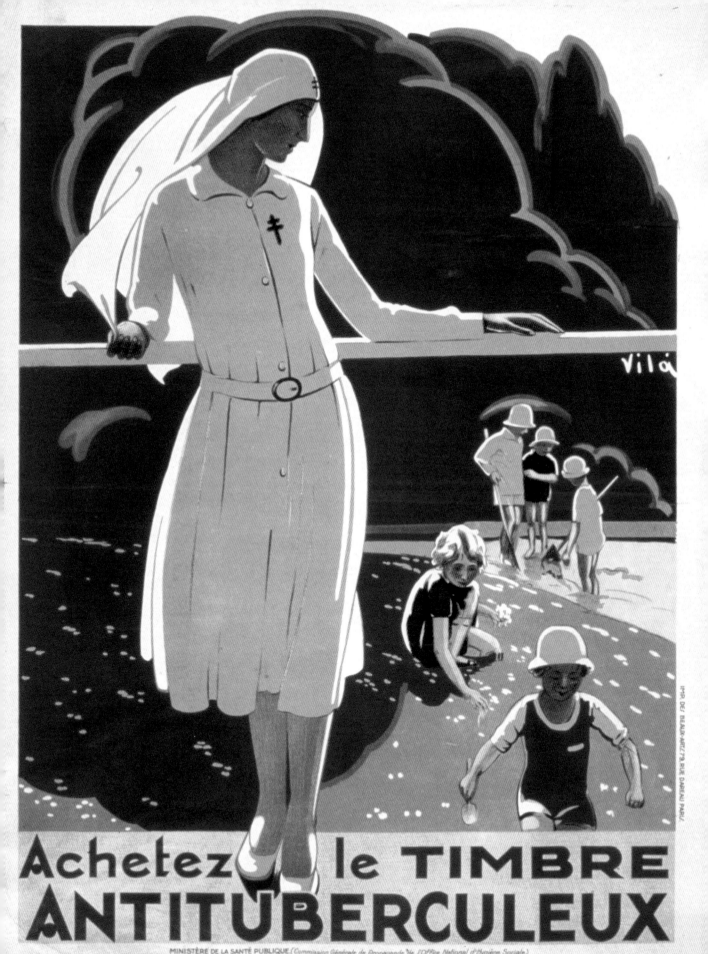

Achetez le **TIMBRE ANTITUBERCULEUX**

MINISTÈRE DE LA SANTÉ PUBLIQUE. (Commission Générale de Propagande de l'Office National d'Hygiène Sociale)
Campagne nationale du Timbre antituberculeux organisée par le
COMITÉ NATIONAL DE DÉFENSE CONTRE LA TUBERCULOSE, 66, Bd St-Michel, PARIS. Reconnu d'Utilité Publique.

39. INFLUENZA A

A mutating virus

Dorothy Crawford & Ingo Johannessen

*… immediately upon the Queene's arrivall here, she fell acquainted with
a new disease that is common in this towne, called here the newe acqayntance,
which passed also throughe her whole courte neither sparinge lordes, ladies
or damoysells, not so much as ether Frenche or English.*
Account of influenza affecting the court of Mary Queen of Scots at
Edinburgh in 1562

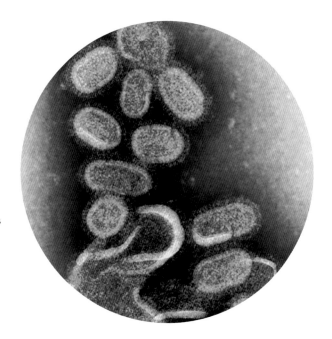

Influenza A virus is one of our greatest infectious
threats. While global surveillance monitors its progress
and scientists generate vaccines and antiviral drugs to
prevent and control it, history has taught us caution in
the face of this deadly killer.

NATURAL HISTORY OF A VIRUS

Flu virus naturally infects aquatic birds, and with
hundreds of virus strains multiplying in their guts
and excreted in their droppings, it is not surprising
that humans occasionally become infected through
handling these animals. However, not all bird flu
strains can infect humans. Infection depends on the
combination of haemagglutinin (H) and neuraminidase
(N) molecules in a particular viral strain, and with 16
H and 9 N subtypes, many different strains exist. These
strains are named after the H and N combination they
contain, such as H5N1 bird flu and H1N1, the currently
circulating swine flu.

Flu has a long history of causing pandemics.
While we experience 'seasonal flu' outbreaks each
winter, flu pandemics arise every 10 to 40 years.
Pandemics occur when an entirely new strain

Virologists have re-created the 1918–19 Influenza A virus in order
to identify the characteristics that made this organism such a deadly
pathogen: it killed around 40 million people worldwide in the
pandemic at the end of the First World War.

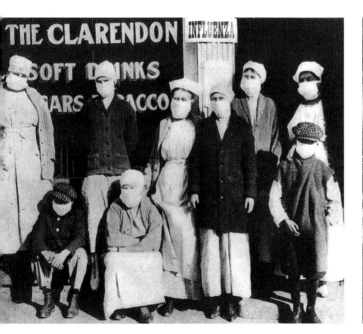

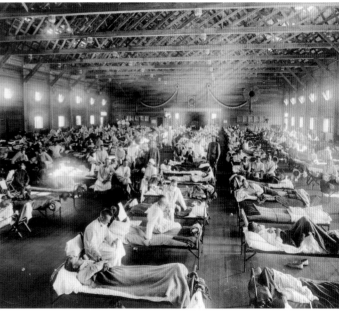

People did what they could to protect themselves during the 'Spanish flu' epidemic of 1918–19, such as donning surgical face masks. Nearly half of those who died in these two years were young, previously healthy adults.

Medical facilities struggled to cope with the vast influx of patients during the 'Spanish flu' outbreak. Temporary civilian hospital accommodation was established and military units cared for the sick troops, as seen here.

arrives to which no one is immune and it can therefore sweep round the world unimpeded. During the 20th century, the world experienced three flu pandemics: 'Spanish flu' (1918–19); 'Asian flu' (1957); and 'Hong Kong flu' (1968). Beginning towards the end of the First World War, the first of these was the biggest killer: around 40 million people died, considerably more than in the conflict itself. The 'Spanish flu' virus probably jumped to humans directly from birds, but other viruses, such as the current swine flu, jumped from pigs.

DRIFT AND SHIFT

The genetic material of flu virus is organized as eight separate segments or 'chromosomes'. This unique feature allows mixing to occur when a single cell in an animal is infected with two (or more) virus strains. This 'genetic re-assortment' occurs often in birds, although these viruses may have to infect a pig, the so-called 'mixing vessel', before they can successfully jump to humans. Both human and bird viruses can infect pigs, allowing for genetic mixing between the two and the possible production of an entirely new flu virus.

This process is called an 'antigenic shift' and has the potential to cause a pandemic.

H5N1 bird flu first emerged in geese in Guangdong province, China, in 1996, and by 1997 was causing outbreaks in poultry farms and live animal markets in Hong Kong. In May 1997 a three-year-old boy died of H5N1 pneumonia, and that year there were 17 further human cases resulting in five deaths – a 29 per cent fatality rate. Mass culling of poultry contained the outbreak, but the virus re-emerged in Southeast Asia in 2003, with more human fatalities. Since then H5N1 flu has spread widely in Asia, Europe and Africa; but as scientists tracked its progress, a new flu threat from Central America took the world by surprise.

Swine flu causes respiratory disease in pigs and occasionally jumps to pig handlers. But the current pandemic swH1N1 that emerged in pigs in Mexico and spread to humans in 2009 contains a mixture of avian, human and swine flu genes. Now that the virus has spread globally we know that most infections are mild, but (similar to seasonal flu) swH1N1 can be a danger for pregnant women, young children, the infirm and the elderly.

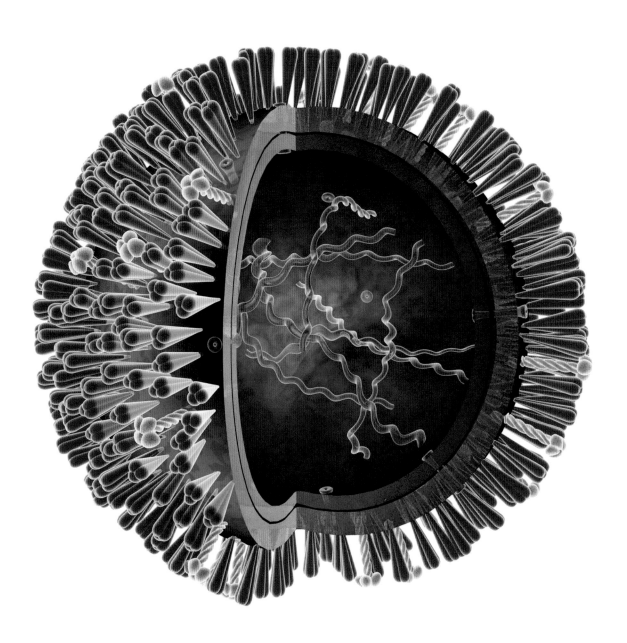

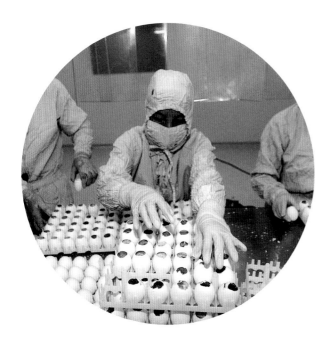

Once a flu strain is circulating in the community it slowly accumulates mutations affecting H and N proteins (antigenic drift). With these minor modifications the virus can overcome host immunity and re-emerge as winter 'seasonal flu'. Each new seasonal flu virus can then infect those who were immune to the previous strain.

PREPARING FOR THE UNEXPECTED

Flu spreads in airborne droplets generated by coughing and sneezing as well as by direct or indirect contact with sufferers, for instance via hands and door handles. After an incubation period of one to four days, a typical infection causes chills, headache, dry cough, fever, muscular aches, malaise and loss of appetite lasting for five to ten days, with the main complication being pneumonia. Complications of pandemic flu can be especially severe and (in contrast to seasonal flu) often arise in previously healthy young adults.

Vaccines [63] are key to flu prevention, but because of antigenic drift seasonal flu vaccine must be prepared every year from the strains in circulation. The challenge for developing a pandemic vaccine is that the process takes up to six months and cannot begin until the pandemic strain is identified. Antiviral drugs are therefore currently the mainstay of flu pandemic plans.

With the recent pandemic swine flu being relatively mild, attention has again focused on H5N1 bird flu. This flu strain has all the attributes of a pandemic strain except that it does not transmit efficiently between humans. But the virus has recently increased in virulence and expanded its host range to include chickens and wild birds, and domestic and wild cats. H5N1 has also been found in pigs in Southeast Asia, so increasing the chance of re-assortment with human strains. This may suffice to enhance H5N1's ability to transmit between humans.

Such a formidable adversary has great capacity to outmanoeuvre us. In the face of this invisible enemy, we would do well to be prepared for the unexpected.

40. SMALLPOX
Eradicating a disease

Sanjoy Bhattacharya

The eradication of smallpox shows that with strong mutual resolve, teamwork and an international spirit of solidarity, ambitious global public health goals can be attained.
Dr Margaret Chan, WHO, 2010

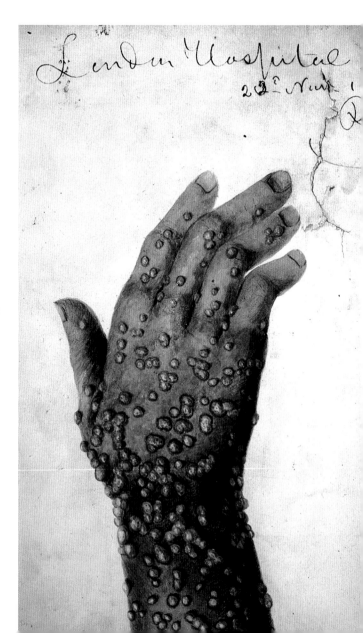

Smallpox was once a dreaded disease: its more virulent avatar, *variola* major, which was widely reported throughout history across Asia and Africa, could wipe out between 25 and 50 per cent of its victims. Although *variola* minor, the less infective form of the disease, appeared to predominate in Europe and the Americas, *variola* major was occasionally imported along trade and transport routes by land, sea and, later, air. The resulting smallpox outbreaks were generally considered major events, owing mainly to their capacity to kill and maim.

INOCULATION AND EARLY VACCINATION
Inoculation is the transfer of smallpox matter (taken from a pustule) between a diseased and a healthy individual, which aims to transmit a mild case of the disease and thereby render the recipient immune for life. It was sometimes called variolation and in various forms was an ancient practice, used widely across Asia and Africa. Lady Mary Wortley Montagu (1689–1762), the wife of the British ambassador in Turkey, witnessed the practice in that country in 1717 and is considered responsible for the introduction of inoculation

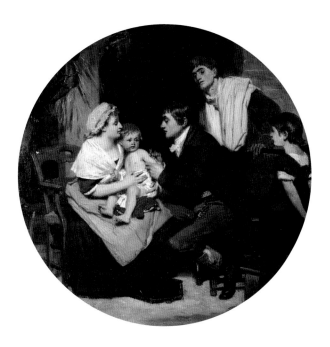

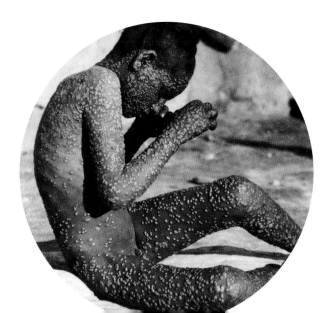

to Britain. Variolation blossomed in Britain, and chroniclers have described many forms of carrying out the operation, some more intricate (and expensive) than others. The practice was sufficiently well established in the 18th century for the East India Company to inoculate its European troops consistently against smallpox. Alternative methods of variolation continued to co-exist in British India well into the 19th century.

Edward Jenner (1749–1823) pioneered vaccination (from the Latin, *vacca*, 'cow') through experiments with the use of cowpox (a closely allied virus) as a method of preventing smallpox [63]. In 1796 Jenner inoculated James Phipps, an eight-year-old boy, with pustular matter from a cowpox sore. A few days later he tried to infect him with smallpox: Phipps was immune. Others, such as Benjamin Jesty (1736–1816), were involved in similar endeavours. Jenner's experiments resulted in products that were not simply replicated; his techniques of vaccine manufacture and vaccination allowed myriad experiments and adaptations that resulted in the creation of a wide range of products.

By the 19th century, European nations were adopting the practice at home and within their colonial possessions. Smallpox vaccination was presented both as a necessity and a powerful example of the benefits of imperial rule. Various nations made vaccination compulsory to control the disease. In some instances re-vaccination was necessary: unlike variolation, vaccination does not provide lifelong immunity. By the mid-20th century smallpox was no longer a problem in the developed world.

AN AUDACIOUS PLAN

As a disease agent the smallpox virus has one major weakness: it has no animal host, making it much easier for those charged with controlling its spread to carry out their work. However, where smallpox was most common – in the tropics – instability in the vaccines was a serious problem. After the introduction of mass-produced freeze-dried vaccines in the 1950s problems of loss of potency were eased. In 1958, following a proposal from the USSR to the World Health Assembly, the World Health Organization (WHO) called for the eradication of smallpox through national programmes. In the 1960s the WHO eradication campaign was intensified. By 1973, transmission remained only in the Indian subcontinent and the Horn of Africa. In May 1980 the World Health Assembly certified that smallpox had been eradicated globally.

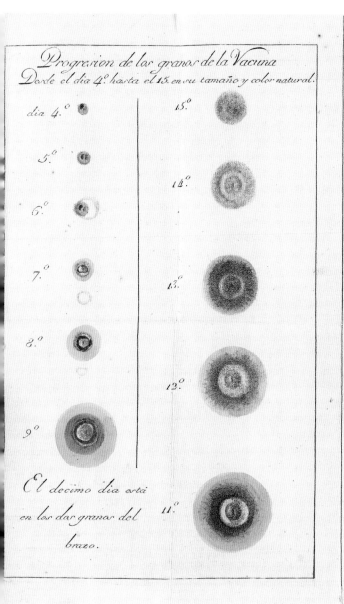

Progresion de los granos de la Vacuna
Desde el dia 4º hasta el 15 en su tamaño y color natural.

dia 4.º

5.º

6.º

7.º

8.º

9º

El decimo dia está
en los dos granos del
brazo.

15.º

14.º

13.º

12.º

11.º

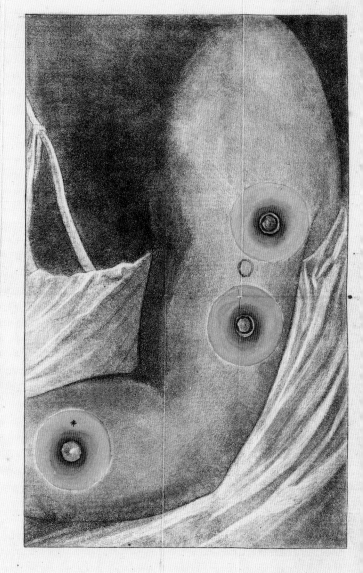

Above
A fold-out plate from the 1803 treatise on the history and practice of vaccination by Francisco Xavier de Balmis (1753–1819), showing the progress of the vaccination site and scar development on a daily basis. Balmis travelled throughout the Spanish dominions practising and teaching vaccination.

Opposite left
A vaccination gun designed to make mass immunization more efficient, delivering a dose of the vaccine through the skin at high pressure without using a needle. It was employed during the smallpox eradication programme, although a simple bifurcated needle was more commonly used.

Opposite right
In 12th-century Japan, the legendary Chinsei Hachiro Tametomo was exiled by his enemies to the small island of Oshima, where he repelled the demon of smallpox with his ferocity. The demon was reduced to the size of a pea and floated out to sea. Woodcut, *c.* 1847–52.

The success of the worldwide smallpox eradication programme cannot be attributed to the ideas and actions of just a handful of individuals and institutions, nor to technical quick fixes. The enormity of the achievement can be appreciated only by acknowledging the great range of input in training, attitude, ability and commitment among those involved in the vaccination campaigns. The global project to limit the spread of *variola*, as it evolved in the 1960s and 1970s, worked simultaneously at both the international and local level, and at each stage had several complex constituents, including mass vaccination programmes as well as a more focused strategy of a combination of surveillance, containment and vaccination (a new tactic, developed in the face of vaccine shortages, which became very popular in Asia and Africa in the late 1960s and 1970s).

Players at all levels, from federal and provincial governments through to members of locally elected urban and rural authorities, cooperated in the eradication programme. Local personnel throughout the campaign countries were vital: they were involved in the house-to-house searches for cases of smallpox, and also served as team leaders, translators, vaccinators, supervisors and guards of lodgings where smallpox cases were being isolated. In the 1970s senior programme managers recognized their importance on the ground, and in hindsight the role of such local personnel is widely regarded as one of the reasons why the eradication programme succeeded. Field experience taught managers that local political and infrastructural conditions needed careful study to avoid tensions, assist in effective negotiations with the target population and allow policy adaptations as required. It provided valuable lessons for other future eradication programmes.

The smallpox virus still exists in laboratories in the USA and the Russian Federation. Debates about the destruction of these stocks have been heated and divisive. Some fear they represent a source of supply for the creation of biological weapons, while others argue that the stored virus is necessary for the mobilization of responses to any attack with a smallpox-based weapon.

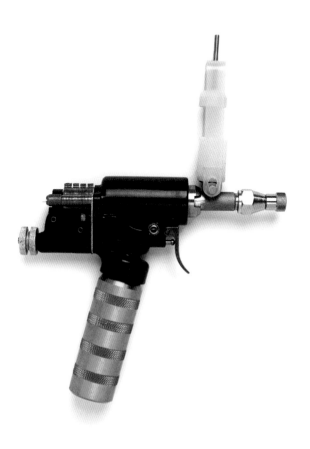

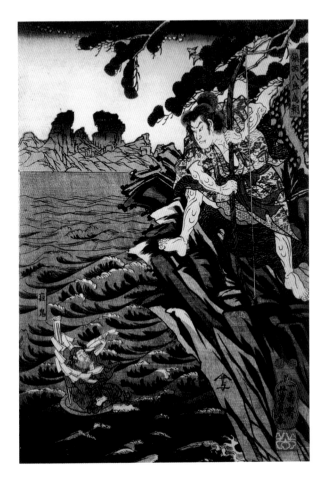

41. POLIO
The summer plague

Dorothy Crawford

Once you've spent two years trying to wiggle
one toe, everything is in proportion.
Franklin D. Roosevelt, 1945

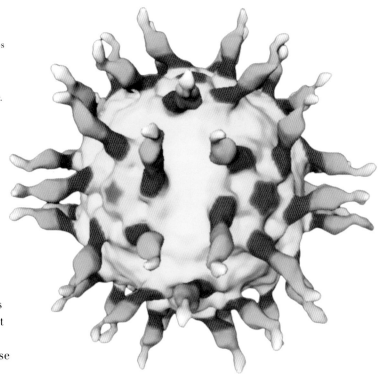

Classic poliomyelitis (polio) is a devastating
disease caused by polio virus attacking the
nervous system. Famous polio victims include
Franklin D. Roosevelt, President of the United States
from 1933 to 1945, who was paralysed from the chest
down and wheelchair bound from the age of 40, and
Scottish novelist Sir Walter Scott, who had the disease
as a young boy and was left with a permanent limp.

The disease, also called infantile paralysis because
it generally affects children and young adults, begins
abruptly with headache, fever, vomiting and stiff
neck, and although some may recover at this stage,
in others the virus targets the nervous system, picking
off the nerves that supply muscles and causing a flaccid
paralysis. Any muscle(s) may be affected, with the
extent of the damage varying from just one muscle to
several whole groups. In the severest cases, accounting
for about 5 per cent of the total, death results from
paralysis of the muscles essential for breathing. Around
10 per cent make a full recovery, but the majority suffer
lifelong paralysis and wasting of one or more muscle.

Interestingly, polio is mainly a disease of modern
times: in the West it rose to prominence in the 1940s and

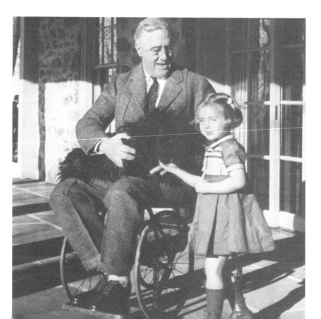

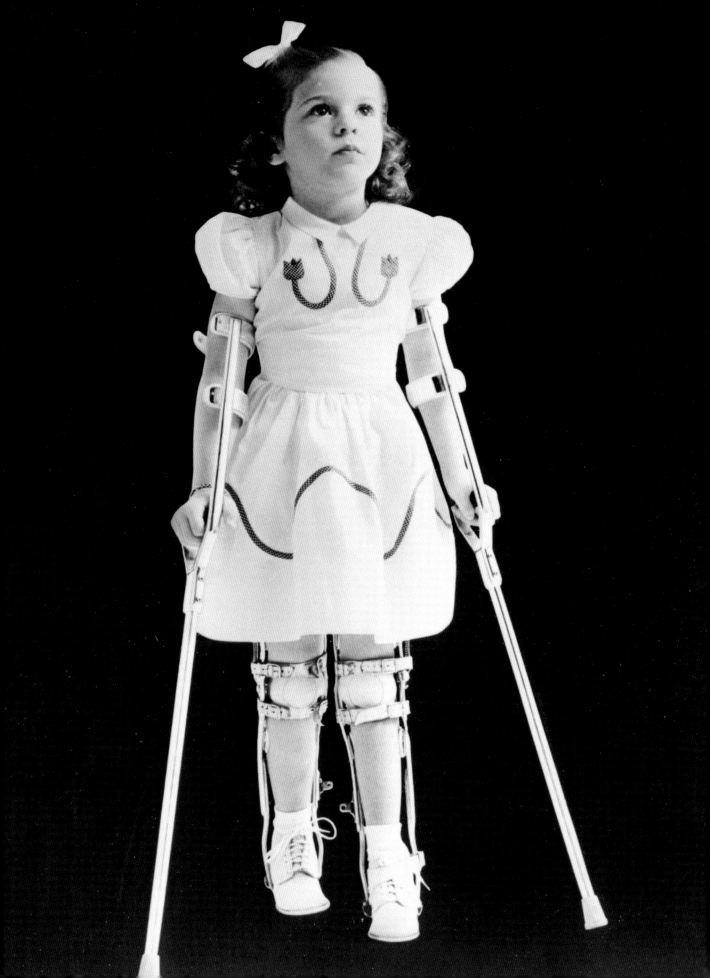

1950s, causing much-feared summer epidemics mainly among the affluent in temperate climates, apparently striking indiscriminately within a community. These outbreaks were only curtailed by the successful vaccine programme beginning in the late 1950s. At that time polio appeared to be rare in developing countries, but its incidence rose from the 1950s onwards as and where standards of living improved.

PATTERNS OF INFECTION

Polio virus was first isolated in 1948 and subsequent antibody studies uncovered the reasons behind its unique pattern of infection. The virus infects cells in the gut and although this does not generally cause any gastrointestinal symptoms, the virus is excreted in large amounts in faeces. It can survive for several weeks in sewage and is mainly spread from person to person by ingestion, often through swimming in contaminated water. In developing countries and poor areas in industrialized nations this spread is enhanced by low standards of living, and so here polio virus is ubiquitous and infects almost everyone by the age of five, but generally without any ill effect. However, where high standards of hygiene prevail, the spread of the virus is severely limited and many young children are protected from infection by lack of exposure. If they

are then exposed to the virus for the first time in later life, they are more at risk of developing the paralytic disease.

The reason for this age-related susceptibility is not known – even among this older age group nervous system infection is rare, only occurring in around one in 100 infections. In the vast majority of cases the virus causes no symptoms, thus giving the impression of targeting just the unfortunate few. But the virus still replicates in the gut during asymptomatic infection and so these people act as silent virus reservoirs that can fuel an epidemic. This phenomenon, known as the 'iceberg effect', is exemplified by an outbreak in an affluent area of New Canaan, Connecticut, USA, in the summer of 1954. The incident centred on a nursery school, with 16 cases of paralytic polio occurring in the school children, their families or friends. Antibody studies showed that almost the entire community was infected with the polio virus, so those presenting with polio symptoms represented the tip of the iceberg.

COUNTERING THE THREAT

The first polio vaccine was a killed virus preparation made by American virologist Jonas Salk (1914–95) and introduced in the West in 1955. It immediately had a dramatic effect, with a ten-fold drop in paralytic polio

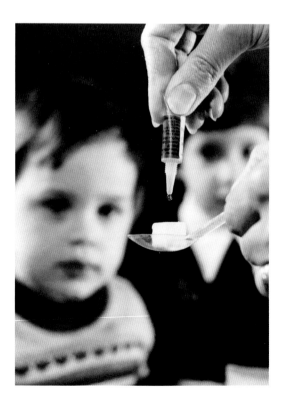

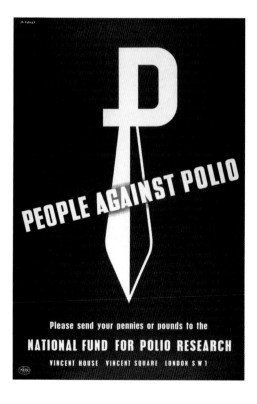

from around 20,000 to 2,000 cases per year in the US. In Scandinavian countries, where vaccination was compulsory, the disease was virtually eliminated. Then in the 1960s another American medical researcher, Albert Sabin (1906–93), made a live attenuated virus vaccine that was non-pathogenic and could be delivered by mouth rather than by injection. This was much more applicable for use in the developing world and had the added benefit of infecting the gut and spreading from the vaccinee to others in the community; it soon replaced the Salk vaccine (see also [63]).

In 1988 the World Health Organization (WHO) announced a global polio eradication programme with the aim of total virus elimination by the year 2000, using the oral vaccine as its main tool. Although the incidence of polio has declined by 99 per cent since 1988, this target has not been met since pockets of virus spread still remain in Afghanistan, India, Pakistan and Nigeria. In addition, some surrounding countries, such as Angola, Chad and Sudan, have experienced imported cases that have spread the virus to the local population. WHO has responded with more intensive vaccine programmes in these countries and it is hoped that the virus will soon be extinct.

There are still some important issues to be considered, however. The live oral vaccine spreads from vaccinees to others, and therefore cannot be used to eradicate completely the virus itself. Furthermore, this usually harmless vaccine virus can occasionally revert to a pathogenic strain and cause polio. And although vaccine-related polio is very rare, occurring in around one in two million infections, it accounts for most cases in countries where polio vaccination prevents the spread of wild polio virus. For these reasons, many countries now use the killed vaccine and this policy will probably have to be adopted globally before complete eradication can become a reality.

Opposite left
A dose of live (but attenuated) polio vaccine was traditionally given on a sugar lump; it can be dropped straight into the mouth. Developed by Albert Sabin and licensed in 1962, it provided an alternative to Jonas Salk's dead but injected vaccine.

Opposite right
A poster from 1954 advertising the National Fund for Polio Research – the British equivalent of the March of Dimes – and asking for donations. By the 1960s the charity had diversified, since the vaccine programme had greatly reduced the incidence of polio.

Below
Hynes Memorial Hospital, Boston, USA, 1955. During polio epidemics iron lungs (mechanical ventilators) kept patients alive while their respiratory muscles recovered. Pumps alter the chamber's pressure to mimic the natural movements of the ribcage and diaphragm.

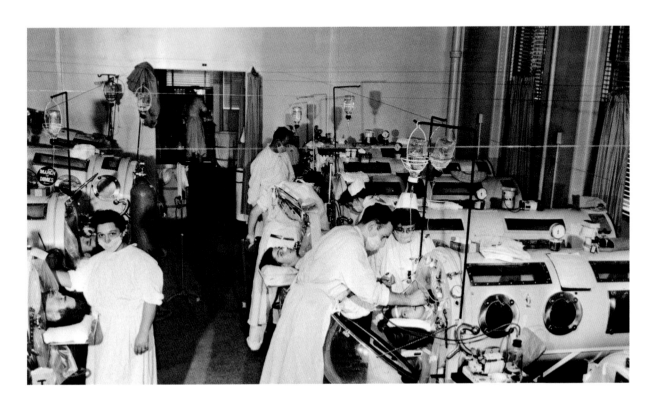

42. **HIV**
A stark reminder

Michael Adler

AIDS continues to challenge all our efforts. Today for every two people who start taking antiretroviral drugs another five become newly infected.
UNAIDS, 2008 Annual Report – AIDS Epidemic Update

In the early 1980s a previously unknown disease gripped the imagination of the world. HIV/AIDS has turned into a global epidemic with profound social and economic effects, particularly in developing countries.

THE FIRST RECOGNIZED CASES

In 1981 two reports appeared in the United States of clusters of cases of a very rare form of pneumonia (*Pneumocystis carinii* pneumonia, or PCP) and an equally rare tumour (Kaposi's sarcoma). These cases occurred in young men who were also both homosexual and immunocompromised and were subsequently described as cases of Acquired Immune Deficiency Syndrome (AIDS). The first UK cases also appeared in 1981. The causative agent, Human Immunodeficiency Virus (HIV), was discovered and isolated in 1983 by a team led by Luc Montagnier at the Institut Pasteur in Paris and almost at the same time by a team led by Robert Gallo at the National Cancer Institute in the US. Major breakthroughs came in 1984 with the development of an antibody test, allowing identification of infected people, and an understanding of the viral transmission dynamics and population prevalence.

Kaposi's sarcoma was the first tumour to be associated with HIV infection. Lymphomas also occur in the brain, gastrointestinal tract, liver and bone, and there are also increases of Hodgkin's lymphoma and anal cancer in infected individuals. And following the association with PCP, it was subsequently realized that a large number of other infections can occur in immunocompromised individuals, especially in the chest, brain and gastrointestinal tract.

TRANSMISSION

The virus is mostly transmitted through sexual intercourse, HIV being isolated in semen and cervical

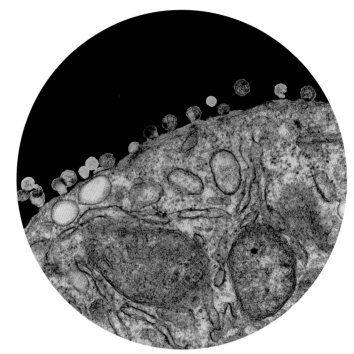

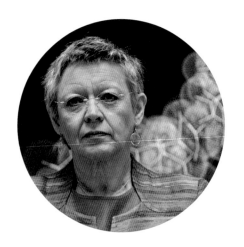

secretions. Whether intercourse is anal or vaginal is unimportant; rarely, transmission occurs as a result of oral-genital contact. The virus has also been isolated from blood, cerebral spinal fluid, tears, saliva, urine and breast milk. Viral load has to be high (as in blood, semen and cervical secretions) for successful transmission and therefore not all of these fluids are sources of infection. Early in the epidemic, before HIV could be isolated, cases resulted through the use of contaminated or infected blood and blood products (for example factor VIII for haemophiliacs). Other modes of transmission occur through donated organs, the sharing or re-use of contaminated needles and from mother to child (within the womb, possibly at birth and through breast milk).

Initially people were also very concerned that HIV was contagious. However, there is no evidence for transmission by casual or social contact, though there are cases of health care workers infected through accidental needle injuries or exposure of their skin or eyes to infected blood or body fluids.

Opposite above
Human Immunodeficiency Virus (HIV) particles (blue) budding from the surface of a T cell (a type of lymphocyte). The viruses replicate inside the cell, with the different components gathering at the cell membrane to be assembled into new virus particles.

Opposite below
Françoise Barré-Sinoussi was awarded the 2008 Nobel Prize in Physiology or Medicine, together with Luc Montagnier, for her role in the discovery in 1983 of the Human Immunodeficiency Virus (HIV), which causes AIDS.

Below
Although there was acrimony at the time of the discovery of the AIDS virus, Robert Gallo (second from the left) and Luc Montagnier (right) have subsequently worked and campaigned together, as seen here in Paris in 1999.

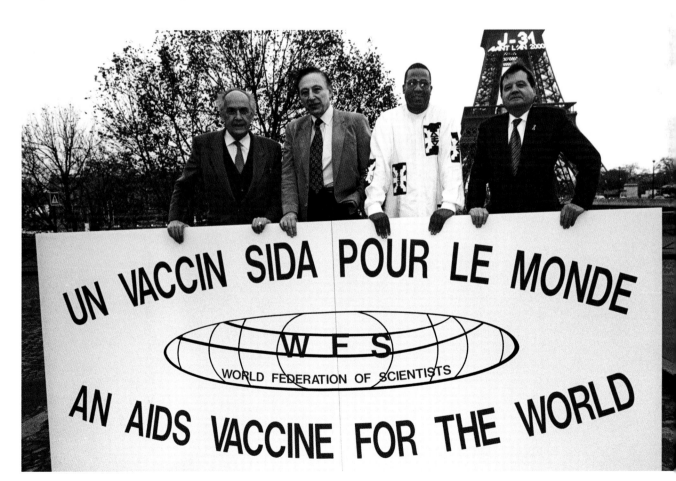

A STAGGERING EPIDEMIC

HIV infection is now worldwide, but the major focus
is in developing/resource poor countries. The United
Nations AIDS programme (UNAIDS) estimates that 33.4
million people are living with HIV/AIDS (31.3 million
adults and 2.1 million children under 15). Currently,
the number of new infections per year is approximately
just under 3 million, with about 5,500 occurring each
day. Ninety-five per cent of all HIV infections occur in
developing countries – the major prevalence is sub-
Saharan Africa and Southeast Asia. Just over 65 per cent
of all adults and children with HIV globally live in sub-
Saharan Africa and two-thirds of HIV infections in that
continent occur in women. Forty-five per cent of new
infections occur in young people aged 15 to 24.

In the UK, an example of the developed world, the
number of cases increases each year. However, the
epidemic's nature has changed considerably since
the early 1980s. Cases of HIV infection diagnosed
among men who have sex with men (MSM) reached
a peak in 1985 before levelling off. In contrast, there
was a rapid five-fold increase in new diagnoses among
heterosexuals between 1996 and 2005, most contracted
outside the UK, predominantly in Africa. Originally,
needle and syringe sharing among drug users was an
important driver, but the early development of needle
exchange schemes essentially curtailed this.

EFFECTS, PREVENTION AND TREATMENT

The HIV epidemic has had a major impact in the
developing world. Life expectancy has been reduced,
particularly in those countries with an adult prevalence
of over 10 per cent. Kenya, Zimbabwe, South Africa,
Zambia and Rwanda face a potential reduction in life
expectancy of over 15 years by 2015, and this will have
a profound effect on their socio-economic development.
Traditional family structures and extended families
are under increasing strain, with a rising number of
orphans. Frequently both parents have died from HIV,
leaving a young child as the breadwinner, whose only
form of income may be commercial sex.

Prevention is better than cure and should start
as early as possible with good sex education before a
person's first sexual contact. The risk of HIV infection
is lessened in several ways: by using condoms for all
penetrative forms of sexual intercourse; by reducing the
number of partners; by adopting safe sexual practices,
for example oral sex, mutual masturbation; by delaying
the age of first sexual intercourse; and by presenting

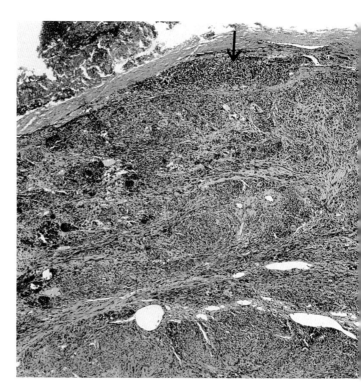

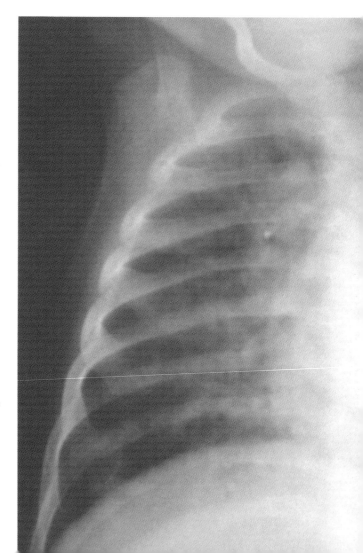

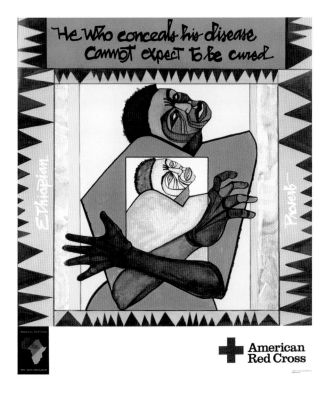

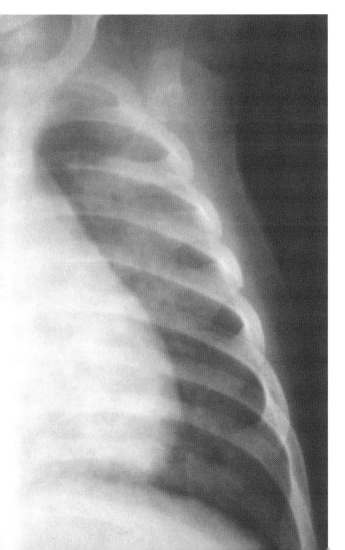

for regular screening and testing for HIV and sexually transmitted infections if the individual is at risk after recently changing partners.

Major therapeutic advances in treatment occurred in 1987 with the development of zidovudine (AZT, an antiretroviral drug), followed in 1996 by the introduction of combination therapy. The latter has had a very profound effect on life expectancy in infected individuals. Antiretrovirals inhibit the replication of the virus, allowing the immune system to repair. The real challenge lies in the developing world where access to antiretroviral treatment is restricted. A number of agencies such as UNAIDS, the World Health Organization, the President's Emergency Plan for AIDS Relief (PEPFAR), the Gates Foundation, and the Global Fund to Fight AIDS, Tuberculosis and Malaria attempt to tackle this. Currently, 60 per cent of infected individuals requiring treatment in the developing world do not have access to therapy. For every two people who start taking antiretroviral drugs, another five become newly infected. Research continues to find a potential vaccine [63].

Although the ultimate origins of HIV are not entirely clear, the human virus shares much with a similar virus that affects chimpanzees. Most scientists believe that accidental contaminations with this virus in Africa, many years ago, are probably the remote sources of the present epidemic of HIV. Tissue samples from people who died in the 1950s contain evidence of the virus, which was probably smouldering for a number of years before it became widespread.

The relatively new epidemic of HIV infection has resulted in global human suffering and represents a major health problem. It would be wrong to view this solely as a medical problem: socio-economic deprivation is a major driver, along with war, migration and sexual inequality.

Opposite above
Kaposi's sarcoma: a lymph node biopsy from an HIV-positive African child. At the top (arrowed) is a small peripheral rim of lymph tissue, but most of the node is now tumour tissue.

Above
'He who conceals his disease cannot expect to be cured.' An Ethiopian proverb is used in this public health poster to try to encourage those who might be at risk of infection with HIV to be tested and treated if necessary.

Left
An X-ray of an infant infected with HIV and *Pneumocystis carinii* pneumonia (PCP). This otherwise rare form of pneumonia is a common co-infection in AIDS and was one of the opportunistic infections first associated with the new disease.

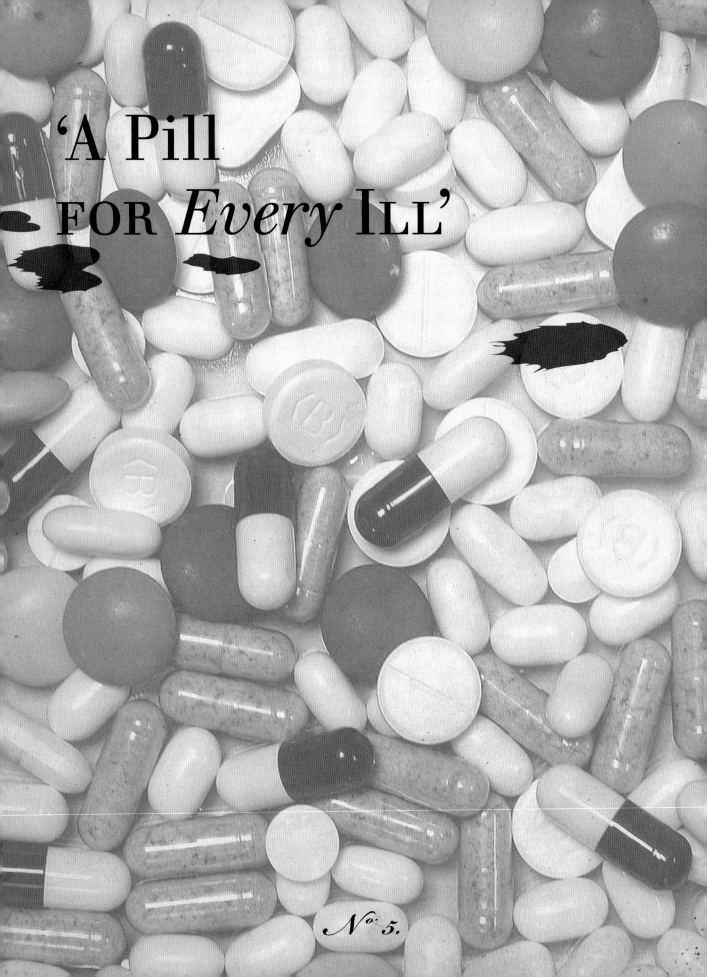

'A Pill
FOR *Every* ILL'

Nº 5.

Almost all the pills we ingest nowadays are of recent development. Pharmacology has transformed what doctors can do to regulate our bodies, keep us functioning normally, improve our chances of survival and, occasionally, cure us of our afflictions.

There are a few drugs of ancient origin that are still used. Opium preparations have a very long history, both for their pain-relieving and mind-altering properties. Quinine was introduced into Europe from South America in the 17th century, and digitalis had been employed in medicine long before William Withering showed in 1785 that it was exceedingly useful in afflictions of the heart. These examples are typical of many early medicines: they come from plants. Plants are still a major source of medicaments, even if modern scientific standards mean that their active ingredients must first be isolated and tested before being used in human beings. After laboratory and animal tests, potential drugs must pass through a rigorous and expensive series of clinical trials to determine their safety and efficacy; when this isn't done properly disasters such as the birth defects caused by the anti-nausea drug thalidomide can happen.

This strategy can be seen in several of the other drugs included here: penicillin, derived from a mould; the first modern oral contraceptive, extracted from the Mexican yam; and even the cholesterol-lowering statins, some of the most widely prescribed drugs of today, which are of fungal origin. In each case, the active principle was eventually isolated so it could be studied more closely, and then chemical modifications were introduced to increase effectiveness, allow an easier mode of administration, or reduce side effects. Much modern pharmacological research now consists of just this kind of systematic investigation and slight modifications of the original compound, with the patent (and profits) that results.

Today's research pharmacologists want to know the chemical structure of the drug, and to understand its molecular mode of action. The discovery of the bronchodilators such as Ventolin, which have revolutionized the treatment of asthma, and the beta-blockers, widely used in the management of several kinds of heart disease, were both rooted in sophisticated knowledge of the physiology of the nervous system's control of certain bodily functions. Beta-blockers are the quintessential 'designer drugs', developed to do at the molecular level exactly what they are supposed to. In contrast to the beta-blockers, many of the drugs that have transformed contemporary psychiatry were chance discoveries. The majority of those that reduce the florid symptoms of schizophrenia and other major psychiatric disorders, calm the anxieties of the neurotic ones, or simply help sufferers cope with life, have side effects and/or are addicting. Nevertheless, they offered an alternative to the institutionalization of psychiatric patients and have been widely prescribed and taken. Prescription antidepressants are fundamental to what has been called the 'Prozac generation', and are another tangible reminder of the centrality of medicine to modern life.

Doctors have an increasingly powerful range of drugs at their disposal, and these medicaments are part of both the achievements and the costs of contemporary health care.

Tablets and capsules are familiar means of ingesting drugs. The tablet – a small flat thin object – began its medical life in the late 16th century as powdered drugs were compressed into a solid. Capsules – small receptacles or cases – were used from the 19th century onwards when nauseous medicines were enclosed in a gelatin sheath for easier administration.

43. OPIUM
Pleasure & pain

Virginia Berridge

Not poppy, nor mandragora, Nor all the drowsy syrups of the world,
Shall ever medicine thee to that sweet sleep.
William Shakespeare, *Othello*, Act 3, Scene 3

Opium and its products have occupied a central place in medical practice and in self-medication throughout history. The substance has played an important role in world trade, and the control of opium and its derivatives in national and international policy today symbolizes the dilemmas of the regulation of mind-altering substances, both licit and illicit.

ANCIENT BEGINNINGS

Opium is the brown resinous substance that dries from the milk obtained from incised seed capsules of the opium poppy, *Papaver somniferum*, which was widespread throughout the Middle East from the earliest times. The pain-relieving and calming properties of the drug have been known for many centuries. References to poppy juice occur in Sumerian texts of about 4000 BC. In both Egypt and Persia, doctors used opium from at least the 2nd century BC. Roman medicine was familiar with it, and Arab physicians [05] used opium extensively.

In Europe the use of opium was revived in the 16th century, helped by the recognition of Galen (AD 129–*c.* 216), who had recommended opium, as an important authority. The Swiss doctor Paracelsus (1493–1541) challenged Galen, but also acknowledged the value of opium; he mixed it with alcohol to make laudanum, taken for reducing pain.

IMPORT, EXPORT

Opium was an important trading commodity, especially in China, although its use had been banned there in the early 18th century. The smoking of opium in China was initially linked to tobacco smoking, but it was then smoked on its own and its use spread throughout society. In addition to considerable domestic production, supply also came through trade. The British

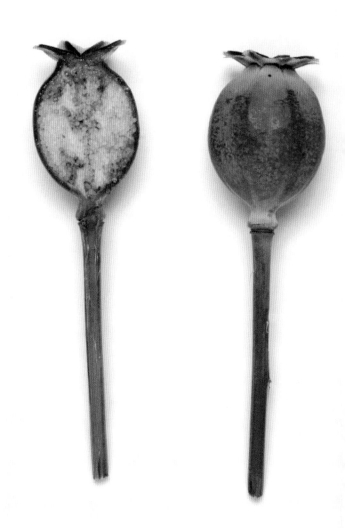

Unripe seed capsules of the opium poppy *Papaver somniferum*. After the flower's petals fall, the central seed-containing capsule swells. Opium is extracted from the latex of unripe seedpods.

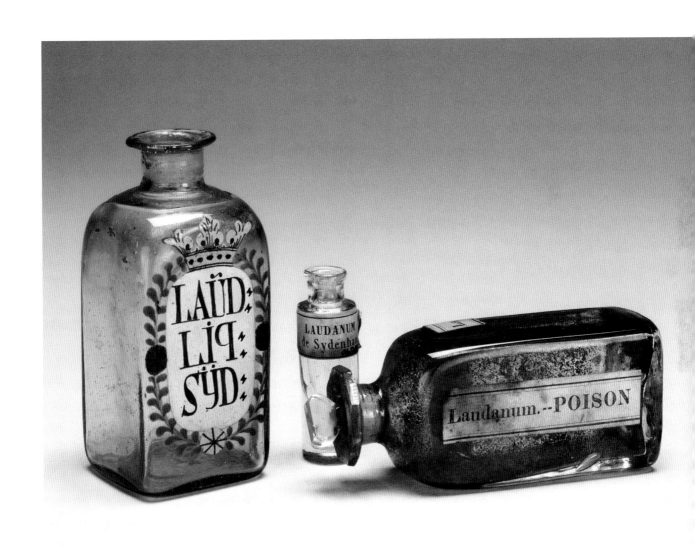

Laudanum, or tincture of opium, is opium dissolved in alcohol.
It was widely used in the 19th century (the date of these bottles)
as a painkiller; note that one bottle is marked POISON.

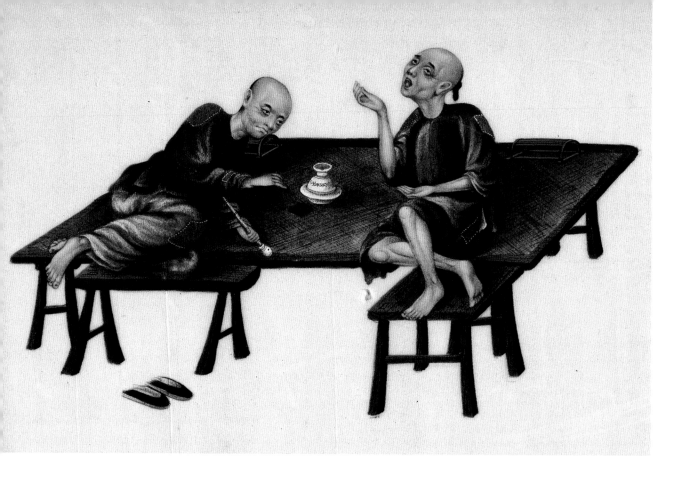

imported large amounts of Chinese goods and solved the resulting balance of payments deficit by exporting Indian opium to China. British merchants dominated the trade, but the Americans also participated. The two Opium Wars (1839–42, 1856–60), in which Britain used force against Chinese attempts to suppress the trade, led to the legalization of the import of Indian opium. The traffic peaked towards the end of the 19th century and declined thereafter, ending in the early 20th century.

PROLIFERATION OF USE AND RESPONSES

Britain and other Western countries also experienced a growing demand for opium in the 19th century. The lack of access for most of the population to proper medical care, and opium's reputation as a 'cure all' and a supreme remedy for pain, ensured its central role in both official and self-medication. It was available over the counter in various forms – pills, penny sticks, laudanum – and there was a growing sector of patent, commercial medicines. Products such as Godfrey's Cordial or Collis Browne's chlorodyne were used for self-medication for a great range of ailments.

New pharmaceutical discoveries enhanced opium's reputation and brought increased medical use. The isolation of the alkaloids in opium, its active principles, began with the discovery by Friedrich Sertürner (1783–1841) of morphine (named after Morpheus, the Greek god of sleep and dreams) in 1806. Codeine followed in 1832, and the Bayer company began marketing heroin in 1898. From the 1850s the introduction of the hypodermic syringe [24] provided a means of administering these drugs that produced faster effects and was initially considered to be safer than 'old-fashioned' oral consumption. The belief that the newer opium products carried fewer risks was also widespread.

From the late 19th century, opium became less central to medical practice. New theories of 'inebriety' (later, addiction) were advanced in Britain and the US. Initially developed to explain alcoholism, they also encompassed liquid forms of opiates, outlining the problems and dangers of their consumption. With strong links to temperance and campaigning organizations, anti-opium groups such as the British Society for the Suppression of the Opium Trade took on an international perspective.

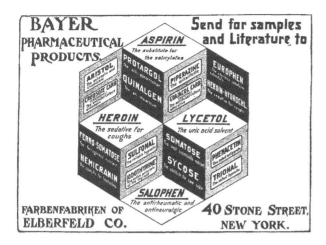

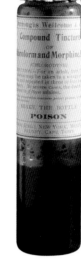

Anti-opium agitation focused on the Indo-Chinese opium trade and was driven by American moral concerns, trade imperatives and the desire to expand US commercial interests and political hegemony in the Far East. International agreement was delivered through a series of treaties signed at Shanghai and The Hague between 1909 and 1914. The post-First World War peace settlement introduced a full-scale, enforceable international system of control, organized through the League of Nations.

Countries subsequently adopted different approaches. In the US, caring for addicts by continuing drug use under medical supervision (addiction maintenance) was prohibited in the 1920s, and addiction was criminalized until the 1970s: anti-drug enforcement was dominant. In Britain, the greater power of the medical profession underpinned the role of addiction maintenance therapies. This 'British system' applied only to addicts who could afford treatment: the overall framework was also one of criminalization and punishment. Earlier colonial systems of regulation of the opium trade through excise, licensing, 'farms' or monopolies, were largely abandoned.

After World War Two, the newly formed United Nations took the lead, with the US assuming dominance and promoting its punitive model. Communist China also seemed to eradicate opium use through punitive measures. However, an illicit international market now flourished, with the location of production and distribution shifting, depending on the political situation. In the 1970s production in Southeast Asia was linked to the Vietnam War; in the 1990s Afghanistan became the world's leading producer of opium. The advent of HIV/AIDS [42] in the 1980s among injecting drug users brought dilemmas which were resolved in some countries, notably the UK, through the adoption of harm reduction policies based on addiction maintenance with methadone (a synthetic opiate) and needle exchange. Such policies were under strain by 2010. Opium continues to be a central issue in national and international policy-making in the early 21st century.

44. QUININE
The bark against the bite

Tilli Tansey

*Cinchona revolutionized the art of medicine
as profoundly as gunpowder had the art of war.*
Bernardino Ramazzini, 1717

Quinine is a naturally occurring drug derived from
the bark of the cinchona tree, which is native to South
America. Now little used medically, quinine was a
treatment for malaria in particular for nearly 400 years
until the middle of the 20th century.

The properties of cinchona bark, ground into a
powder and drunk as an infusion, were known to
the indigenous populations of Peru and Bolivia as a
treatment for fevers, including the disease we now
call malaria. The tree was first named *Cinchona* in
1742 by the Swedish botanist Carl Linnaeus (1707–78),
possibly in memory of the Countess of Chinchón, wife
of a viceroy of Peru, who according to legend had been
treated for malaria with a bark extract. In the 17th
century Jesuit missionaries noted the native use and
the efficacy of the bark, also known as *quinquina*,
the 'bark of barks', and introduced the remedy into
medical practice back in Europe. Subsequently, regular
shipments of the bark were made to Europe, although it
was not universally accepted; in Protestant England it
was viewed with suspicion as a 'Popish' remedy.

UNRAVELLING THE CHEMISTRY, SELLING THE PRODUCT

At the beginning of the 19th century a Portuguese
surgeon, Bernardino Gomez, attempted to isolate the
purely therapeutic component, or active principle,
of the bark. He produced crystals of a substance he
called 'cinchonin'; this did not have the bitter taste of
the bark extract, and because he could not completely
replicate the effect of the bark, he suspected that there
was another key component. In 1820 two French
chemists, Pierre Joseph Pelletier (1788–1842) and
Joseph Bienaimé Caventou (1795–1887), repeated
Gomez's work, and isolated a more potent alkaloid
they called quinine. This became the first effective

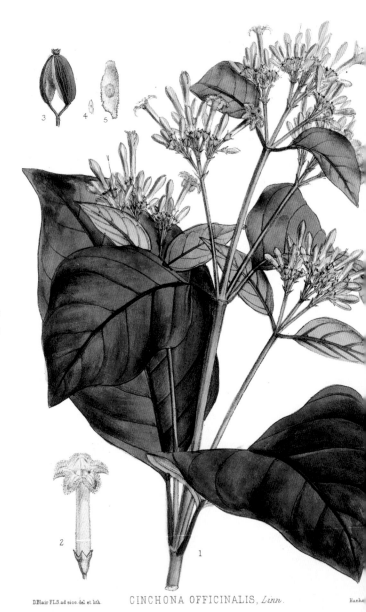

D.Blair FLS ad vice. del. et lith.   CINCHONA OFFICINALIS, *Linn*.   Hanhe

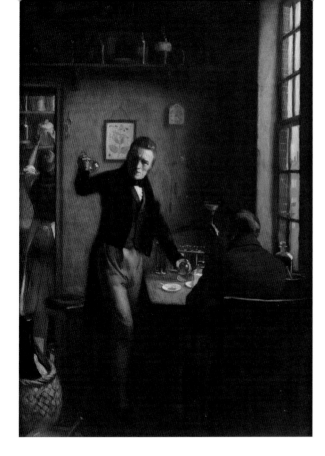

Opposite
The flowers and seedpod of *Cinchona officinalis*, the bark of which yields quinine, the first specific antimalarial drug. Long used by the natives of Peru and Bolivia for fevers, it was introduced into Europe in the 17th century.

Left
Ernest Board's depiction (early 20th century) of the Frenchmen Joseph Bienaimé Caventou and Pierre Joseph Pelletier isolating the highly active alkaloid of cinchona bark in 1820, which they named quinine.

Below
Original samples of quinine hydrochloride (left), quinine (centre) and quinine acetate (right) from the early to mid-19th century. The bitter powder was used against fevers, including malaria, and as flavouring for bitters – alcoholic aperitifs and mixers.

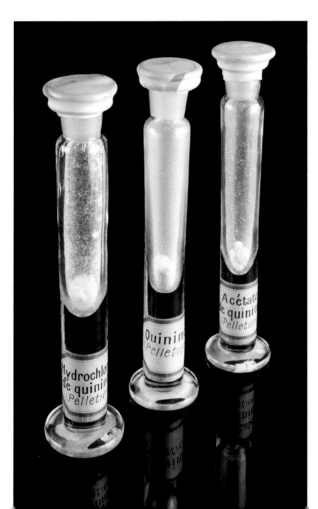

treatment for malaria. As a result of their work, Pelletier and Caventou stimulated the use of such pure extracts, rather than whole plant preparations, marking a significant change in therapeutic practice. Their discovery provoked an immediate demand for quinine, and by 1826 Pelletier's own factory was processing more than 150,000 kg (over 330,000 lb) of cinchona bark.

The increasing popularity of quinine raised concerns about the sustainability of the South American cinchona forests, especially among the European colonial powers. Peruvian authorities tried to bar foreigners from their forests in an attempt to preserve their monopoly, but in 1860 the British government sponsored a series of expeditions to identify different species of trees that could be transplanted to India. In Calcutta, Madras and Bombay cinchona commissions were established to determine the chemicals each species contained, in order to find the most effective combination to treat malaria. Likewise, the Dutch experimented with growing different species of cinchona in their East Indies colonies, especially Java in Indonesia, finally achieving spectacular success with seeds obtained from an Englishman living in Peru, Charles Ledger. The Dutch cinchona forests effectively broke the Peruvian monopoly and established their own. The Netherlands had an 85–95 per cent world monopoly on the production of quinine until the Second World War.

Demand for quinine grew throughout the 19th century and by 1880 it was the most commonly prescribed medicine for treating fever. Several companies followed Pelletier's example (and his methods of quinine extraction, which he had published openly) to manufacture and market quinine. Among these was the British pharmaceutical firm, Burroughs, Wellcome & Co. The American-born Henry Wellcome

(1853–1936) had started his pharmaceutical career searching for cinchona trees in Ecuador, and quinine preparations were among the first that the company manufactured and marketed worldwide. Quinine was an important component of the company's travellers' medical chests, and large contracts from British and foreign armies, missionaries and plantation owners contributed to Burroughs, Wellcome & Co.'s success. In 1916, during the First World War, they issued over 21 tons (nearly 65 million doses) of quinine for military use in malaria treatment. However, quinine was not solely taken for malaria; during the 1920s and 1930s in particular, a Dutch 'Bureau for increasing the use of quinine' promoted its use to treat conditions as diverse as acute lumbago, hearing loss, heart disorders and as a local anaesthetic.

PARASITOLOGY AND PROBLEMS

The identification of the protozoa, *Plasmodium,* that causes malaria [15] prompted experiments to investigate quinine's mode of action. It was discovered that quinine caused disruption of the parasite itself and its reproductive cycle. Various attempts were made to synthesize quinine and to develop new anti-malarials, but it was the Japanese invasion of the Dutch East Indies in 1942, which cut the supply line of quinine to Allied forces, that really stimulated such efforts. By 1944 chloroquine, first synthesized in 1934, was used as a malarial prophylaxis for troops, and was introduced into civilian practice after the Second World War.

Mepacrine, then mefloquine, synthesized during the Vietnam War in the 1970s, and malarone followed over the next 40 years. However, these drugs have all become less useful as parasite resistance has increased. In the final decades of the 20th century artemisinin, a modern extract from an ancient Chinese remedy, also plant-derived, came into worldwide use, although always in combination with other drugs (ACT – artemisinin combination therapy) to prevent resistance developing.

Thus quinine's role has been largely supplanted, although it continues to be used in specialized cases of drug resistance. It is also still added in minute amounts to tonic water – for its characteristic bitter flavour, rather than its anti-malarial properties.

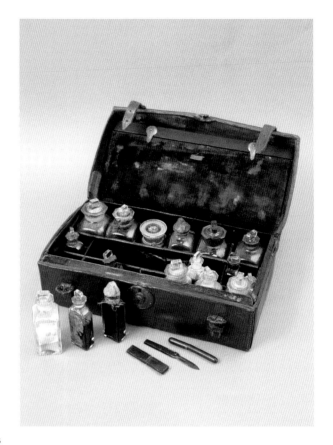

The medicine chest of the explorer and missionary David Livingstone (1813-73), from his last expedition in the African interior. Quinine was one of the drugs Livingstone wanted to have included. He was a keen advocate of the drug for malaria, combining it with jalap, rhubarb, calomel and tincture of cardamoms in pills known as 'rousers' because of their ability to get his fevered companions back on their feet.

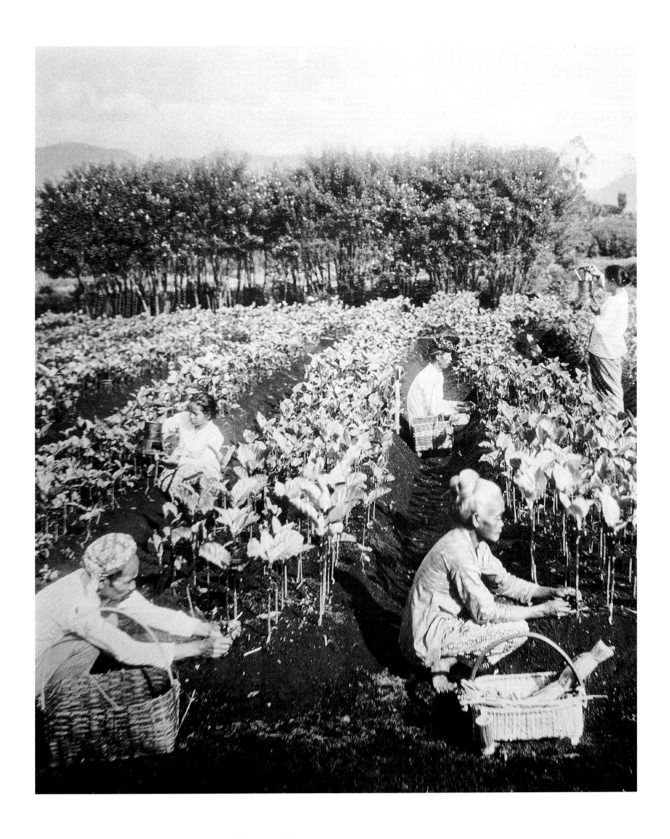

Grafting *Cinchona ledgerina* to *Cinchona succirubra* in Java. These
two species of cinchona give the highest yields of quinine. The Dutch
established plantations in the East Indies, eventually dominating the
global supply of quinine before the islands fell to the Japanese in 1942.

45. DIGITALIS
Tonic for the heart

William Bynum

The active herb could be no other than the foxglove.
William Withering, 1785

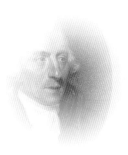

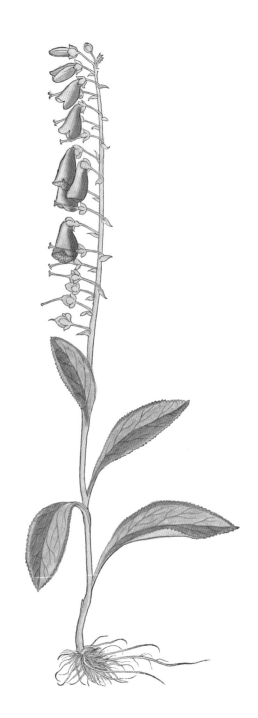

The introduction of digitalis was one of the triumphs of 18th-century therapeutics. It derives its name from the purple foxglove (*Digitalis purpurea*), a common and beautiful woodland flower, from which it is extracted. One of many important medicines of botanical origin, it had its immediate origins in folk medicine. Earlier medical writers had described it as too toxic to be useful, but in 1775 William Withering (1741–99), a prominent physician and botanist, learnt that an old lady in Shropshire, in western England, could cure the dropsy with a mix of plant extracts. He examined her mixture and determined that the active ingredient was digitalis. In 1785 he published his treatise on its medicinal uses in cases of dropsy.

Dropsy (today called oedema) is an accumulation of fluids in the body. Doctors now consider it as a sign of a disease such as heart failure or liver cirrhosis. Withering and his contemporaries thought dropsy a disease in itself, but he recognized that only some of his patients were helped by digitalis, which he believed acted through the kidneys. He also noted that the drug influenced the heart rate and described what happened when patients received too much of the drug. Withering

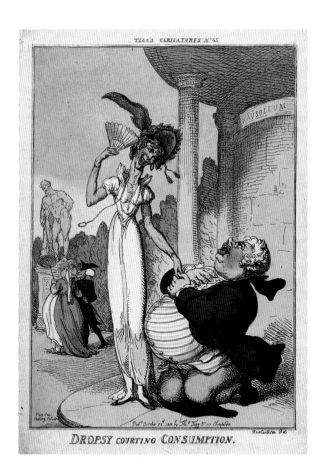

TEGG'S CARICATURES N.º 45

MAUSOLEUM

DROPSY COURTING CONSUMPTION.

Rowlandson Del

provided instructions on how to prepare the plant's leaves for administration.

Withering's treatise encouraged other doctors to use digitalis, and the drug has remained an important remedy. During the 19th century, however, it also began to be used for many other diseases – epilepsy, tuberculosis, insanity, for example – in which it had no benefit. This is a common theme in medical therapeutics: a therapy good for one disorder is indiscriminately tried for other conditions. (More recently, cortisone and penicillin [46] were also too widely used in a fit of early enthusiasm.) Because digitalis can cause serious side effects, its inappropriate use led many 19th-century doctors to abandon it altogether.

Around 1900 pharmacologists began to examine its actions more carefully. Karl Benz (1832–1912) in Germany and Arthur Cushny (1866–1926) in Britain investigated the drug's effects on the heart beat, and showed how potent it is in controlling atrial fibrillation, a common disorder in which the heart beats irregularly. This distressing complication is experienced by many people with heart failure, which also leads to accumulation of fluid (oedema) in the lungs, abdomen

and extremities. Digitalis can control the irregular beating, thus improving the efficiency of the failing heart and helping the body to expel the excess fluid. In 1970 digitalis was the fourth most commonly prescribed drug in the US. The clinical management of patients with heart failure was immeasurably aided by the development of the electrocardiograph (ECG) in the early 20th century, and the machine is familiar today in hospitals and medical centres.

Physiologists have now elucidated many cellular aspects of the mode of action of digitalis, relating it to its effects on essential chemicals, especially calcium and sodium, vital for the efficient action of the heart.

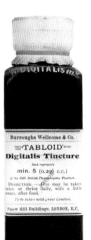

Burroughs Wellcome & Co.

'TABLOID'
Digitalis Tincture

min. 5 (0.200 c.c.)
of the 1898 British Pharmacopoeia Tincture

DIRECTION.—One may be taken twice or thrice daily, with a little water, after food.

To be taken with great Caution.

Snow Hill Buildings, LONDON, E.C.

46. PENICILLIN
The healing mould

Robert Bud

One does not need a crystal ball to predict that, within this generation, medical science will have overcome, and controlled, all man's external enemies.
Ritchie Calder, 1958

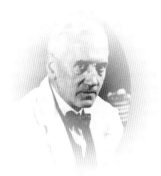

Alexander Fleming made the initial discovery of the antibacterial properties of the penicillin mould at St Mary's Hospital, London, in 1928.

Medicine was transformed from the late 1930s. In scarcely more than a decade, infections that had been feared as a source of misery and often inevitable death came widely to be seen as curable. The greatest reason was the ready availability of penicillin. We are today both the beneficiaries of the science that yielded this unprecedented advance and victims of the propaganda that promised miracle cures.

Anecdotes about the benefits of moulds in fighting infections go back millennia, if with marginal, hard to reproduce, results. In 1928, however, Alexander Fleming (1881–1955), working in London's St Mary's Hospital medical school, made an observation that he carefully followed up and published. About to discard a dish contaminated with a *Penicillium* mould, he noticed that the bacteria which prospered elsewhere on the plate had either failed to grow at all or had died around the intrusion. Investigating the phenomenon further, he discovered that the mould exuded a small amount of yellow liquid that affected some feared strains of bacteria. Fleming could not find a way to purify the yellow liquid in order to extract the active principle. So, in a paper describing his painstaking

experiments, he named the impure liquid itself penicillin, after the mould.

EXTRACTION AND PRODUCTION
It was not until the end of the 1930s that new techniques made possible substantial further advance. At Oxford University, the German refugee biochemist Ernst Chain (1906–79) had discovered Fleming's old article on penicillin. Provoked by the scientific challenge of the difficult separation, he adopted the new process of freeze-drying being used in Cambridge to make blood products. In March 1940 he succeeded in producing a dry, albeit still impure, material. Immediately, a colleague, Norman Heatley (1911–2004), suggested an entirely different approach to extracting penicillin, by moving it successively between two solvents which themselves would not mix. The combination of these two methods made possible the systematic if slow extraction of the medicine. A test on eight mice in May 1940 showed the efficacy of the chemical in saving animals from otherwise fatal infection.

Medical promise and wartime need now transformed penicillin from academic curiosity to

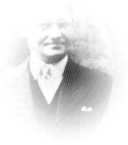
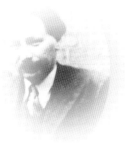

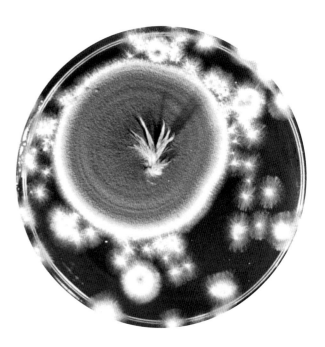

Above
Howard Florey (left) and Ernst Chain (right) shared the Nobel Prize in Medicine with Alexander Fleming for their different roles in developing penicillin from an experiment in a Petri dish to a mass-produced drug. As only three can share the prize, the essential work of Norman Heatley was overlooked.

Right
A Petri dish with a culture of *Penicillium notatum*.

Below
A scanning electron micrograph of *Penicillium* (from Latin *penicillus*: paintbrush) mould producing chains of spores. *Penicillium* moulds are soil fungi favouring cool, moderate conditions where organic material is present.

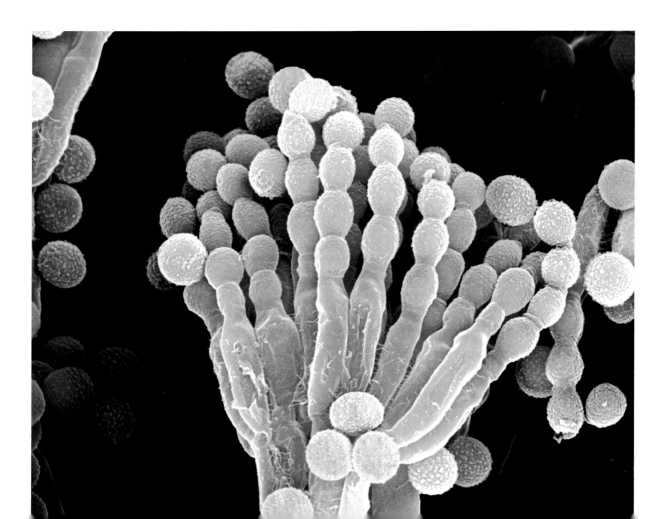

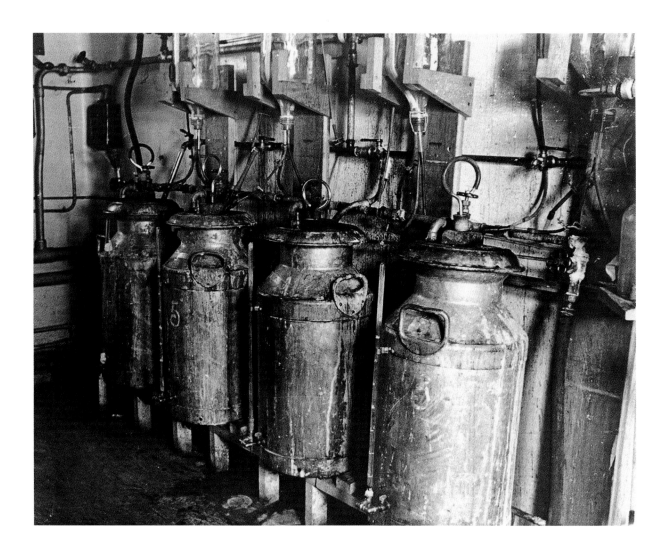

Above
Norman Heatley solved the basic problem of how to extract and purify penicillin, and his technical ingenuity automated the multi-stage process using an unlikely assortment of 'equipment' including baths, petrol cans, biscuit-tin lids and milk churns.

Right
Sketches by Heatley for the ceramic 'bedpans' that were used in the Dunn School of Pathology at Oxford University for *Penicillium* cultures. Staffed by a team of six 'penicillin girls', this improvised factory produced just enough of the drug to begin testing in people.

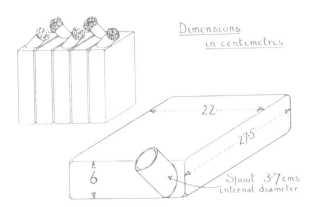

Dimensions in centimetres

22

27·5

6

Spout 3·7 cms. internal diameter

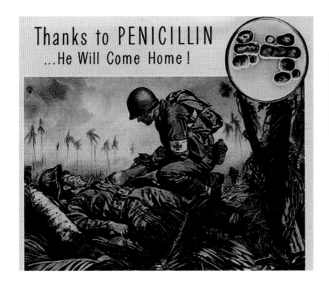

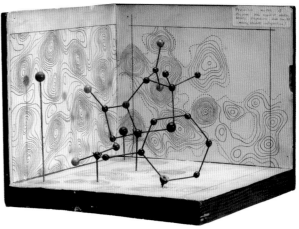

An adequate supply of penicillin was taken into consideration in the timing of the D-Day landings, such was the power of this drug to save the lives and limbs of the injured servicemen in the ensuing conflict.

Dorothy Hodgkin's model of the atomic structure of penicillin. After suitable crystals of penicillin were produced in 1944 she determined the structure in 1945 with the aid of a punch card calculator, one of the earliest examples of computing in X-ray crystallography.

scientific obsession. By the beginning of 1941 the team of Oxford scientists, under the leadership of Howard Florey (1898–1968), successfully showed the potential value for a human patient. Unfortunately, their supplies proved inadequate to prevent a relapse, and their first patient died. A few more successful outcomes raised hopes over subsequent months. But however committed, the team could hardly match the urgency of wartime demand.

For every ton of liquid, only 2 g of penicillin were produced. A few companies produced mould-juice for them to extract, but British manufacturers had little expertise in this area and such marginal work had low priority in wartime. To obtain better supplies for their research, Florey and Heatley flew to the US in July 1941. A coordinated response was immediately organized by the Americans, now preparing for war themselves.

A scientist at a Department of Agriculture laboratory in Indiana briefed by Heatley worked out how to grow the mould far more efficiently in the body of a vat, fed by air bubbles and food based on waste corn. Some still-small companies such as Pfizer in Brooklyn and Merck in New Jersey applied their considerable expertise in

engineering and microbiology to converting academic innovation into industrial product.

Over the next two years the British and Americans made enough penicillin to test on numerous wounded soldiers and some civilians, demonstrating that here indeed was a revolutionary product. Their success underpinned wartime propaganda proclaiming a wonder drug. Leading doctors and newspaper proprietors saw the benefits to Britain and to their organizations of promoting a great good news story. Against a background of criticisms of a lack of British commercial benefits and visible US dominance, a simple story was shouted. Here was a British-discovered medicine that cured syphilis, pneumonia and gangrene in days, and was itself no more toxic to most people than salt water.

A WONDER DRUG

By the end of the war, penicillin was being produced in sufficient quantities to meet American, then British and soon European needs. Doctors anxious to help patients where they could, and patients desperate to get hold of the wonder drug, used large quantities. Little regard was

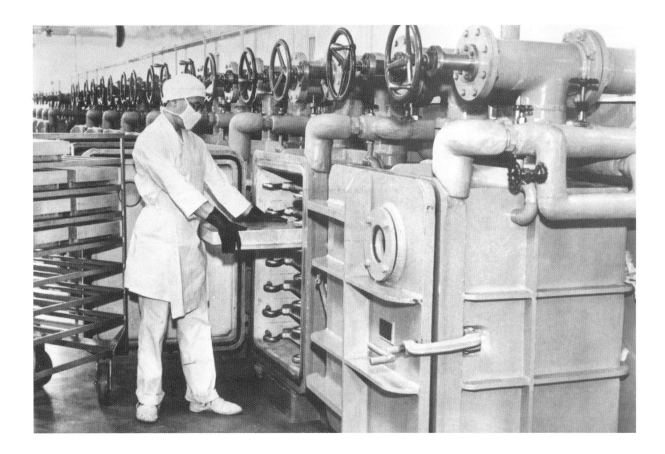

paid as to whether infections such as colds and influenza would really be affected, and often basic hygienic practices were substituted by penicillin use. The hope of even more effective natural products led to a huge search for new antibiotics. The families of the tetracyclines and products of the streptomycetes vindicated these hopes.

However, the 1950s saw the emergence of bacteria that appeared to be able to resist even the newer drugs. Once more, a penicillin-based technical solution seemed to be all that was needed. Several chemically similar penicillins had been discovered even in wartime. Ernst Chain, who had moved to Rome, built up a major new research group devoted to improving fermentation and its products. Two young scientists sent by the Beecham pharmaceutical company developed their skills in Chain's laboratory. They also brought back to Beecham an observation which, they quickly realized, meant they had inadvertently isolated the common core of all penicillins. Now they could easily engineer alternative penicillins rather than relying on nature. By 1960 methicillin, capable of resisting the dreaded *Staphylococcus aureus,* had been prepared and was quickly launched.

Other ways of making new penicillins were soon developed, and such familiar products as ampicillin and amoxycillin were discovered and widely disseminated. Again, bacteria resistant to methicillin – methicillin-resistant *Staphylococcus aureus* (MRSA) – were shortly discovered, but it was only in the 1990s that they became widespread. It was soon clear that the attitude towards penicillins as wonder drugs, and the abuse that had accompanied it, had fostered the growth of these feared organisms. It also showed that infections could be managed by antibiotics such as penicillin, but never eradicated.

Above
It was in America that large-scale production of penicillin was achieved using deep vat fermentation. Here, further down the production line, an employee at the Pfizer factory places a tray containing vials of frozen penicillin solution into a dryer preparatory to vacuum evaporation of the water.

Opposite
Clusters of methicillin-resistant *Staphylococcus aureus* (MRSA) bacteria. One of many bacteria that have evolved antibiotic resistance, they remind us that our apparent mastery of pathogenic microorganisms may have been spectacular but has also been short-lived.

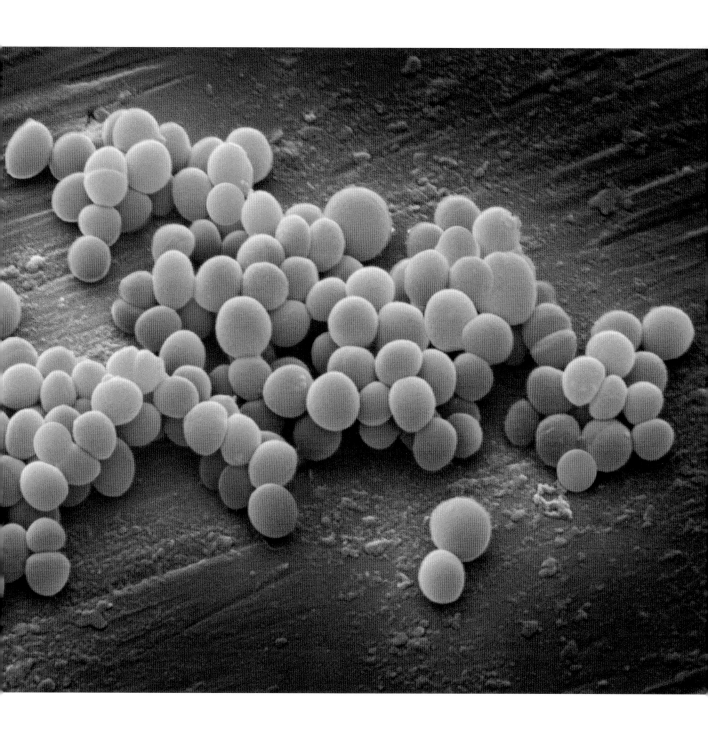

THE PILL
A woman's choice

Lara Marks

*Not since the sulfa tablets emerged in the 1930s to conquer
pneumonia and a host of other infections, has a little tablet
exerted such far-reaching influence upon the world's people.
It may, in fact, be the most popular pill since aspirin. It is
certainly relieving bigger headaches – both family and global.*
S. M. Spencer, 1966

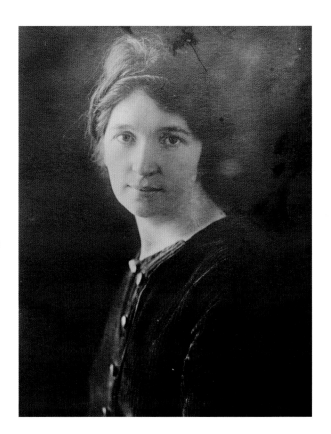

One of the 20th century's most radical medical
inventions, the oral contraceptive has transformed our
lives over the past 50 years. Heralded as a catalyst for the
sexual revolution and the solution to global population
growth in the 1960s, the pill was one of society's first
'lifestyle' or 'designer' drugs. Over 300 million women
have taken the pill worldwide since its first appearance
in 1960, with profound impacts on society.

As early as 1912 the American birth-control activist
and nurse Margaret Sanger (1879–1966) advocated
a 'magic pill' for contraception to improve women's
health and social status. This, however, was not an
easy task. From antiquity humans had experimented
with various plants and mineral sources to find an
oral contraceptive, but still the most effective means
of contraception in the early 20th century remained
barrier methods, such as the condom and diaphragm,
which could interfere with the spontaneity of sex.

In 1921 an Austrian physiologist, Ludwig Haberlandt
(1885–1932), first proposed that sex hormones might
be utilized for a contraceptive pill. This was difficult
to achieve, however, because of the high costs and the
absence of cheap and effective sex hormones. Part of the

Above
Margaret Sanger, the American advocate of birth control, believed that
a woman's ability to control her pregnancies would facilitate greater
sexual equality, as well as preventing the health risks associated with
frequent childbirth and attempted abortions.

Opposite left
A Marie Stopes diaphragm, the 'Clinocap', in its box. Stopes
(1880–1958) was a pioneer birth-control advocate in Britain, founding
the first birth-control clinic in London (1921), which advocated barrier
methods of contraception such as the diaphragm.

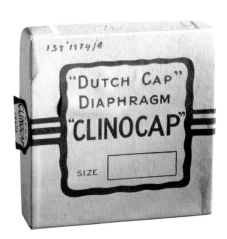

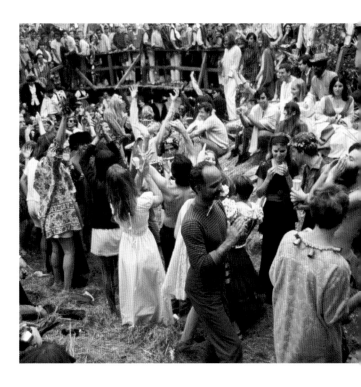

problem was overcome when Russell Marker (1902–95),
an American chemist investigating a Mexican wild
yam in the 1940s, made a breakthrough in steroidal
chemistry, paving the way for large-scale production
of cheap sex hormones.

EARLY TRIALS

While the supply and efficacy of hormones improved
over the years, few scientists exploited their oral
contraceptive potential. One reason was that
contraception was extremely taboo, even illegal in
many places, making it a highly unattractive subject
for funding or research. Despite the obstacles, by 1950
Sanger had secured financial help and support for her
pill project from the American philanthropist Katherine
Dexter McCormick (1875–1967). Both believed that such
a pill would not only empower women, but also become
a weapon to fight population growth, a phenomenon
many then feared threatened world peace.

From the early 1950s McCormick began funding
Gregory Pincus (1903–67), a reproductive biologist, to
devise a contraceptive pill. Pincus was well placed: he
possessed vital expertise and the networks necessary

to source potential compounds, and he also co-headed
an independent institution, which had greater freedom
to pursue such controversial research than other,
more established institutions whose funding might be
cut if associated with such work. In 1951 Pincus and a
Chinese-born colleague, Min Chueh Chang (1908–91),
began testing various hormones on animals. By
1953 they had identified two possible compounds for
human trials: one developed in 1951 by the chemists
Carl Djerassi and Luis Miramontes at the Mexican
pharmaceutical company Syntex; and one synthesized
by the chemist Frank Colton at the American
pharmaceutical company G. D. Searle in 1952.

Pincus, with the help of John Rock (1890–1984),
a Boston-based obstetrician and gynaecologist, began
the first clinical testing in women in 1953. Initial
small-scale tests, launched on the pretext of looking
to solve infertility, included volunteer nurses and
infertile women in Massachusetts. Necessitating a
high degree of cooperation from the women, these
tests indicated a contraceptive pill was possible.
Larger trials were needed, but this could not be done
in Massachusetts because of the state's draconian

laws against contraception. The major problem Pincus and his colleagues faced was finding places where contraception was not illegal and where there would be large groups of women who would comply with the complicated rules and intense medical investigation necessary. In 1956 two large-scale Puerto Rican trials were started among low-income women with large families. This was followed by trials in various American states and other parts of the world.

CHALLENGES AND SUCCESS

The first pill approved for market was Colton's compound, known as Enovid. Initially approved in 1957 for the treatment of gynaecological disorders, Enovid received its first official licence as an oral contraceptive in America in 1960 and in Britain and other countries the following year. Uptake was rapid: by 1965 nearly 11 million women globally were taking the pill. While greeted by many with great enthusiasm, not everyone welcomed the arrival of the contraceptive. Some of its strongest critics were the Catholic Church and the Indian and Japanese governments, who regarded the pill as unnatural. From the early 1960s criticism also began to surface from others in the wake of concerns about its possible cardiovascular and carcinogenic complications, raising questions about the degree

to which women should shoulder responsibility for contraception and stimulating a search for the means to develop a male contraceptive pill, a goal which to this day has not been achieved.

Unlike most drugs before it, the pill was unique in that it was designed to be taken by healthy individuals for long periods of time. Challenging the limits of drug monitoring and regulation, the pill prompted some of the largest medical investigations ever undertaken of a drug. The pill not only raised new questions about the risks and benefits of medicine, but also radically raised the standards by which other contraceptives were to be judged in terms of efficacy and their interference in sexual intercourse. Providing the ability to control fertility on an unprecedented scale, the oral contraceptive enabled women and men to pursue higher education and further their careers on a magnitude unforeseen.

The social and economic benefits of the pill, however, have been mostly confined to the developed world, where its uptake has been greatest. In the developing world, a key target for Sanger and McCormick in the 1950s, the pill's impact has been less dramatic. Here, limited access to contraception and health-care provision mean women's reproductive health continues to be poor.

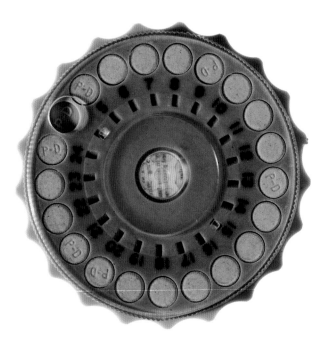

Left
An early combined (oestrogen and progestogen) monophasic (the same amount of each hormone every day) contraceptive pill, c. 1960. The transparent plastic disc rotated, releasing a daily pill for 21 days. A new pack was started after a 7-day break.

Below
Enovid was initially approved in 1957 for gynaecological disorders, before being licensed as the first commercial combined oral contraceptive in 1960.

Opposite
Making the news: a *Daily Herald* feature included this photograph of a packaging line for Ovulen at the pharmaceutical firm of G. D. Searle in High Wycombe, southern England, which produced 8 million contraceptive pills each week in 1965.

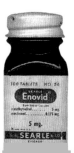

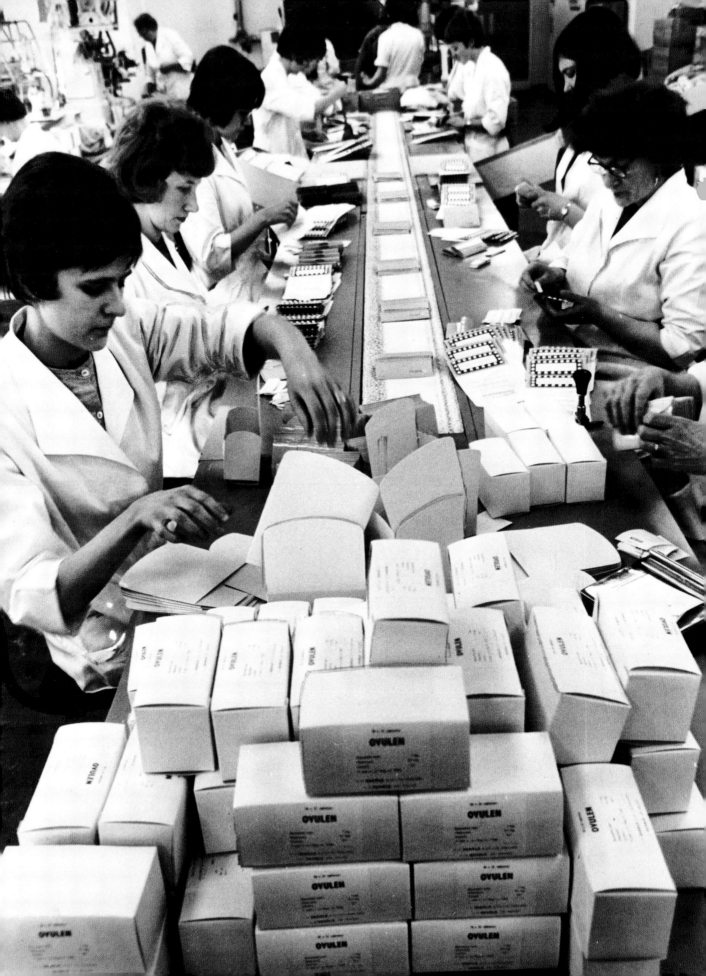

48. DRUGS FOR THE MIND
Treating mental suffering

Andrew Scull

In time, I suspect we will come to discover that modern psychopharmacology has become, like Freud in his day, a whole climate of opinion under which we conduct our different lives.
Peter D. Kramer, 1993

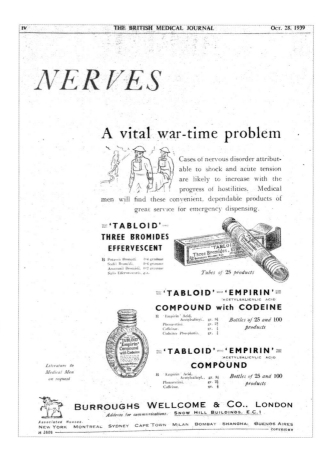

Drugs have long been used to alleviate psychiatric symptoms. Some 19th-century psychiatrists experimented with giving their patients marijuana, though most soon abandoned it. Opium [43] was mobilized as a soporific in cases of mania. Later, chloral hydrate and the bromides had their enthusiasts, though bromides in excess caused psychotic symptoms and their widespread use outside the asylum produced toxic reactions that saw substantial numbers of patients admitted to mental hospitals [12], diagnosed as mad; and chloral, though effective as a sedative, was addicting, and with long-term use led to hallucinations and symptoms akin to delirium tremens.

Lithium salts seemed to calm the agitation of manic patients, and some hydrotherapeutic establishments used them in the treatment of their nervous patients. But lithium could easily prove toxic, producing anorexia, depression, even cardiovascular collapse and death. The Australian psychiatrist John Cade (1912–80) later championed its value after the Second World War, and the existence of calming effects in mania prompted some continuing clinical interest in such compounds in Europe and North America.

Potassium bromide was used as a specific anti-epileptic drug but more generally was a popular sedative in the late 19th century. In the First World War there was a veritable epidemic of 'nerves' among troops, who experienced both highly stressful situations and long periods of boredom in the trenches: bromide was seen as one of the solutions.

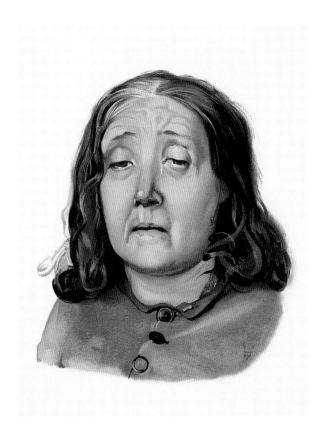

A portrait of 'Georgina W.', aged 46 years. Georgina, a domestic servant, was admitted to the Royal Edinburgh Asylum, Morningside, aged 20 (1864). Twenty-two years later she was transferred to the Craiglockhart Poorhouse, where this portrait was painted. It was used to illustrate 'melancholia' in an *Atlas of Medicine* (by B. Bramwell, 1892–96).

The 1920s saw experiments with barbiturates, including attempts to place mental patients in chemically induced periods of suspended animation in the hopes of a cure. But barbiturates, too, had major drawbacks: they were addicting; overdoses could easily prove fatal; and, when they were discontinued, withdrawal symptoms were highly unpleasant, even dangerous. Besides, like the earlier drugs used by psychiatrists, they produced mental confusion, impaired judgment and an inability to concentrate, as well as a whole spectrum of physical problems.

THE ARRIVAL OF THE ANTIPSYCHOTICS

In the early 1950s a new class of drugs entered psychiatry, which were initially thought to cause fewer complications. Over time these so-called antipsychotics, the phenothiazines, of which the first was Thorazine (known in Europe as Largactil), prompted a revolution in psychiatry, establishing drug treatment as the dominant therapy for all manner of psychiatric ills and persuading the majority of the profession and the public to view mental illnesses as rooted in biology. Yet Thorazine's psychiatric

usefulness was discovered serendipitously, after the drug companies exploring its clinical applications, first Rhône Poulenc in France and then Smith, Kline and French in the United States, had experimented with it as a way to reduce the dosage of anaesthetic needed during surgery, as an anti-nausea drug and as a treatment for skin irritations.

When given to psychiatric patients, Thorazine (chlorpromazine) reduced florid symptomatology and calmed patients down, producing an indifference that some observers at the time likened to a 'chemical lobotomy' – then seen as a positive development. It did not seem to be addictive, or to have many of the prominent negative effects of the other drugs. Introduced in 1954, Thorazine was an enormous commercial success. Thirteen months after it first came to market, it was being given to an estimated two million patients in the United States alone. By 1970, US pharmaceutical houses sold over half a billion dollars worth of psychiatric drugs, of which phenothiazines as a class accounted for more than $110 million. In a pattern that would become familiar in the drug industry, Smith, Kline and French's competitors

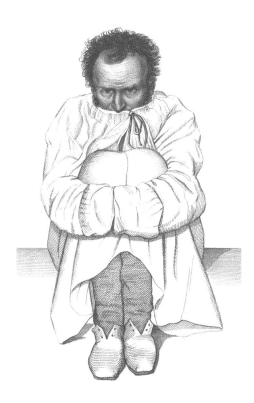

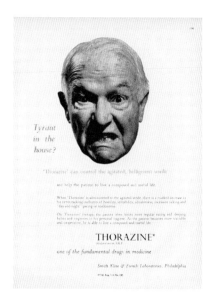

immediately rushed to develop marginally different versions of the original drug that they could patent – and profit from – as their own.

For the first time, Thorazine and its derivatives gave psychiatry a therapeutic method that was easy to dispense and closely resembled the approach to treating disease that increasingly underpinned the cultural authority of medicine at large. For all the initial excitement surrounding their introduction, however, they were at best a treatment that reduced psychiatric symptoms. They did not cure the underlying disease. Over time, too, reports surfaced of disturbing side-effects – restlessness, movement disorders, serious and often permanent neurological complications, most notably a disorder known as tardive dyskinesia, whose associated involuntary movements, facial tics and grimaces are deeply stigmatizing. For some patients these costs were offset by demonstrable benefits, alleviating their psychic distress, but for others the drugs worked poorly, if at all.

DRUGS AND MOOD DISORDERS

Long before these problems emerged as a major source of concern, the pharmaceutical industry had brought other classes of psychoactive drugs to market. First, there were the so-called minor tranquillizers: Miltown and Equanil (meprobamate), which made

users drowsy, and, later on, Valium and Librium (the benzodiazapines), which didn't. With their advent, the troubles of everyday life were effortlessly redefined as psychiatric illnesses. Here were the pills that proffered a solution to the boredom of the trapped housewife and the blues of overwhelmed mothers and of the fading middle-aged. As early as 1956, statistics suggest as many as one American in 20 was taking tranquillizers in any given month. Anxiety, tension, unhappiness – all could seemingly be smoothed away by medication. Once again, however, these advantages were secured at a price: many of those taking the drugs became physically habituated to them, finding it difficult or impossible not to continue using them, for to abandon the pills was to court symptoms and psychic pain worse than those that had driven the decision to use them in the first place.

Other compounds that changed people's moods were developed in the late 1950s, beginning with Iproniazid (a monoamine oxidase inhibitor), in 1957, and Trofranil and Elavil, so-called tricyclic antidepressants, in 1958 and 1961 respectively. Perhaps in part because many depressed people suffer in silence, the belief persisted that depression was a comparatively rare condition. The belated success of Prozac in the 1990s changed that mind-set completely. Depression has become a disease of epidemic proportions.

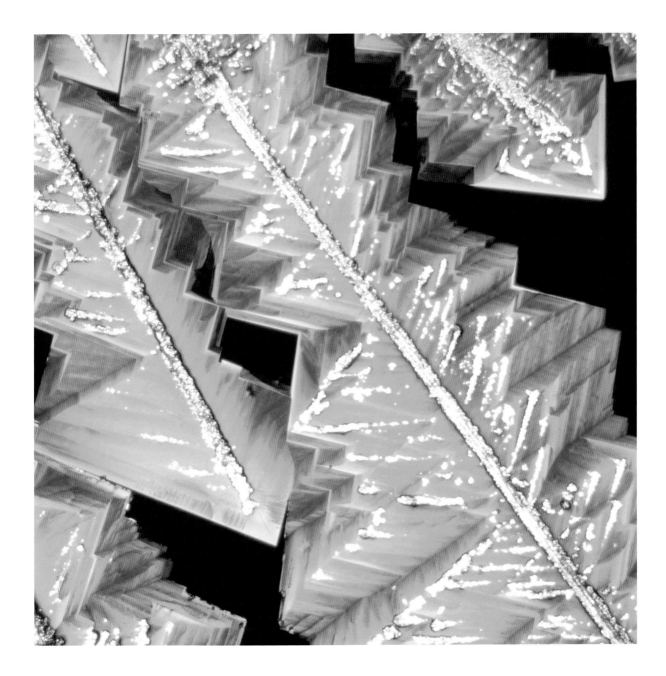

Opposite left
A patient restrained in a strait-jacket in a French asylum in the 1830s. Although there was a progressive trend away from physical restraint in the 19th century, in some cases involving extremely violent patients it remained a necessity. Critics argued that the antipsychotic drugs that appeared in the 1950s corralled the mind as the body had once been.

Opposite right
Thorazine was one of the earliest antipsychotic drugs. In this advert from 1957 it offers help with the symptoms of senility, when the formerly mild-mannered elder becomes agitated, angry, violent and therefore unmanageable in the home. Acting on a variety of receptors in the central nervous system its unwanted side effects included constipation, excessive sedation and low blood pressure.

Above
Crystals of the neurotransmitter serotonin. In depression and seasonal affective disorder (SAD) serotonin levels may be reduced. Drugs such as Prozac are selective serotonin reuptake inhibitors (SSRIs) and are thought to increase the amount of serotonin available because at the synapse they stop the donating cell from reabsorbing it.

49. VENTOLIN
Breathing easier

Mark Jackson

The most used bronchodilator in the world.
Sir David Jack, 1996

The launch of salbutamol by the British pharmaceutical company Allen & Hanburys in the late 1960s constituted a watershed in the treatment of asthma. Marketed as Ventolin and dispensed in a distinctive hand-held blue inhaler, salbutamol rapidly became the principal means by which asthmatics and their doctors attempted both to relieve the suffocating symptoms and to prevent the potentially fatal consequences of an acute asthma attack.

Recognized as a distinct disease since antiquity, asthma was traditionally regarded as a type of difficulty in breathing accompanied by wheezing and coughing. In the 20th century, it was increasingly defined as reversible airway obstruction, often triggered by allergic reactions to dust mites, pollen and animals, or by emotional stress. For many centuries, asthmatics had experimented with a variety of herbal remedies in order to reduce the production of phlegm, relax the airways and ease their breathing. During the early years of the 20th century, the range of treatments for asthma was expanded by discoveries within the pharmaceutical sector: ephedrine, derived from the Chinese herb *ma huang*, and adrenaline were administered to relax bronchial smooth muscle; and aminophylline, oral steroids and antihistamines were ingested or injected to reduce inflammation and widen the airways. In spite of these developments, however, morbidity and mortality from asthma increased during the middle decades of the 20th century.

The introduction of salbutamol depended on two critical scientific insights. In the first place, developments in inhaler technology were necessary. Inhalation had been employed by most ancient cultures to relieve asthma attacks and had become commercially and clinically more important during the 18th and 19th centuries. The introduction of the metered-dose inhaler in the 1950s, however, made it

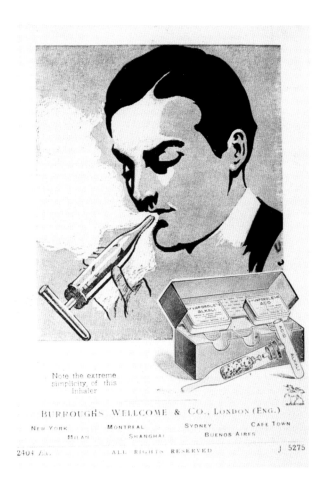

possible for the first time to deliver precise quantities of active compounds to asthmatic lungs. Secondly, the discovery of salbutamol was dependent upon increasing scientific understanding of the physiology of adrenergic receptors, that is the cell surface receptors that initiate responses to adrenaline and noradrenaline (referred to in North America as epinephrine and norepinephrine).

Early bronchodilators, such as isoprenaline, had stimulated receptors in both the lungs and the heart, leading occasionally to fatal cardiac complications. Differentiation between beta-1 receptors in the heart [50] and beta-2 receptors in the lungs in the early 1960s stimulated David Jack and his colleagues at Allen & Hanburys to develop a selective bronchodilator that relaxed the airways effectively but had little action on the heart: salbutamol was the result.

Administered either via an inhaler or in nebulized form, Ventolin rapidly became the most effective means of relieving an acute asthma attack both at home and in hospital. In addition to improving the lives of patients, the drug also transformed the fortunes of Allen & Hanburys: by 1985, annual sales of Ventolin had reached £171 million and by 1995 they exceeded £500 million. In 1973 David Jack and his team received a Queen's Award for Technological Achievement and Jack himself was awarded a CBE in 1982 and knighted in 1993.

The successful production of Ventolin encouraged further discoveries in the treatment of asthma. In 1972 Jack's team marketed Becotide, an inhaled steroid used for preventing asthma attacks, and during the closing decade of the 20th century longer-acting beta-2-agonists, such as salmeterol, were introduced. Long-acting bronchodilators, often administered in conjunction with an inhaled steroid such as fluticasone, have partially replaced salbutamol in asthma management. However, Ventolin remains the most important and most iconic means of relieving the respiratory distress associated with asthma.

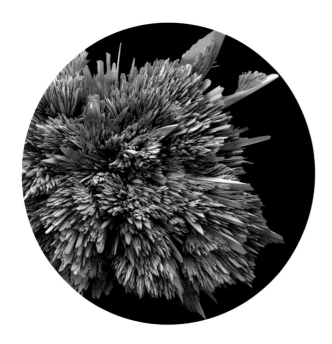

Above
Salbutamol (Ventolin) crystals: used as an inhalant where there is a narrowing of the airways, such as in bronchitis, asthma and emphysema, salbutamol is a short-acting beta-2-agonist that acts on receptors in the lungs. When stimulated by the drug, these receptors cause the airway muscles to relax and open. The cluster of crystals is about 600 micrometres in diameter.

Right
A modern inhaler used to deliver medication such as salbutamol (Ventolin). As a variety of drugs can be administered in this way the outer plastic surround is colour coded to help patients use the correct medication. The inner pressurized container contains the drug; when it is depressed a measured dose of the drug is released.

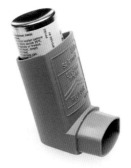

50. BETA-BLOCKERS
Designer drugs

Tilli Tansey

... saving the lives of millions of people worldwide ...
Obituary of Sir James Black, *The Times*, 2010

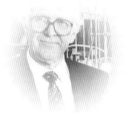

Left
Sir James Black shared the Nobel Prize in Medicine in 1988 for his development of beta-blockers.

Opposite
An illustration of sections of a diseased heart (above) and lungs (below), *c.* 1843, showing blood clots and haemorrhage. Blood clots in the coronary arteries cause heart attacks. Beta-blockers dilate the arteries and increase blood flow while reducing the heart rate and its force of contraction to help prevent further morbidity.

Beta-blockers are used to affect the control of the heart in the management of conditions such as cardiac arrhythmia, to protect the heart after a heart attack (myocardial infarction) and to control high blood pressure. Strictly speaking they were not 'discovered', but were rather specifically designed in the 1950s by a chemical pharmacologist, James (later Sir James) Black (1924–2010), building on the scientific discoveries of others.

Beta-blockers act by disrupting or blocking the effects of chemicals called the catecholamines, such as noradrenaline. These are used by the involuntary, or autonomic, nervous system in the control of routine, involuntary functions such as breathing, heart beat and gland secretions, as opposed to actions such as running, speaking etc, which are controlled by the voluntary nervous system.

THE BASIC SCIENCE
It was known by the early 1900s that the autonomic nervous system itself comprised two anatomically and physiologically distinct parts: the parasympathetic system, which predominantly promotes slowing down;

and the sympathetic system, which promotes what is called the fight or flight response, in which the heart rate increases and the pupils dilate, and blood flow diverts from non-essential organs to skeletal muscle.

Investigations then revealed that the parasympathetic system mainly used the chemical acetylcholine as its neurotransmitter (a substance that conveys information from one nerve cell to another, or from one nerve cell to a final 'effector' cell such as a gland or heart cell), and that the sympathetic system used a chemical similar to, but not identical with, adrenaline, then known as a hormone released by the adrenal gland [17]. However, the chemistry of the sympathetic system was more complicated than the parasympathetic, and scientists who studied the effects of adrenaline and chemically related compounds, including noradrenaline, synthesized in the laboratory, discovered that these drugs could cause either contraction or relaxation of smooth muscle, depending on the chemical, dosage and site of action.

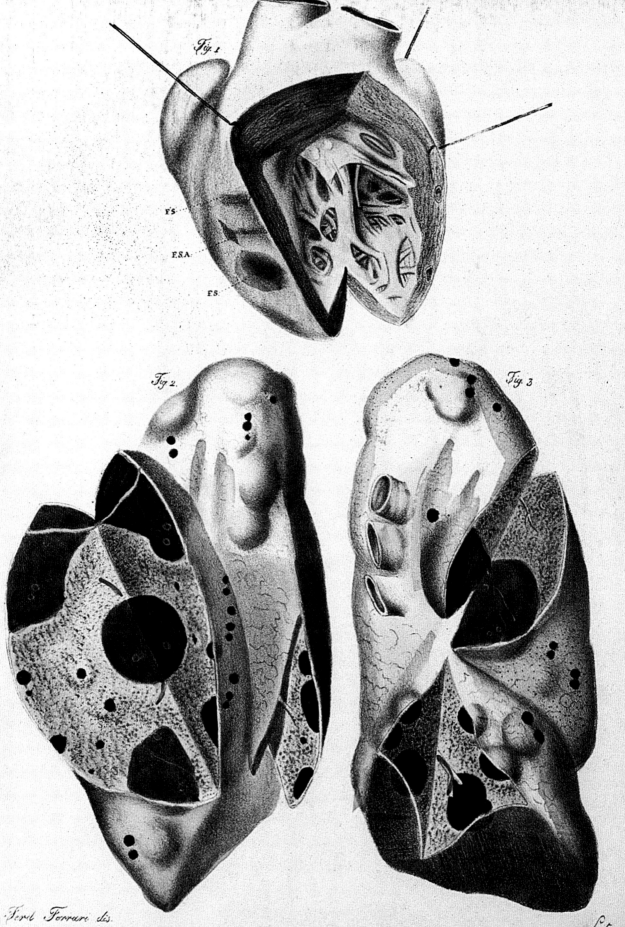

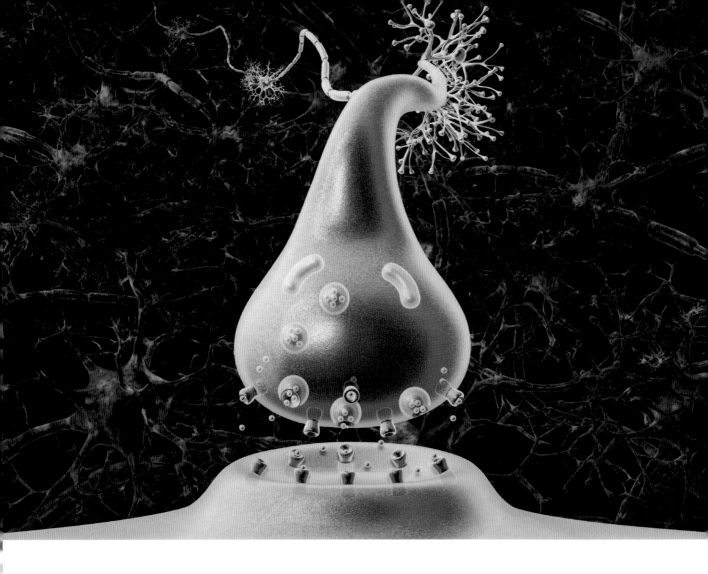

A digital image illustrating the action of neurotransmitters such
as noradrenaline in the synaptic cleft – the gap between a nerve
cell (above) and its target receptors on muscles, other nerves or
glands (below). Vesicles containing the neurotransmitter (green) move
towards the pre-synaptic membrane where they fuse with the cell
membrane before releasing their contents into the synaptic cleft.
The neurotransmitter molecules act on the target cell by binding
to specific receptors on the cell surface (purple). The nerve cell
can reuse the neurotransmitter molecules, taking them up by
other receptors (orange).

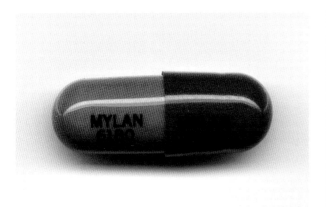

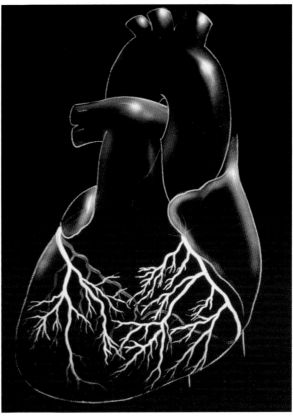

ADVANCES

In the 1940s, two major advances were made. First, the Swedish pharmacologist Ulf S. von Euler (1905–83) discovered that noradrenaline was a natural component of the body. The second was the proposal by the American pharmacologist Raymond Ahlquist (1914–83), initially much resisted, that the sympathetic system contained two different receptor types, which are distinguished by their responses to different catecholamines. He classified alpha-receptors as responding most to noradrenaline, then to adrenaline, and then to isoprenaline, and suggested that these receptors were involved in smooth muscle relaxation; while beta-receptors responded most to isoprenaline, and then equally to adrenaline and noradrenaline, and were associated with heart and smooth muscle contraction.

THE BLACK DESIGN

James Black was inspired by this hypothesis to design molecules that could block the unwanted effects of chemicals associated with disorders such as angina pectoris. His father had suffered for years from this condition, at a time when the only 'treatment' for anginal chest pains was to take a tablet of nitroglycerine, believed to increase temporarily the blood flow to a diseased heart. Black wondered if, rather than increase the blood flow, the energy demands of the heart were decreased, the same effect could be achieved. Armed with Ahlquist's proposal, he sought to design a selective blocker of the beta-receptors on the heart. Working at ICI, Black produced pronethalol, the first clinically used beta-blocker. It was soon replaced by propanolol.

These were the first drugs to be rationally designed rather than discovered empirically. Although now largely superseded by more refined, selective blockers, propanolol remains in clinical use, and like other beta-blockers is banned in the Olympics because it can control stage fright and tremor. The first beta-blocker thus both revolutionized the medical management of angina pectoris, and marked a major turning point between drug discovery and drug design. It was one of the most significant contributions to clinical medicine and pharmacology of the 20th century.

51. STATINS
Lowering cholesterol

Akihito Suzuki

... the penicillin of arterial sclerosis.
New England Journal of Medicine, 1981

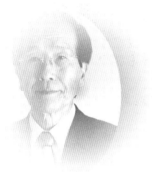

Left
Akira Endo: his long-term interest in the biochemistry of fungi resulted in the discovery of the statins and their action in the metabolism of cholesterol. In 2008 he received the Laskar award for clinical medicine.

Opposite
A section of an atherosclerotic artery: the arterial walls (purple) surround the lumen, or channel (white), containing several cholesterol clefts (red), spaces left as the cholesterol crystals dissolve in the sample's preparation. In life such crystals would obstruct the artery; statins reduce their size and number.

Statins are a group of drugs that lower the cholesterol level in the blood. They are used to prevent arterial sclerosis, also called arteriosclerosis or atherosclerosis, a major cause of heart diseases. Hailed as a new wonder drug in 1981, statins have largely lived up to their promise: they are now given to 40 million patients every day around the world and annual sales amount to about $2.6 billion. The discovery of this successful drug reads like a microcosm of contemporary medicine, involving epidemiologists, research scientists, clinicians and pharmaceutical companies around the globe.

NEW DISEASES
The epidemiological transition – the decline of infectious diseases and the increase of degenerative disorders – started in the 1920s in economically developed countries. It has been repeated in many countries since. With the rise of living standards and effective drugs against infectious diseases, the developed world faced the new 'diseases of civilization'. Arterial sclerosis is one of them.

Research in the mid-20th century, such as the Framingham Heart Study, begun in 1948 with 5,209

residents of Framingham, Massachusetts, identified risk factors that contribute to developing coronary heart diseases. Other large-scale and often international studies followed. In addition to age, family history and smoking, these investigations demonstrated a positive relationship between raised blood cholesterol level and the likelihood of developing heart diseases.

Pathological and experimental studies of cholesterol reinforced these epidemiological findings. In the 1950s, scientists elucidated how cholesterol is synthesized in the body, mainly by the liver, a breakthrough for which Konrad E. Bloch and Feodor Lynen received a Nobel Prize in 1964.

NEW SOLUTIONS
The actual discovery of an effective drug to reduce the cholesterol level came from a relatively obscure source. Akira Endo (1933–), a Japanese scientist working for Sankyo Pharmaceutical Company, was investigating the possibility of finding a fungal metabolite that could block cholesterol synthesis by inhibiting the enzyme, HMG-CoA reductase, that is involved in the process. He and his team spent two years examining 6,000

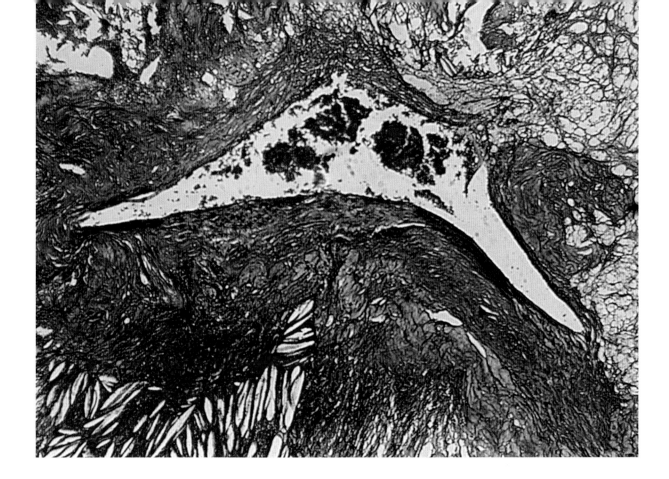

fungi looking for HMG-CoA inhibition, before his discovery in 1973 that *Penicillium citrinum*, a mould isolated from rice from a vendor in Kyoto, made a substance inhibiting *in vitro* synthesis of cholesterol. This was the first statin, mevastatin, known as compactin. In 1975 scientists at Beecham Laboratories independently discovered the same substance, but did not develop it further.

At Sankyo compactin was almost abandoned several times. First, it was found that it did not lower the cholesterol level of rats; however, Endo showed it was effective in hens and dogs. Then other scientists at Sankyo feared that compactin might cause liver disorders in animals; this time, university clinicians rescued the drug. In 1977 Akira Yamamoto of Osaka University asked Endo for compactin to treat severe cases of high cholesterol. Endo did not tell Sankyo about the clinical experiment, and secretly handed the substance to Yamamoto. Fortunately for Endo and Yamamoto, this gamble succeeded. Sankyo started formal clinical trials in 1978.

An international pharmaceutical giant, Merck & Co. in the US, soon noticed the news of Sankyo developing

a wonder drug for arterial sclerosis. Merck secured the collaboration of Sankyo and developed the drug in systematic and efficient ways. Other scientific research also progressed, and in 1985 Joseph L. Goldstein and Michael S. Brown received the Nobel Prize for their research on low-density lipoprotein receptors that extract cholesterol from the bloodstream.

In 1987 the first group of Merck statins was approved by the US Food and Drug Administration (FDA). The controversy over the efficacy of statins lingered until, in the 1990s, several large-scale, multi-centred clinical surveys showed that statins could prevent heart attacks and strokes and generally prolong life.

Surgical
Breakthroughs

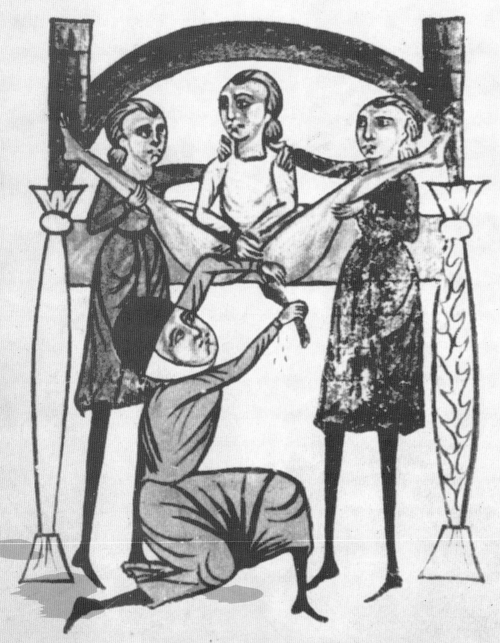

N.º 6.

S urgery is an ancient craft and a modern discipline. Before the 19th-century innovations of anaesthesia and antisepsis, surgeons were severely limited in what they could do for their patients. Infection and shock limited their cutting to the extremities and superficial parts of the body. They could lance abscesses and boils, set simple fractures, and treat lacerations and contusions. They also dealt with skin diseases and let blood. Amputation and the removal of bladder stones were the most substantial operations they generally performed. Within this context, the French surgeon Ambroise Paré stands out as an enlightened exponent of the surgeon's craft.

Anaesthesia, to control pain, and antisepsis, to counter post-operative sepsis, gradually changed all this. They allowed surgeons to be more deliberate and to try to avoid the often fatal infections that frequently attended earlier operations. They also enabled them to open up the body cavities – abdomen (including for caesarean section), thorax and brain – that had been effectively closed to them. Because operating to remove a tumour, gallstones or an inflamed appendix could cure definitively, whereas other medical treatment had less immediate effect, surgeons became the vanguard of modern medicine. They could offer cure, not simply care, and although many of the pioneering operations had horrific mortality rates, surgeons persisted and frequently made once dangerous operations routine.

Modern surgery relies on teamwork, and much innovation rests on technological and scientific research. The support – assistants, surgical nurses, anaesthetists, recovery rooms, monitoring equipment, blood transfusion – means that surgeons no longer work alone. The proportion of science and technology in evolving surgical capability varies. Neurosurgery, an early surgical sub-specialty, rested on basic physiological research on the localization of brain function to allow the surgeon and neurologist to pinpoint the lesion. Transplant surgery would not have been possible without a fundamental understanding of the body's immune system, and the development of drugs to suppress the natural tendency of the body to reject foreign tissues and organs.

Contemporary cardiac surgery could not have taken place without the technological invention of the heart-lung machine, which allows the surgeon to stop the patient's heart while circulation and respiration are maintained externally. Heart transplantation also requires the immunological backup that all transplant operations need, with the special circumstance that if the heart fails, the patient dies. If the kidney transplant does not take, however, dialysis is a fallback therapy. Hip replacement, a life-enhancing operation for many in an ageing population, relies on the inert material for the new hip joint – durability and the capacity to escape the body's natural immunological reactions being key. Hip replacement was a technological solution to a common problem.

Cataract surgery has also been transformed by technological innovation, both in the way that the operation is done and the materials used. However, no area of modern surgery relies more heavily on technology than keyhole, or minimally invasive, surgery. Improved visualization, robotic controls, fibre optics and scanning equipment allow the contemporary surgeon to do more with less violence to the integrity of the patient's body. Surgery is becoming increasingly an outpatient specialty.

Lithotomy, the surgical removal of a stone from the bladder, is shown here in an illustration from a 14th-century surgical manuscript. In the absence of anaesthesia, the patient's hands would be tied and the surgeon's assistants further restrained him. Unsurprisingly, the speed at which a surgeon could operate was part of the way his expertise was judged.

52. PARÉ & WOUNDS
Innovation on the battlefield

Simon Chaplin

I dressed him and God healed him.
Ambroise Paré, 1585

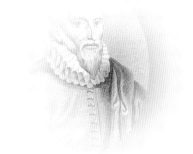

Ambroise Paré (1510–90) is often seen as the archetypal surgeon. Trained through apprenticeship and schooled in war, he is fêted for challenging medical dogma. He opposed the use of boiling oil on gun-shot wounds, applied arterial ligation (tying vessels to stem blood loss) to amputation and developed new treatments for burns. Although he had little formal education, Paré became one of the most influential medical practitioners of his time.

Born near Laval, in the province of Maine in northwest France, Paré began his career as a barber-surgeon. At the age of 22 he moved to Paris, where became a resident surgeon at the Hôtel-Dieu, the city's public hospital. During this time he undertook anatomical dissections and gained valuable experience in clinical and surgical practice. On leaving the hospital in 1536 he entered the service of the Mareschal de Montjean and accompanied him to Italy with the French army.

MILITARY SURGERY

Military campaigning exposed Paré to cases not usually encountered in civilian practice, notably gun-shot injuries. Unlike those caused by swords, guns left ragged wounds more likely to include foreign matter and hence prone to what are now recognized as bacterial infections. Sixteenth-century surgeons blamed the effect on gunpowder's 'venomous' nature. To combat it, boiling oil was applied to wounds – a method popularized by the Italian surgeon Giovanni da Vigo (1450?–1525). Paré initially used this method, but on campaign near Turin in 1537 he ran out of oil, and improvised a cold dressing made of egg yolk, oil of roses and turpentine. After spending a night fretting about the consequences he returned to discover that those treated with his new mixture were recovering well,

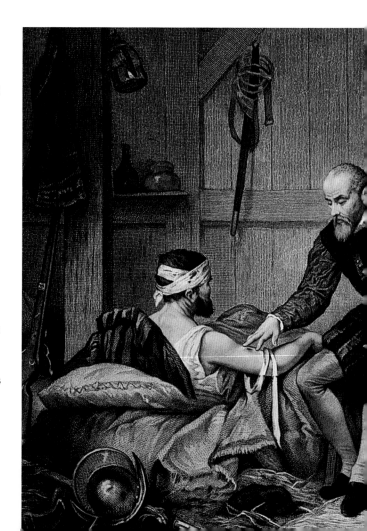

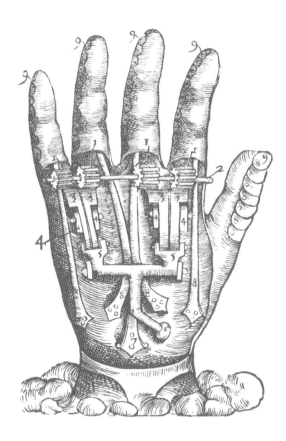

while others who had received hot oil were feverish and in pain. Paré described his experiences in his first book, *La Méthode de Traicter les Playes* (The Method of Treating Wounds; 1545). As well as the dressing of wounds, it described a method of locating and removing projectiles based on careful anatomical study. Written in French in an engaging and accessible style, it helped bring Paré's ideas to a much wider audience than traditional Latin texts.

BEYOND THE BATTLEFIELD

Many more military campaigns followed, interspersed by spells in civilian practice. Paré's success led to his appointment as surgeon to King Henri II of France in 1552. He went on to serve three more French kings over a period of almost 40 years. He continued to publish, writing not only on surgery, but also on anatomy and midwifery, teratology (fetal malformations), and on the treatment of tumours and diseases such as plague and measles. His surgical treatises included descriptions of many instruments. Among them was the bec-de-corbin or 'crow's-beak' used to grip arteries so they could be ligated during amputation – a technique Paré preferred to the use of a hot cautery. Like many of Paré's ideas, this was not wholly novel but was an adaptation of an existing practice.

Although Paré was admitted as a master-surgeon to the College of St-Côme in 1554, he was not universally admired. He was involved in a number of disputes, especially when his work strayed into matters of physic rather than surgery. Paré used his later books to answer some of these criticisms, notably in his *Apologie et Traité* (1585), a mixture of autobiography, travelogue and surgical treatise that helped cement his posthumous reputation.

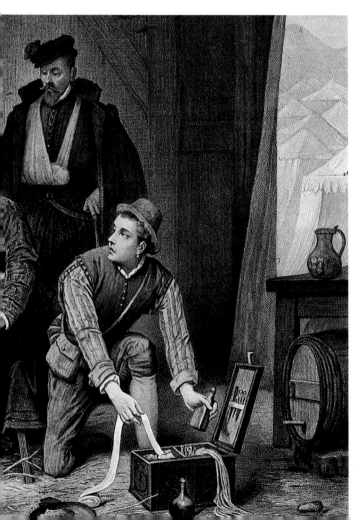

Opposite above
Ambroise Paré had little formal education or training but was renowned for his innovations in the treatment of wounds on the battlefield.

Above
An illustration of a mechanical hand designed by Paré, one of several replacement prostheses he designed and had illustrated in his texts.

Left
Paré attending to the sick after battle. The military tents are visible through the door to the right. There is no boiling oil in this depiction – Paré abandoned this ill-fated technique of wound treatment and encouraged others to follow him. His demeanour is that of the caring and careful observer, the image he created through his surgical practice and writings.

53. ANAESTHESIA
Revolutionizing surgery

Stephanie Snow

It is the grandest & most blessed of discoveries.
Charles Darwin, 1850

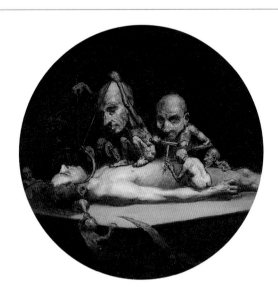

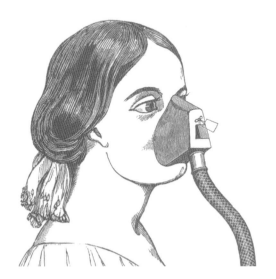

Anaesthesia was at the same time one of the most important and controversial discoveries of the 19th century. Surgeons had long searched for a method of pain-relief, but the first anaesthetics – ether and nitrous oxide – were discovered by chance by American dentists in the 1840s. Nitrous oxide had been known since the 1790s, when Humphry Davy experimented with the gas. By the 1840s it was known as 'laughing gas' and was used at fairs. In 1844 in Hartford, USA, the dentist Horace Wells (1815–48) noticed how a young man under its influence seemed impervious to the pain of an injured leg. Wells successfully used nitrous oxide on dental patients, but his demonstration at Massachusetts General Hospital in Boston in 1845 failed, and the procedure was dismissed as a sham.

ETHER AND CHLOROFORM
Only 12 months later, fellow dentist William Morton (1819–68) experimented with ether, a highly pungent chemical, widely available and used to relieve bronchial disorders. Crawford Long (1815–78), a doctor in the southern American state of Georgia, used ether in operations but never reported his results. He

was unsure whether the anaesthetic effects had been produced by the ether or the patient's imagination. Morton had no such qualms and successfully demonstrated ether in Boston on 16 October 1846.

The news crossed the Atlantic to Britain and Europe and spread worldwide within six months. Ether was immediately taken up in London. The surgeon Robert Liston (1794–1847) used it successfully in a leg amputation on 21 December 1846. Anaesthesia's benefits were indisputable, but many doctors struggled to administer it effectively. Patients who received too small a dose grew excited, struggled and lost their sense of propriety. 'Now we'll dance the Polka', a respectable solicitor told his dentist. The serious business of surgery became a farce. The writer Charlotte Brontë noted: '[I] would think twice before I consented to inhale; one would not like to make a fool of oneself.'

The difficulties occurred because few doctors understood the scientific basis for anaesthesia; most simply tried it out. But John Snow (1813–58), then a general practitioner in London and later to become famous for his work on cholera [**36**], researched the physical and chemical properties of ether. He

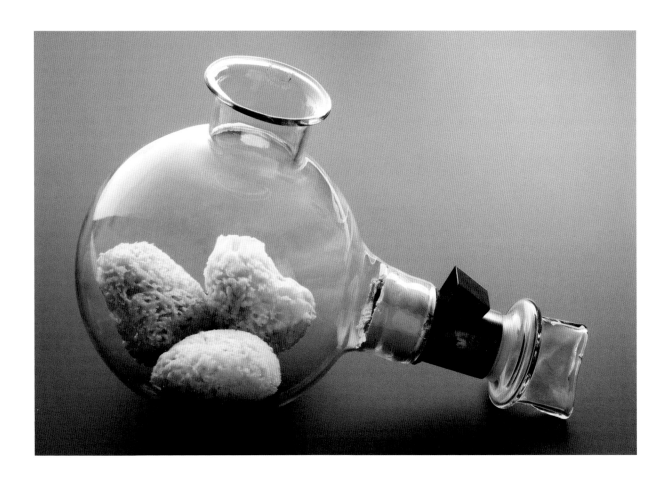

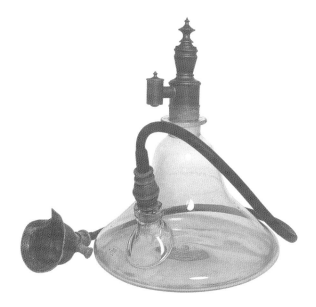

Opposite left
A macabre realization of the effects of chloroform on the human body, by Richard Cooper, c. 1912. An anaesthetized man lies on the table being attacked by little demons wielding an array of surgical instruments to which he is insensible.

Opposite right
John Snow's anaesthetic inhalation apparatus for delivering chloroform, from the mid-19th century. Snow's careful research resulted in an inhaler in which he could accurately measure the dose he gave to his patients.

Above
A replica of the inhaler used by William Morton in his pioneering operation in 1846. The ether was placed on the sponges in the glass vessel. Tubing connected it to a face mask (neither shown) placed over the patient's mouth.

Right
William Squire was a medical student who assisted Robert Liston at the first use of ether anaesthesia, at University College Hospital on 21 December 1846. This replica of his apparatus was made by the pharmacist Peter Squire (William's uncle).

POETRY.

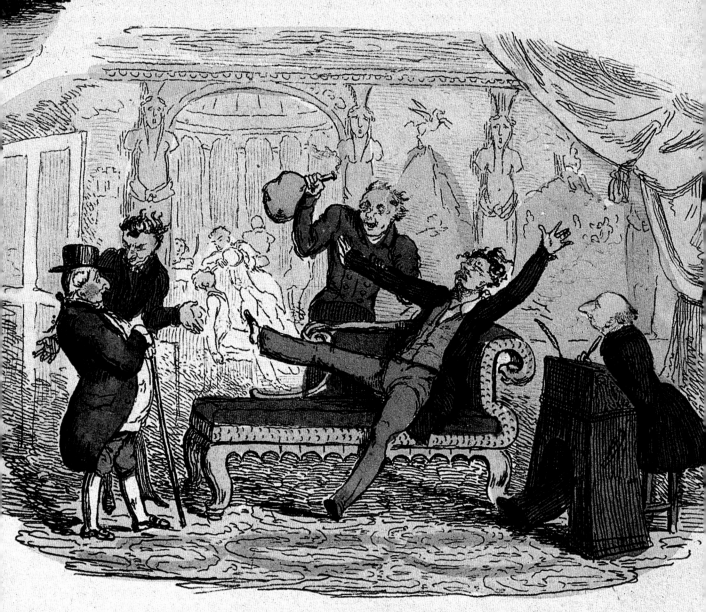

This is not the Laughing, but the Hippocrene or Poetic Gas, Sir, the Gentleman you see inspired here is throwing out the rough materials for an Heroic Poem, we have various sorts as the Terrific much in request, the Simple by which all the new Songs are done, and many others.

discovered that the degree of anaesthesia was determined by the concentration of ether in the blood, which in turn depended on temperature. He designed an inhaler with a water bath to control the temperature of the air and thereby the amount of ether given to patients.

Snow deduced that ether produced its anaesthetic effects by being absorbed into the blood and acting on the nervous system. Ether initially affected the higher, more subtle brain functions, and as the concentration in the blood increased, sensibility was suspended and the more important functions such as respiration were steadily depressed.

In November 1847 the Edinburgh physician James Young Simpson (1811–70) discovered the anaesthetic properties of chloroform. Worldwide, chloroform rapidly replaced ether. But in January 1848, 15-year-old Hannah Greener died within two minutes of inhaling chloroform while having a toenail removed at her home in Newcastle upon Tyne. An intense debate broke out. Had chloroform killed through the respiration, or had an overdose poisoned the heart? The questions remained unresolved until 1911, when the physiologist A. Goodman Levy (1866–1954) showed how low doses of chloroform could cause death by inducing ventricular fibrillation of the heart [28].

MORAL AND MEDICAL DILEMMAS

Patients were immediately enthusiastic about anaesthesia, but chloroform fatalities inflamed debates about its risks. And although medical practitioners had always sought to relieve pain, within Western medicine it was understood to be of physiological and moral value. In surgery, pain was thought of as a stimulant helping to preserve life during the stress of an operation.

In 1853, a spate of chloroform fatalities caused the *Lancet* to condemn the risks of anaesthesia as too great, even in amputations. In childbirth, doctors feared chloroform could complicate births: labour pains were 'natural and physiological forces that the Divinity has ordained us to enjoy or to suffer', stated obstetrician Professor Charles Meigs (1792–1869). However, mothers persisted in demanding pain-relief, and chloroform's most famous advocate was Queen Victoria (chloroform was administered to her by John Snow during the births of her last two children). Over time, the success of anaesthesia in countless operations, including those on the battlefields of the Crimean War (1853–56),

strengthened the arguments that the risks of pain were more dangerous to a patient's physiology than the risks of anaesthesia.

By the end of the 19th century, together with antisepsis techniques to control infection [54], anaesthesia had revolutionized surgery. A range of inhaled anaesthetics – chloroform, ether and nitrous oxide – were in use, much apparatus had been invented and a new medical specialty created. But the risks remained: best estimates suggest a ratio of one fatality to every 2,500 or so chloroform administrations. In some countries doctors had returned to ether as a safer anaesthetic, but in Britain chloroform remained popular well into the 1950s.

PAIN CONTROL TODAY

During the 20th century, new techniques such as intubation – placing tubes in the trachea to aid control of breathing – and new agents, including intravenous barbiturates, which put patients to sleep without the unpleasantness of inhalation, improved patient experience and safety. The risk of fatalities fell to around one per 100,000 anaesthetics; the use of muscle relaxants also enhanced operating conditions. Anaesthetists now combine a raft of drugs with different functions – analgesia, amnesia, muscle relaxation, sedation – to create balanced anaesthesia, and manage a wide range of medical services, including Intensive Care Units and chronic pain clinics. Millions of patients worldwide benefit from anaesthesia, a 19th-century innovation that changed ideas about pain irrevocably.

Opposite
A coloured print by Robert Seymour, 1829, showing a laughing gas (nitrous oxide) party. After the discovery of the intoxicating properties of nitrous oxide by Humphry Davy, a group of doctors, scientists and poets in Bristol experimented with it and the phenomenon spread during the first third of the 19th century among intellectuals of all stripes.

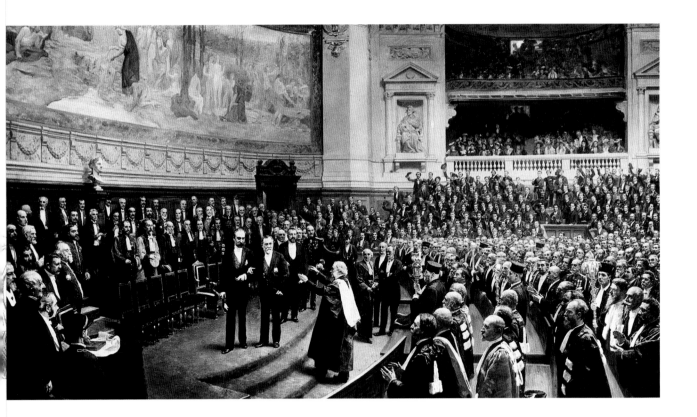

By the time he first published his experience with the substance in 1867, Lister had found an explanation of why his method should work. He had heard of the germ theory proposed by Louis Pasteur, who stated that microscopic organisms were ubiquitous in the environment and could lead to fermentation in certain foodstuffs. Lister claimed that these germs could also get into wounds, where they would live on dead tissue and cause putrefaction, and that the wound therefore had to be protected against the microorganisms that invaded the body at every disruption of the continuity of its surface. Lister tried to perfect his antiseptic technology by introducing a special spray technique in 1871: an aerosol of carbolic acid was designed to kill microorganisms even before they reached the wound.

Seeking to convince his colleagues of his new technique, Lister reported that between 1864 and 1866 16 of his 35 amputation patients (46 per cent) had died, whereas in 1867–69, after the introduction of antisepsis, this figure was reduced to 6 out of 40 (15 per cent). But not everyone believed that antisepsis was the cause of this improvement. Many of his colleagues, for example, challenged Lister's theory of the ubiquity of living

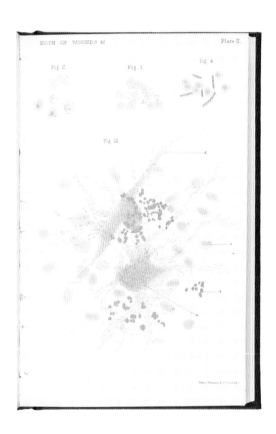

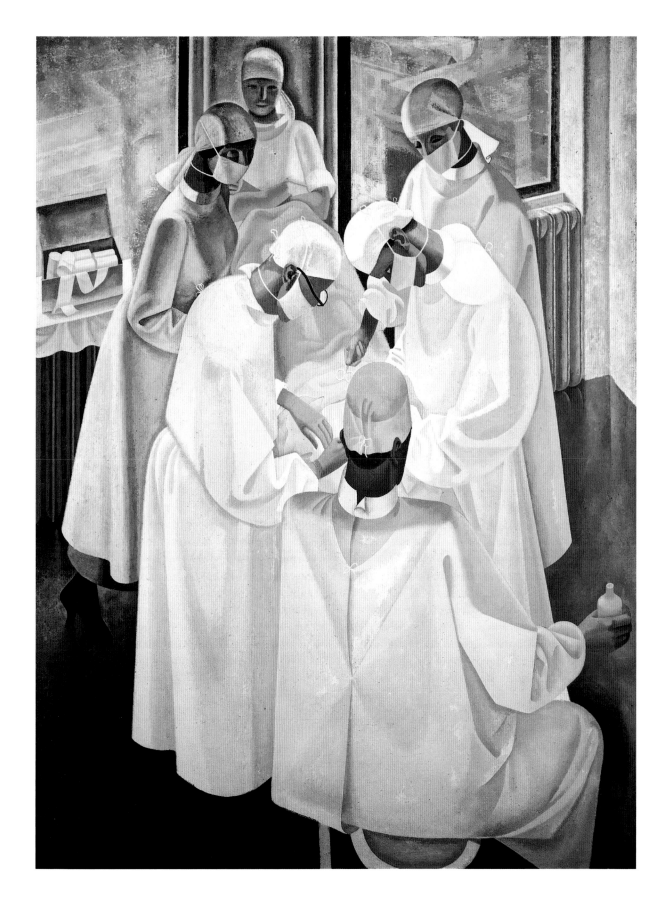

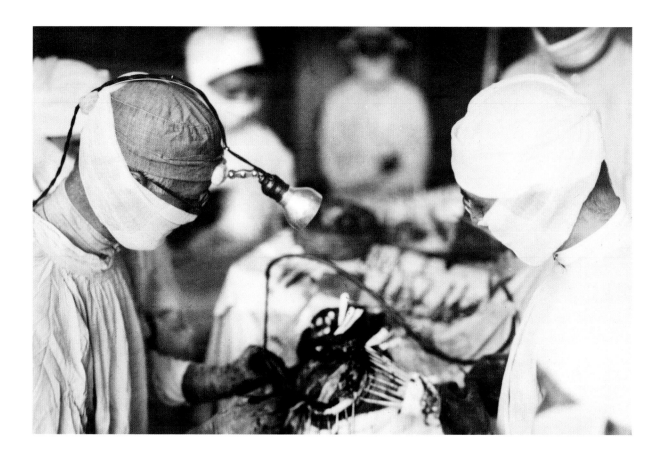

of successful neurological surgery – unsuccessful brain surgery had had many parents – Cushing moved to the Peter Bent Brigham Hospital in Boston, where for the next 20 years his operating room was a mecca for the surgical world, the place where young men came to witness and learn the amazing new procedures.

SCHOOLS OF BRAIN SURGEONS

Cushing's students spread out across North America and Europe, treating patients and training their own successors. Even today, most neurosurgeons in the Western world can trace their 'lineage' through three or four generations back to Harvey Cushing. The American Association of Neurological Surgeons, which has several thousand members around the world, was founded in 1931 as the Harvey Cushing Society.

Cushing was a driven workaholic, a tough taskmaster, who stayed on the frontier of his specialty to the end of his career (while also finding time to win a Pulitzer Prize for his biography of his medical mentor, Sir William Osler, and become a famous figure in endocrinology for his description of Cushing's disease, a pituitary disorder). In the 1920s he developed the

Harvey Cushing (left) operating: in the pre-antibiotic era, Cushing was utterly scrupulous in maintaining aseptic operating conditions and in haemostasis, or stopping blood flow. The clamps (visible in the centre bottom of the photograph) were used to seal the many blood vessels within the cranium.

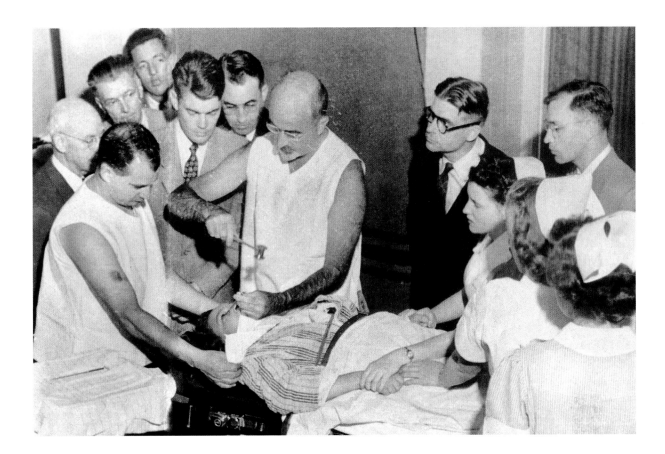

histological classification of brain tumours still in use, and was the first to apply techniques of electrosurgery to the brain. None the less, a group of younger brain surgeons, led by Cushing's former student and successor at Johns Hopkins, Walter Dandy (1886–1946), became much more aggressive than their mentor in attempting difficult tumour removals, and began learning how to treat aneurysms, epilepsy and cases of hydrocephalus.

Neurosurgeons tended to divide into those who favoured either conservative or radical approaches to brain problems, and traces of that divergence remain to the present. In the 1930s and 1940s the most radical neurosurgeons attempted 'psychosurgery', the removal of the frontal lobes of mentally disturbed patients.

Lobotomies fell out of favour in the 1950s, but at the beginning of the 21st century some neurosurgeons are still experimenting with radical, invasive techniques to attack depression. Others are pioneering noninvasive and microsurgical approaches to tumours and other brain conditions. In many hundreds of medical centres around the world, successful operative treatment of brain conditions has become routine. Most

neurosurgeons still open and close the human cranium with the basic instruments and techniques Harvey Cushing had mastered a hundred years earlier. Seldom in the history of surgery has one individual been so far ahead of his time or had such a dominating influence.

Cushing's precision was in stark contrast to the crudeness of lobotomy. Here, Walter Freeman (1895–1972) uses an instrument resembling an ice pick, which he had designed. He inserts the lobotomy tool under the upper eyelid of the patient, severing the nerve connections in the front part of the brain.

57. CATARACT SURGERY
Restoring lost sight

John Pickstone

Age-related cataract is responsible for 48 per cent of world
blindness, which represents about 18 million people.
World Health Organization, 2010

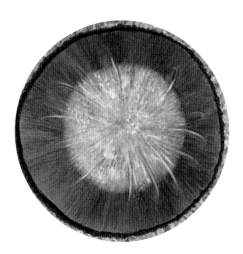

Cataracts – the progressive clouding of the eye's crystalline lens – are the most frequent cause of defective vision in later life. 'Couching' (pushing the clouded lens out of the line of sight) was a traditional operation practised in ancient India, whence it spread around the world. In the 18th century itinerant 'oculists' were well known, and eye surgery was an early field of specialism as medicine assumed its modern form in the 19th century. Before the Second World War the standard surgical 'cure' was removal of the lens (usually with its capsule) so that light could pass to the retina but without being focused as a clear image. The only corrective method was to use 'pebble glasses' – which, at best, provided poor, distorted, post-operative vision. The risk of infection and of collateral operative damage made this generally a procedure of last resort.

DEVELOPING THE INTRA OCULAR LENS
Soon after the Second World War, Harold Ridley (1906–2001), senior surgeon at Moorfields, London's major eye hospital, began to experiment with plastic lenses which might be inserted within a lens capsule after a clouded lens had been removed. He knew that

plastic contact lenses, invented in the 1930s, seemed to be tolerated, and that wartime injuries to pilots had indicated that Perspex 'shrapnel', like glass, would lie 'inert' in the eye. He joined forces with John Pike of Rayner, a small ophthalmic company, and John Holt of ICI (the giant British chemical company) to develop 'Perspex CQ' (Clinical Quality).

Ridley implanted the first Intra Ocular Lens (IOL) on 29 November 1949, at St Thomas's Hospital, London, but waited until July 1951 before announcing his eight results. The response was largely hostile. In the early years the lenses were thick and heavy, variable and difficult to sterilize, and about 15 per cent of patients had to have their new lenses removed. Though many surgeons shunned the operation, Ridley attracted a following, and some experimented with lenses placed in the anterior chamber, or with iris-supported lenses, but all were problematic, even with super-skilled surgeons. Indeed, in the 1970s, American consumer groups protested about untested lenses, leading to FDA regulation under the 1976 Medical Devices Amendments.

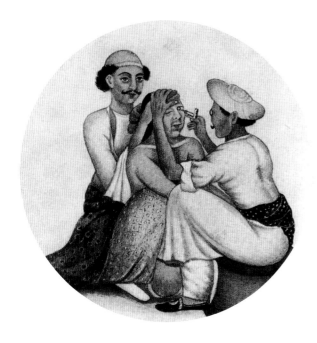

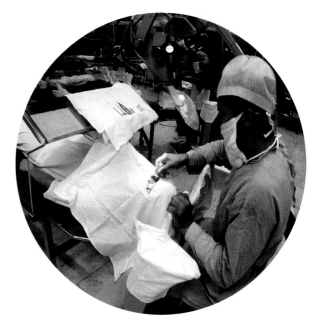

EMULSIFICATION AND UNFOLDINGS

Of all the developments that have transformed Ridley's innovation and operative method into a mass procedure, the most important was the adoption of phakoemulsification techniques for cataract extraction. These were developed by Charles Kelman (1930–2004), a professor of clinical ophthalmology in New York, who had tried to reduce the size of the incision in the lens capsule. Rotating mechanical cutting devices proved fruitless for the hard cataracts found in old people, but Kelman chanced upon a possible solution in an ultrasound device. He then used a vibrating needle to fragment a cataract, which could be sucked clear of the eye through a very small incision.

Improvements followed quickly, with the first crude machines available in 1970, signalling the shift of commercial cataract innovation towards the USA. But it is pointless to make a small incision to remove the cataract if a larger one then has to be made to insert a conventional, rigid or semi-rigid plastic lens. So commercial companies experimented with various materials to produce foldable lenses, which proved satisfactory by the mid-1980s. They can now be injected into the eye, unfolding within the intact capsular bag.

By the end of the 20th century the IOL had become the standard complement to cataract surgery, which itself had become one of the most frequently performed outpatient operations in the advanced industrial world. The procedure is now standardized, can be done quickly and in some countries is performed by nurses.

Opposite
Most cataracts are age related, and malnutrition, dehydration, diabetes, and perhaps exposure to sunlight can accelerate the process. A zonular (or perinuclear) cataract seen here is a rare inherited disorder: a clear area in the centre of the lens is surrounded by a ring of opacity.

Above left
Couching the cataract – pushing the opaque lens out of the sight line with a curved needle – originated in India. The coucher must have a steady hand and his assistant hold the head absolutely still.

Above right
Sviatoslav Fedorov (1927–2000), a flamboyant Russian ophthalmologist who pioneered the plastic lens, performing an operation. He also introduced a conveyor belt system, carrying the patients past a series of surgeons who each specialized in part of the operation. His team treated 150 patients a day.

58. CAESAREAN SECTION
'from his mother's womb/Untimely ripped'

Janette Allotey

Through this ring of bones [the pelvis], every child which comes into the world must pass, except they come by the caesarean operation.
Margaret Stephen (midwife), 1795

Greek myths recount the 'pulling out' of babies through abdominal incisions and, more amazingly, of fetal extractions from various parts of women's and even men's bodies. References are also found in Hindu, Jewish and Muslim writings to the caesarean operation being performed on the living and the dead. Caesarean after the mother's death was sanctioned in Egyptian and Roman law (the *lex Caesarea*), to allow the infant a chance of survival. Julius Caesar has also been linked (tenuously) with the operation. The medieval Christian church placed great importance on delivering and baptizing babies that risked dying in the womb. Those few that survived such an operation were regarded as possessing great strength or special powers, although during the medieval period this type of 'unnatural' birth was linked to the birth of the antichrist and viewed with suspicion.

Until the Renaissance, post-mortem caesareans were performed by midwives. The first successful operation on a living woman was reportedly carried out in 1500, by Jacob Nufer, a Swiss pig-gelder, on his wife. From the 16th century onwards the operation was extensively documented and discussed in European medical writings. In the 17th and 18th centuries cases were reported of abdominal piercings by the horns of livestock that subsequently led to 'opportunistic' abdominal births. In the 18th and 19th centuries there were reports also of women performing the operation upon themselves. Its performance on living women was always a subject of considerable controversy because of the very high number of fatalities.

EARLY ATTEMPTS
Women in obstructed labour – sometimes caused by a small or distorted pelvis, usually the result of childhood rickets, congenital deformity or osteomalaciac-type

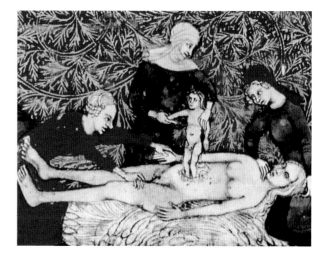

Above
During the medieval period the myth of Julius Caesar's life and miraculous birth were embellished and featured in popular epics, as seen in this 14th-century French manuscript illustration.

Opposite
A drawing of a caesarean section being performed in Central Africa (now Uganda), from the 1880s.

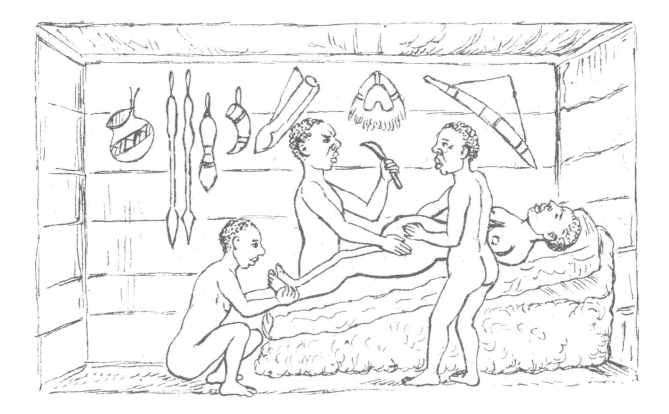

disorders (soft bones) – often struggled for days. If the fetus could be accessed by the vaginal route a hand or, in more severe cases, wooden or metal instruments could be applied to the fetus to remove it whole or piecemeal. Less popular means devised in the 18th century also included dividing the pubic bones to widen the pelvic exit (symphysiotomy) and, where problems were foreseen, early induction of labour.

Women were invariably exhausted and suffered from infections before the caesarean began; their weakened state, combined with deficiencies of surgical technique, inadequate anaesthesia and the inherent risks of haemorrhage [55] and sepsis [54], led to poor outcomes, and many medical men were reluctant to jeopardize their reputations by attempting it. The debate was complicated by ethical and theological issues concerning the priority of life for the mother or the child.

PIONEERING THE OPERATION

Mary Donelly, a midwife, performed the first successful (with the mother surviving) caesarean operation in Ireland in 1738. During the 19th century, obstetricians sometimes resorted to its use in industrial areas of England and Scotland where cases of severe pelvic contraction leading to maternal death were more commonly encountered.

Overall, though it very slowly became more popular, the caesarean remained relatively rare until the late 19th century. In 1876 an Italian obstetrician, Eduardo Porro (1842–1902), pioneered a technique in which haemorrhage and sepsis were minimized through removal of the mother's uterus during the operation, thereby reducing maternal mortality at the cost of subsequent fertility.

FROM LAST RESORT TO EVERYDAY OCCURRENCE

Significant improvements during the late 19th and the 20th centuries in public health, including antenatal care, refinements in surgical techniques, anaesthesia, the advent of antibiotics, intravenous therapies and blood transfusions, and the use of oxytocic drugs (which induce uterine contraction and reduce bleeding), have contributed to making the operation safer and more effective. Continued economic growth, leading to improvements in transport and

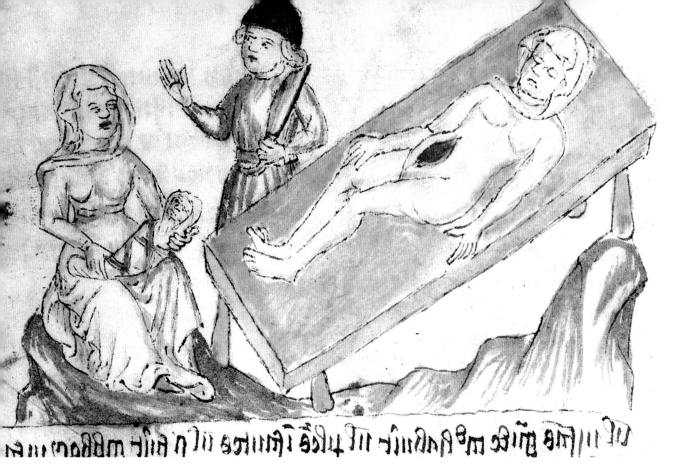

communications, and to increasing urbanization and the development of large maternity units, has meant that fewer women in childbirth are far from an operating theatre. This is reflected in significant reductions in maternal and infant mortality across the developed world.

The popular impression of a caesarean birth today is one of a quick, safe alternative mode of delivery when labour becomes complicated or, in some cases, simply inconvenient. Despite improvements in its effectiveness, however, the operation still constitutes major abdominal surgery, and the procedure is not entirely risk-free, for either mother or baby.

VICTIM OF ITS OWN SUCCESS?

In an increasingly litigious environment, obstetricians, who historically had to justify their resort to caesarean section now more frequently have to justify its non-use. The caesarean rate has climbed from around 3 per cent in the 1950s to as high as 23–33 per cent in parts of the UK and the US, and 98–99 per cent in private clinics in South America. The World Health Organization has determined that a caesarean rate of over 10–15 per cent does not improve maternal and infant outcomes. Although for numerous women it is a life-saving operation, the high rate of caesarean sections in parts of the world today has become an international problem and a cause of concern to many health care professionals and health economists.

Above
An illustration from *Apocalypsis S. Johannis* (The Apocalypse of St John), *c.* 1420–30. The dead mother lies on the bench while the surgeon wields his knife and a woman holds the swaddled child: possibly a depiction of the birth of the antichrist.

Opposite
A plate from Hermann Friedrich Kilian's *Geburtshülflicher Atlas* (Obstetrical Atlas), 1835–44, showing procedures for caesarean section: making the incision; delivering the baby using forceps; and binding the abdomen after the operation.

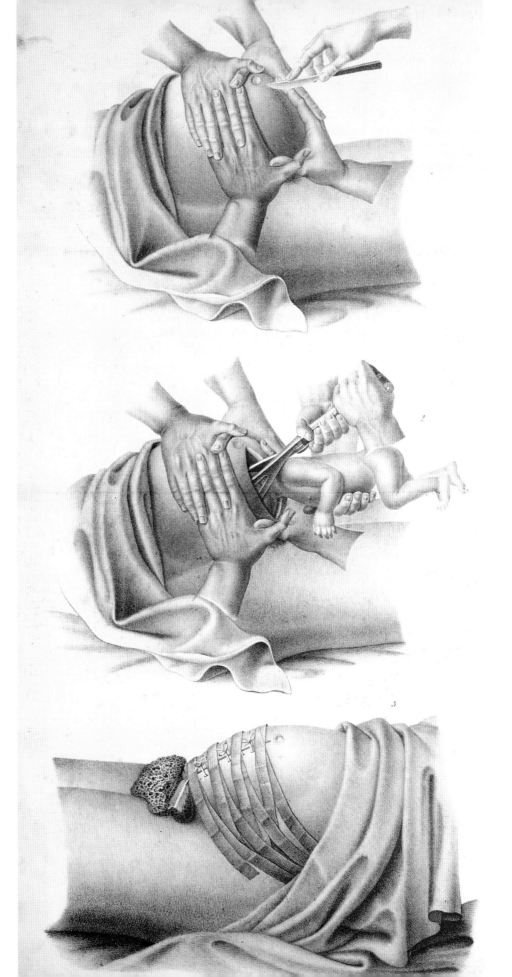

59. CARDIAC SURGERY
Pushing the limits

Tom Treasure

Surgery of the heart has probably reached the limits set by
Nature to all surgery: no new method, and no new discovery, can
overcome the natural difficulties that attend a wound of the heart.
Stephen Paget, 1896

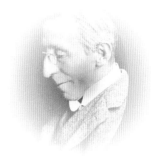

Right
Stephen Paget, surgeon and animal experimentation campaigner.
Paget thought the heart beyond the reach of the surgeon's knife
at the end of the 19th century.

Opposite
A plate from Robert Carswell's *Pathological Anatomy: illustrations*
of the elementary forms of disease (1833–38) showing the changes in
the heart wall that precede and accompany the formation of dilations
in its muscle.

It remained a widely accepted truth among the medical
profession for more than 50 years after the statement
quoted above that the heart was beyond the bounds
of surgery. Stephen Paget (1856–1926) was a surgeon
working in London, and in his 460-page textbook, *The*
Surgery of the Chest, he described the state of the art
at that time, including how chest surgery should be
performed and the outcome that might be expected for
a range of injuries and diseases. He could not find any
account of even a simple suture to the heart such as
would be needed to close a stab wound. His statement
reflected his times. The heart beat defined life; the
technical and conceptual barriers to operating seemed
insurmountable. Yet today heart surgery is routine.

TENTATIVE BEGINNINGS
In Paget's time physicians had a clear understanding
of the mechanics of the heart. They perceived how the
pumping chambers (ventricles) push blood out into the
arteries, to the lungs and to the body [11]. By correlating
what they heard through the stethoscope [22] and what
they saw in the heart when their patients died, they knew
that the valves might either be narrowed and obstruct

blood flow, or leak and make the heart inefficient. In
the 19th century when rheumatic fever was rife they
were all too familiar with the damage done to the heart
valves by this disease, and in particular the narrowing
of the mitral valve, called mitral stenosis. Two London
physicians, D. W. Samways in 1898 and Sir Thomas
Lauder Brunton in 1902, suggested that a surgeon might
be able to open the valve. The idea was firmly rebutted.
Only in 1923 in Boston, USA, and in 1925 in London, did
Elliot Cutler and Henry Souttar do as they suggested,
both with initial success in that the patient survived and
symptoms were relieved. There followed a number of
failures, and no further attempts were made for more
than 20 years, during which time the opposing medical
views became more firmly entrenched.

GREATER CONFIDENCE
Two things changed. Surgeons developed both skills and
confidence in operating within the chest, including on
the large blood vessels delivering blood from the heart.
From the late 1930s isolated successful operations were
reported in children with birth defects affecting the
main vessels outside the heart. Then, during the Second

Plate III.

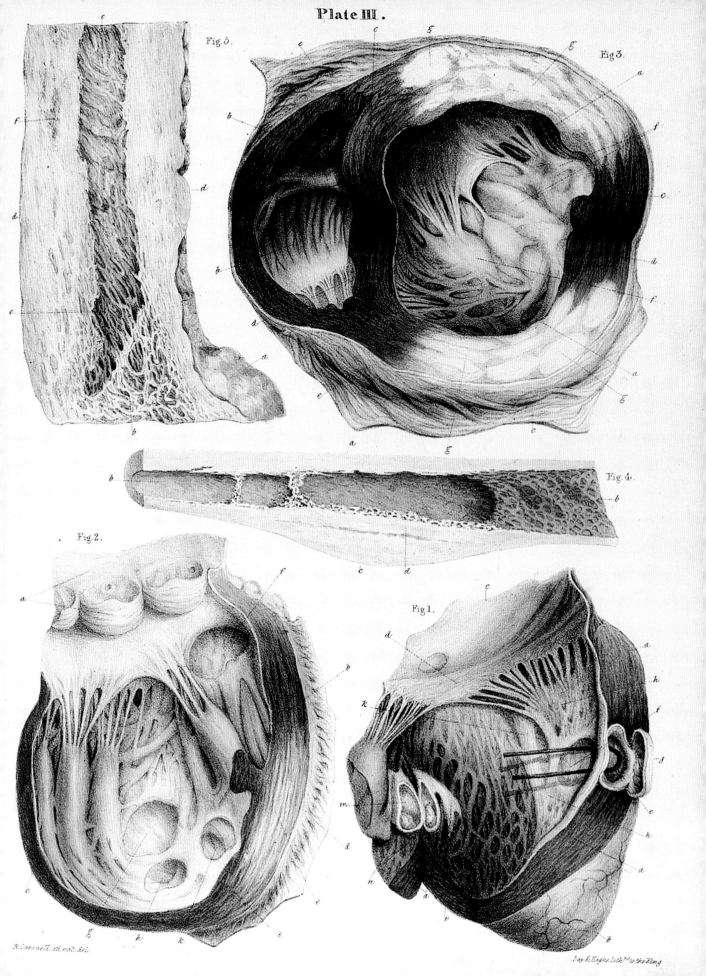

Fig. 5.

Fig. 3.

Fig. 4.

Fig. 2.

Fig. 1.

R. Carswell ad nat. del.

Day & Haghe lith. to the King.

World War, Dwight Harken (1910–93), an American surgeon working in a US military hospital in Cirencester, England, performed 139 operations to remove bullets and shrapnel in and around the heart, without a death. If it was possible to reach into the beating heart with instruments to retrieve a bullet, then why not to open a narrowed valve? In 1948 Harken was one of three surgeons successfully to perform the operation of mitral valvotomy, to open up the mitral valve.

The landmark that established mitral valvotomy was a publication by Russell Brock (1903–80), a British chest and heart surgeon, who did not report his efforts until he had performed nine operations, with seven surviving successes. Two of the operations were performed in Johns Hopkins Hospital, Baltimore.

AN EXPANDING REPERTOIRE

Brock had set up a fruitful collaboration with Alfred Blalock (1899–1964), who had come to Guy's Hospital in London to share experience in operating on 'blue babies' – children with birth defects resulting in deoxygenated blood not being routed to the lungs but perfusing the body. Various operations were devised by them and others that ameliorated this problem, but they were severely limited in what they could do because the child's heart had to be kept beating to sustain life throughout any attempts at surgery. This was the next obstacle to be overcome.

Four possible solutions were considered. One was the exploration of ingenious ways of working within the beating heart. Thanks to modern radiology and catheter-tip devices this has now been realized for a number of heart problems. Another was to connect the child to the mother's circulation with pipes. Though this was indeed performed in a few instances, the quip that it provided an opportunity to have an operation with 200 per cent mortality sums up the limitations. The third, cooling the patient to below 20°C (68°F), was an established technique, and is still used as a means of protecting the brain if the blood flow has to be halted.

The fourth solution, and the method that is now standard practice, is cardiopulmonary bypass, in which all the blood is diverted to a machine, oxygenated and redelivered to the patient beyond the heart. John H. Gibbon (1903–73), of Jefferson Medical College, Philadelphia, began work on an artificial heart-lung machine in the late 1930s, but routine success only finally came in 1953 at the Mayo Clinic.

In the early days cardiopulmonary bypass was a major hazard in itself, but many incremental refinements in materials and design from the 1960s to the 1990s mean that in expert and practised hands

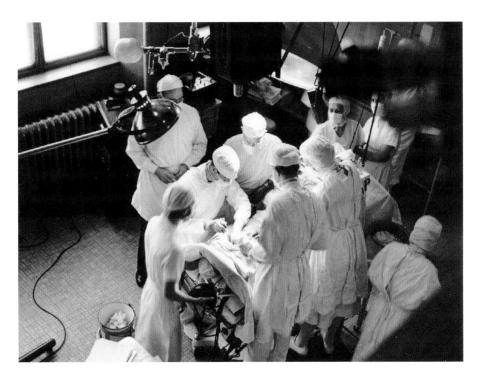

Left
Alfred Blalock operating on a 'blue baby' in 1945. His technician Vivien Thomas, standing behind him, offered advice on suturing. The operation created a Blalock-Taussig shunt – an alternative path for the passage of deoxygenated blood back to the lungs.

Opposite
A plate from Henry Souttar's paper in the *British Medical Journal* (1925) in which he reported his operation for opening the mitral valve in the heart after its narrowing as a consequence of rheumatic fever.

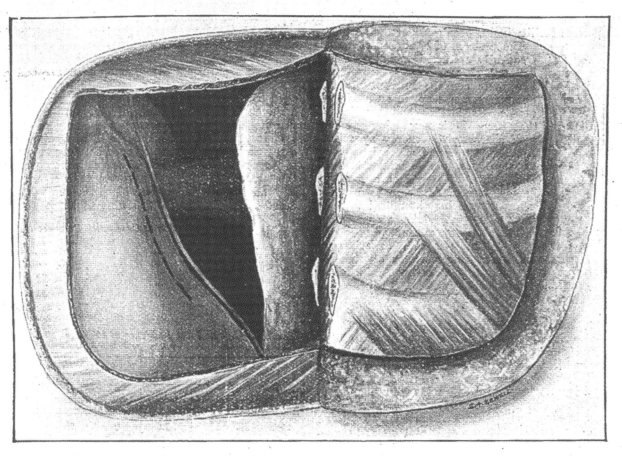

FIG. 2.—Ribs divided, and flap, formed by cutting through muscles and costal cartilages, turned back; left side of pericardium exposed.

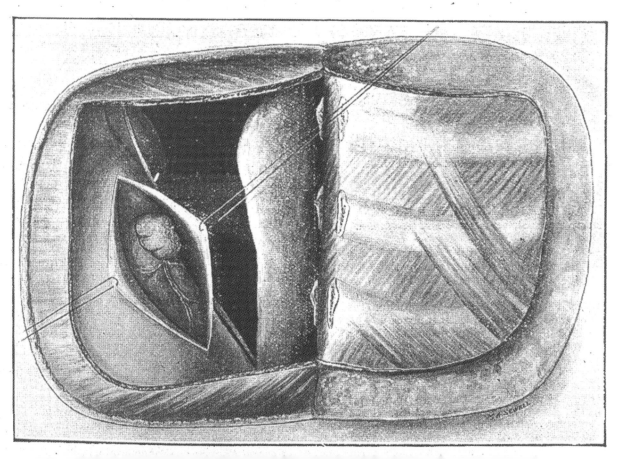

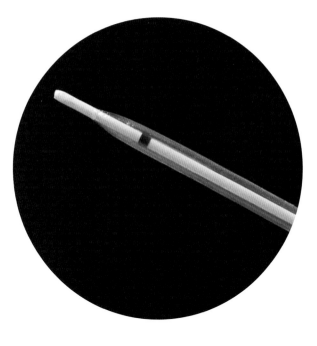

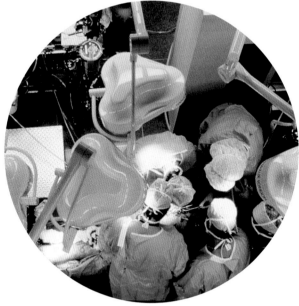

the inherent risk is now very low. Thanks to this technology there are now few structural abnormalities of the heart, whether resulting from birth defects or acquired disease, that cannot be corrected. It is interesting that coronary artery surgery at its inception in the late 1960s depended on cardiopulmonary bypass to allow the surgeon to open and suture blood vessels of 2–3 mm. By the 1990s, surgical skill, experience and the development of stabilizing devices meant that this surgery could be performed on the beating heart.

A variety of mechanical and animal tissue valves became available from the 1960s and it was possible to replace any one or several of the heart valves. There are serious limitations to their use, however. Animal tissue valves have so far all been prone to fail in time, typically after 7–12 years, leading to the need for repeat operations, often in old age. Mechanical valves rarely escape problems of blood clotting, so life-long anti-coagulation is mandatory. Here, too, there is an interesting reversal: conservation of the native valves is performed when possible in current practice – although the techniques are considerably refined compared with mitral valvotomy within the beating heart.

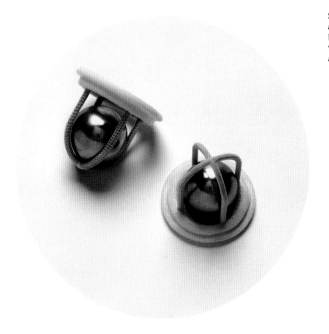

Starr-Edwards replacement heart valves (made of plastic and metal and contained in sterile cases) were the product of collaboration between a young surgeon (Albert Starr) and an engineer (Miles 'Lowell' Edwards) in the USA. The first human replacement of an aortic valve for stenosis was performed in 1960.

AUDACITY REWARDED?

Heart transplantation took the world by storm when it was first performed by Christiaan Barnard in Cape Town in 1967 [60]. Over the next three to four years about 150 hearts were transplanted, many of them by quite unprepared teams and with almost universal short survival. To ensure success, a new definition of death, based on brain death rather than cessation of the heart beat, was needed. As a result of the rather reckless uptake, clinical failure and an outcry about the ethics of removing what were ideally still-beating hearts, there was a worldwide moratorium, imposed in some countries and negotiated in others.

A resurgence in the 1980s was associated with much improved short-term survival, although the unresolved problems of tissue rejection and the inescapable fact that someone has to die to provide a heart for transplantation limit the number of operations performed. The resulting use of hearts from executed prisoners and health tourism allowing those who can afford it to avail themselves of these resources has opened a debate about ethics and medicine in a global marketplace.

By far the greatest impact of heart surgery in the last 30 years has been for atherosclerotic heart disease. The developed world led an epidemic in arterial disease related to a diet high in animal fats, smoking and a more sedentary lifestyle. Coronary artery surgery is highly effective and can be performed with remarkably low risk. Changes in lifestyle and the development of cholesterol-lowering drugs [51] have reduced the incidence of such operations, and since the 1980s a progressively improving, minimally invasive technique of reopening coronary arteries with balloons threaded into the circulation (percutaneous angioplasty) has reduced the numbers of patients receiving this surgery.

60. TRANSPLANT SURGERY
Diseases & organs, self & non-self

Thomas Schlich

One should not prematurely ridicule a therapy that aims at replacing an organ that has become dysfunctional.
Otto Lanz, 1894–97

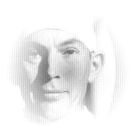

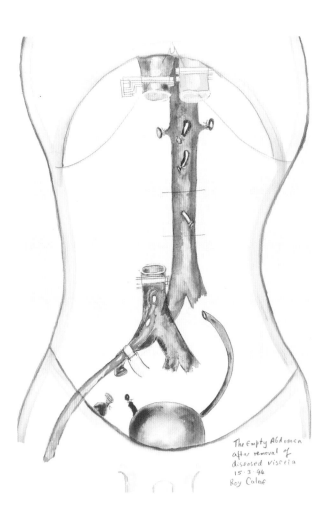

The Empty Abdomen
after removal of
diseased viscera
15·3·94
Roy Calne

On 2 December 1967 the surgeon Christiaan Barnard (1922–2001) took the heart of Denise Larvall, a brain-dead road accident victim, and put it into the chest of Louis Washkansky, a patient with end-stage cardiac disease [59], where it continued to beat for 18 days. Contemporary commentators saw this operation as a milestone in modern history that changed the world forever – on a par with the first moon landing a couple of years later. And indeed, organ transplants were a radical break both with the way diseases were traditionally treated, and with how the human body had been understood for centuries.

Transplant surgery is based on two assumptions. According to the first assumption – the concept of organ replacement – doctors can cure a complex internal disease by replacing an isolated organ of the body, such as a heart, a liver or a kidney. The second assumption – the concept of exchangeability – is that it is possible to use someone else's organ to perform a function one's own cannot, in other words that the difference between self and non-self can be overcome [18]. Both ideas did not exist before the 1880s. Until well into the 19th century the body was seen as an individual

Above left
Christiaan Barnard in his operating clothes: he became a surgical icon and celebrity after the 1967 heart transplant, appearing on the cover of *Time* magazine a couple weeks after performing the operation.

Above
A watercolour by British liver transplant pioneer, Sir Roy Calne. Here he has captured the abdomen of a patient awaiting the transplantation of several organs to replace diseased ones, a symbol of transplantation's unique ability to treat internal diseases by surgical means.

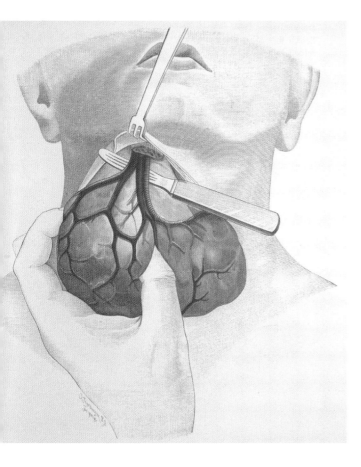

and functional whole, interacting with its external environment. People believed that diseases were caused by disruptions in the balance of the body's fluid constituents, its 'humours' [04], resulting from the sick person's way of life or some other environmental factor. Disease could be treated by changing an individual's environment or lifestyle, or by restoring the humoral balance through vomiting, purging and blood-letting. Replacing an organ would have appeared ridiculous to many people, even in 1894, as the quote above shows.

THE FIRST STEPS

Modern surgeons, by contrast, treat the body as a composite of individual organs and tissues with particular functions. Disease can affect their structure or their function, and surgery can cure these problems by removing the diseased structures or restoring function. In the second half of the 19th century the strategy of cutting out the disease proved to be particularly successful, for example in cases of cancer or tuberculous joints. Another of these diseases was goitre – a potentially life-threatening enlargement of the thyroid gland.

In the hands of the brilliant Swiss surgeon Theodor Kocher (1841–1917) the removal of the goitre became a safe procedure. Kocher was so good at the operation that he could take out the whole thyroid gland without risking his patient's life. This radical solution seemed to be sensible in those cases in which the goitre tended to grow back, so that the patients had to submit themselves to the complicated operation several times. At that time, the role of the gland in the body was completely unknown. In fact, it only became apparent as a consequence of Kocher's radical operations. After the removal of their thyroid, patients developed a characteristic clinical picture, which included physical weakness, mental sluggishness, swollen hands and feet, a puffy face and anaemia – all symptoms we associate today with impaired thyroid function [17].

As a reaction to the unexpected consequences of his operation, Kocher tried to reverse the removal. In July 1883 he took thyroid tissue from a patient's goitre and transplanted it to another patient who was suffering from the effects of complete thyroid removal. This attempt to cure a complex of symptoms by replacing an organ constituted the first organ transplantation in our modern sense. It became the prototype for all other organ transplants and the starting gun for research into organ replacement.

Above
'Surgical removal of a goitre': this plate from Theodor Kocher's *Chirurgische Operationslehre* (a textbook on surgical operations) illustrates what became the first part of his revolutionary transplantation of thyroid tissue from those with too much to those with too little. This was a byproduct of his surgical cure of goitres and an eventual component of his surgical research programme into the function of the thyroid, its disorders and treatment.

Researchers performed thyroid removal on animals, meticulously documenting the effects and subsequently checking their findings by reinserting the organ. Soon the same technique was adapted to other organs, starting with other endocrine glands – pancreas, testes, ovaries, suprarenal glands. By creating and then stopping disease symptoms at will, physiologists and surgeons were able to determine the function of particular organs and bring about a better understanding of a number of hitherto mysterious diseases and their treatment, such as diabetes, which was redefined as a lack of the function of a certain portion of the pancreas [65]. Kocher became the first surgeon to be awarded the Nobel Prize in 1909 for his discovery of the thyroid gland's function.

THE PROBLEM OF REJECTION

In parallel to such transplant experiments on animals, surgeons also started to use transplantation in the treatment of human patients. Among many other transplants, in 1905 Alexis Carrel (1873–1944) in New York City carried out the first heart transplant in a dog, and in 1906 Mathieu Jaboulay (1860–1913) in Lyons performed the first kidney transplant in a human being. It seemed only to be a question of time before all diseased organs and tissues could be replaced by healthy ones, and surgeons were busy developing techniques to make that possible. Now that the idea

of organ replacement was generally acknowledged, the second assumption of transplant medicine, the exchangeability of body parts, appeared on the agenda.

This issue became obvious after the French-American Carrel, who in 1912 was the second surgeon to win a Nobel Prize (for his work on blood vessel surgery and transplantation), had perfected his surgical technique to such an extent that he noticed that the success of transplants between individuals was blocked by a problem that could not be solved by surgical means. His experimental transplants showed that organs survived for an unlimited period of time, as long as they were transplanted within the same animal. If transplanted between different individuals, the organs invariably perished. Apparently, organ tissues possessed some kind of biological individuality.

Some researchers made the immune system [18] responsible for what was increasingly called the 'rejection' of foreign tissues. However, all attempts to prevent transplant rejection by suppressing the recipient's immune reaction or by selecting suitable donors failed. As a result, organ transplantation was gradually abandoned in the course of the 1920s.

Opposite
Alexis Carrel depicted as a magician in the French satirical medical magazine *Chanteclair*. His experiments garnered him the Nobel Prize in Medicine in 1912 and a burlesque fame for what he might achieve through tissue culture and transplantation.

Milestones in Transplant Medicine

1883	first organ transplant (thyroid) to treat a complex internal disease
c. **1900**	organ replacement concept generally acknowledged
1902	first kidney transplant in a dog
1905	first heart transplant in a dog
1906	first kidney transplant in a human
1912	Nobel Prize for Alexis Carrel for his revolutionary technique for suturing blood vessels in organ transplants
1920–45	stagnation of transplant research
1945	new start of transplant medicine; kidney transplant in Boston
1954	first successful kidney transplant between identical twins
1962	first successful kidney transplant from a non-related donor
1967	first successful heart transplant
1968	commission at Harvard University defines brain death as personal death
1969	founding of agency 'Eurotransplant' for transnational allocation of transplants according to compatibility criteria
1982	introduction of new immune suppressant cyclosporine
1980s	increase of transplant survival times, success with heart, lung, liver, pancreas transplants

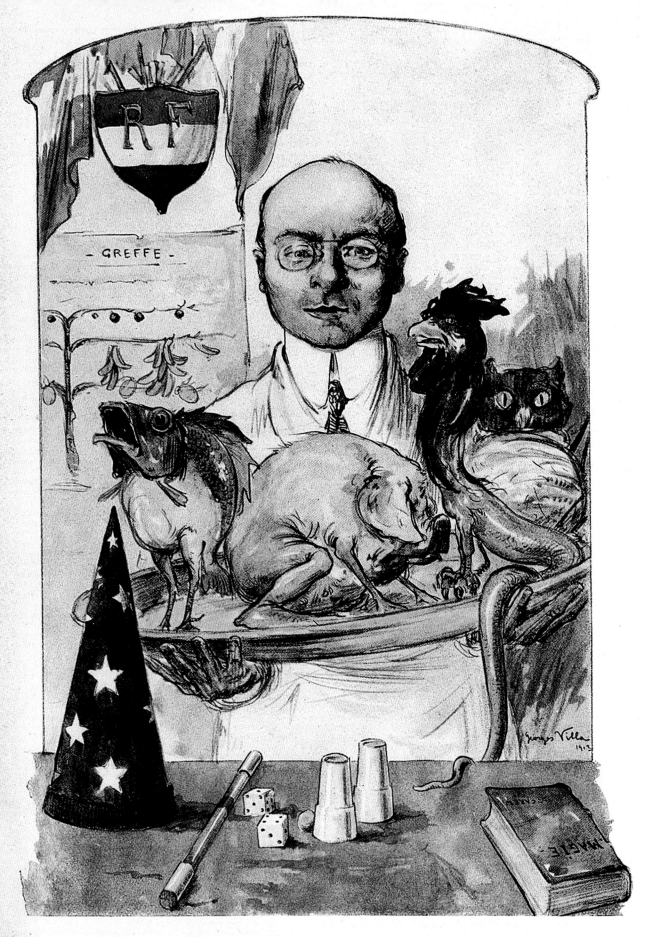

Le Docteur CARREL, de New-York

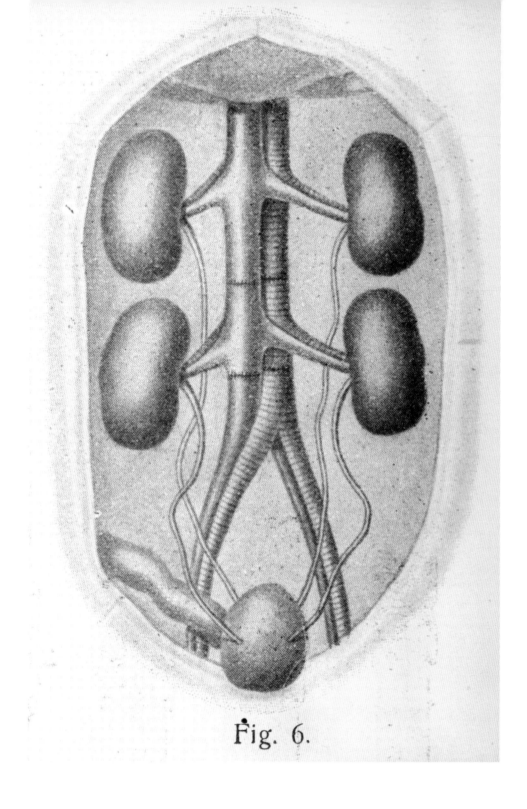

Fig. 6.

Illustration showing the experimental transplantation of an additional
set of kidneys into a dog (1910) in order to try out different surgical
techniques of transplantation.

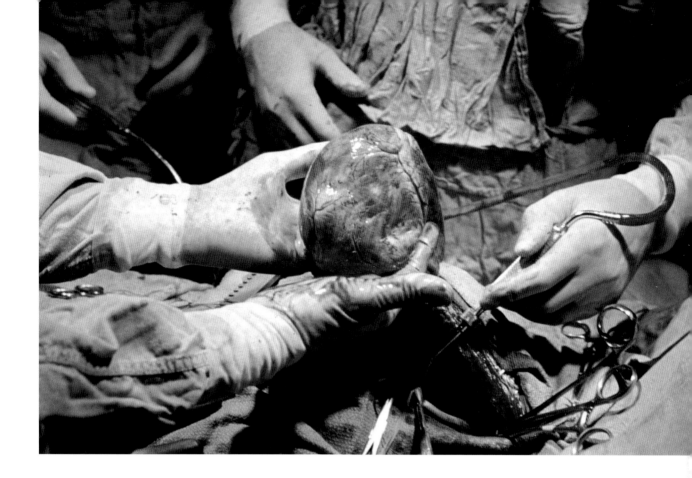

Then in 1945 surgeons at Peter Bent Brigham Hospital in Boston initiated a new phase in the history of organ transplants when they transplanted a kidney from a dead donor to a woman suffering from renal failure. Even though this and subsequent transplants failed, this time the American surgeons did not abandon their efforts. In 1954, at the same hospital, a kidney was transplanted from one healthy identical twin to his brother, who had severe renal disease. The transplant worked and earned the surgeon, Joseph E. Murray (1919–), the Nobel Prize in 1990.

ORGAN EXCHANGEABILITY ACHIEVED

In order to make transplantation applicable on a broader scale, however, surgeons had to discover how to suppress the recipient's immunological reaction to the transplant. In 1962 the first successful kidney transplantation from a non-related donor was performed, again in Boston. Immune suppression had been achieved by the antimetabolic agent azathioprine. This approach was subsequently perfected, so that more effective but simultaneously more selective immune suppression became possible. At the same time, efforts

to select suitable organs from non-related donors were being made with the help of tissue typing using the Human Leucocyte Antigen (HLA) system as a marker of compatibility.

The issue of exchangeability had finally been solved. For all practical purposes organs had become exchangeable. They could now indeed be used for curing a complex internal disease by replacing the particular affected body part – an approach that became self-evident in 1967 when the first heart transplant fascinated the world.

However, transplantation will continue to raise a number of relevant cultural and ethical issues concerning personal identity and the definition of human life. After all, it is a technology that transcends boundaries of the individual body that had previously been taken for granted.

A living heart is held in the hands of one of the surgical team during a heart transplant procedure. This is now a common operation, but is limited by the number of donors.

61. **HIP REPLACEMENT**
New for old

Thomas Schlich

*The man-made replacement, of plastic and metal,
removes all pain and usually results in improved mobility.
There is a 95 per cent success rate for such operations.*
Independent, 17 November 1995

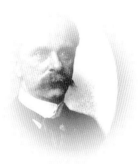

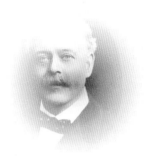

The quote above came from a spokesman for the British
Arthritis and Rheumatism Council in connection with
the first hip replacement that Queen Elizabeth, the
Queen Mother received in 1995, at the age of 95, for a
chronic hip ailment. When three years later the popular
patient underwent a second successful operation
(this time after a hip fracture), the number of total hip
replacements (THR) in England and Wales amounted to
46,601 prostheses. Ten years later, by 2008, the number
had hit the 80,000 mark.

TRIALS

Until well into the 20th century, chronic disease of
the hip joint was a painful and debilitating condition
for which, despite its frequency, medicine had little to
offer. However, there had been a long history of surgical
experimentation to solve the problem. Surgeons tried
to rebuild the hip joint (arthroplasty), sometimes using
artificial material. Themistocles Gluck (1853–1942) in
Germany performed the first operation of arthroplasty
of the hip in 1890; Robert Jones (1857–1933) used gold
foil in his arthroplasty in 1908, and Ernest William
Hey-Groves (1872–1944) replaced the femoral head

Above left
Themistocles Gluck, the orthopaedic surgeon who performed the
first hip arthroplasty – an operation to realign or reconstruct the joint.

Above right
Robert Jones was one of Britain's leading orthopaedic surgeons,
whose work on hip arthroplasty was part of his wider innovative
practice in and around Liverpool. John Charnley, who developed a
standard hip replacement prosthesis, would later train in the hospital
Jones co-founded.

Opposite
A Charnley-type hip replacement made from cobalt alloy by Chas F.
Thackray Ltd. As well as the question of the design of the replacement
hip ball, there were considerable difficulties to be overcome to allow
smooth movement without adverse wear and tear in the replacement
hip socket.

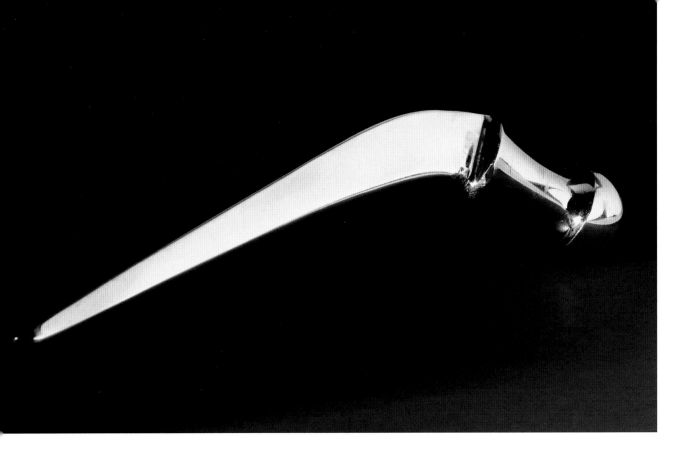

with an ivory prosthesis in 1922. And in 1923 Marius Smith-Petersen (1886–1953), in Boston, introduced the mould or cup arthroplasty, for which he used glass. Essentially, a cup was fitted over the head of the femur, which then moved against that cup rather than the diseased bone socket.

Results were disappointing, however. In 1946 the brothers Robert (1901–80) and Jean (1905–95) Judet of Paris replaced their patients' femoral head with an acrylic prosthesis. Unfortunately, the acrylic wore and broke in many of the recipients, and invariably became loose in the bone. The shape of the prosthesis was modified, and copied in steel, vitallium and other materials, but still the procedure did not provide lasting results.

SUCCESSES

In 1938 Philip Wiles (1899–1966) inserted the first total hip prosthesis into a patient at the Middlesex Hospital in London, although it was not entirely satisfactory. This was a stainless steel device, the femoral and acetabular (socket) parts being fixed to the bones with screws. From the 1950s several surgeons worked on improving

total hip replacement in Britain. The most successful of the British surgical inventors was John Charnley (1911–82), who influenced the development of hip replacement more than any other individual. Charnley created a hospital unit devoted to hip surgery in a sanatorium at Wrightington in Lancashire, northern England, to tackle the various problems of hip replacement.

The first obstacle was the issue of excessive friction within the joint. To deal with this Charnley reduced the size of the femoral head and used stainless steel to make it. For the hip socket he used a low-friction plastic, first Teflon, which turned out to be the wrong material because of wear, and subsequently high-density polyethylene. The other principle introduced by Charnley was the application of dental acrylic cement to fix the prosthesis in the patient's bone. Charnley had learnt of the cement from Dennis Smith, a material scientist in the Dental School of Manchester University. This basic design remained unchanged until the 1980s, though a greater range of femoral replacement lengths, stronger stainless steels and a new finish (Vaquasheen) were developed from the 1970s.

TEAMWORK

Creating a hip prosthesis was not just a surgical challenge – above all it also involved issues of design and materials, which could only be overcome by collaborating with bio-engineers and manufacturers. Though Charnley was in some ways a self-taught engineer – he had his own lathe to make instruments – he collaborated with a series of academic engineers, and at Wrightington he was ably supported by a succession of technicians. In addition, he was in a position to draw on a number of local industrial firms and university departments in Manchester.

For the production of his hip replacement, Charnley chose to work with a small manufacturing company, Chas F. Thackray Ltd in Leeds, which had made instruments for him. In many ways this relationship was the foundation for the development of his prostheses. In 1966 Charnley came to an arrangement with Thackray that, instead of royalties, the firm would pay to his research fund a sum of one pound sterling per complete prosthesis sold by them, thus securing independent funds for his work.

Charnley systematically developed both the prosthesis and the operation and collected excellent data. However, he was concerned that other surgeons would use his prosthesis but not follow his techniques carefully enough, and that if dislocation occurred they would blame the prosthesis and tarnish its reputation. Therefore, Charnley initially restricted the use of his prosthesis to those surgeons to whom he had given his personal approval. Like other contemporary inventors of orthopaedic implants and instruments, he arranged courses to instruct his colleagues and created a global network of surgeons who used his technology. But that did not prevent a much wider and less careful diffusion of his methods. For example, surgeons went to their own manufacturers and asked for copies of the Charnley hip. In the end, the restrictions could not be maintained.

Charnley's prosthesis proved reliable and has been widely used and imitated in all Western countries. With its improvements and derivatives, it remains a standard internationally. With an estimated 959,000 hip prosthesis operations taking place annually in the world in 2010, total hip replacement has become the basis of a major growth in elective orthopaedic surgery and a model for improving the life of older people by surgical means.

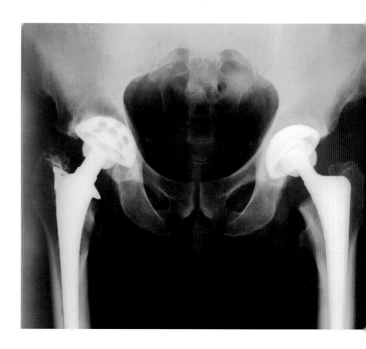

Above
An X-ray showing the replacement of both hip joints. The metal prostheses have to be attached to the femur – the thigh bone – as well as to the hip bone, and Charnley's solution to this problem was to look to the material (poly-methyl-methacrylate) used by dentists for fillings and dentures.

Opposite
A replacement 'ball and socket' in the hip joint, revealed in an X-ray. The acetabular cup replaces the natural socket in the pelvis, the acetabulum. Cartilage and bone are removed from the acetabulum and the cup is attached with cement and temporarily pinned.

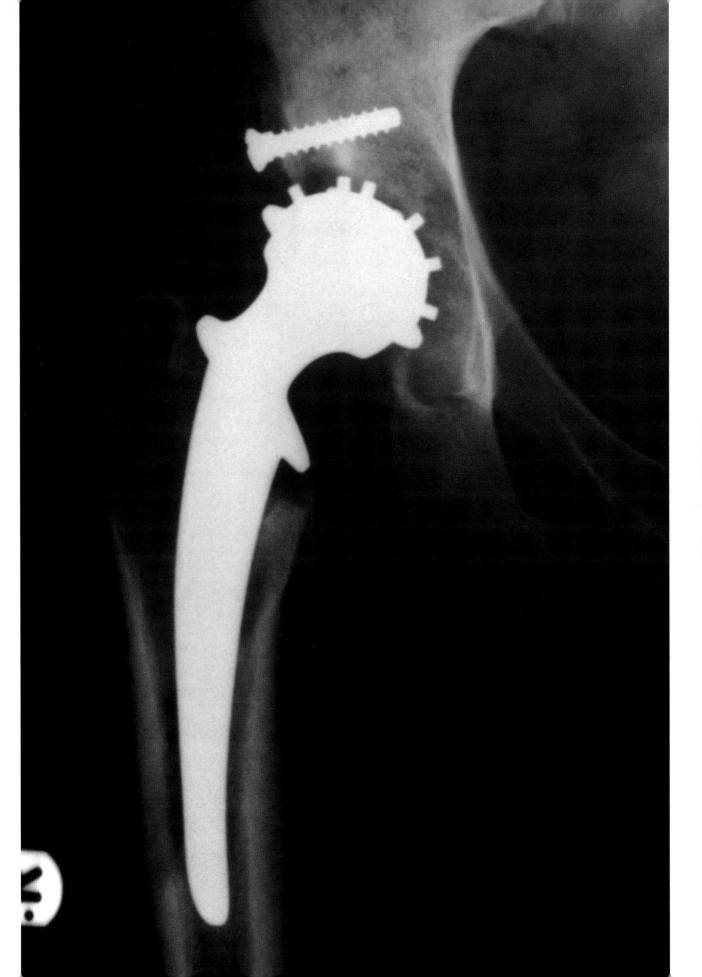

62. KEYHOLE SURGERY
Through the looking glass

Thomas Schlich

We must now acknowledge that the procedure from which
our patients may benefit in the future may not always involve
an incision, sponges, scissors or sutures.
David L. Nahrwold, 1989

Since the 1990s, many open surgical operations have
been replaced by 'minimally invasive surgery' or
'keyhole surgery'. The underlying principle consists
of inserting a miniaturized camera inside a patient's
body, connecting the camera to a television monitor and
viewing magnified images on a screen. Doctors can then
perform complex operations by directing instruments
to anatomical structures through either a natural orifice
(endoscopy) or through small incisions in the abdominal
wall (laparoscopy). Having been developed by internists
(specialists in internal diseases), the concepts of keyhole
techniques were taken up in gynaecology, initially as a
diagnostic tool and then for therapeutic purposes, and
finally were adopted by surgeons.

Over the course of the 19th century, physicians had
started using rigid or flexible tubes to look inside the
living body [30]. The first laparoscopic interventions
through such tubes were attempted around 1900.
In subsequent decades, gynaecologists in particular
began using this approach, and, during the 1970s,
they embraced the scope technique on a massive scale,
most often for laparoscopic sterilizations by tying the
Fallopian tubes.

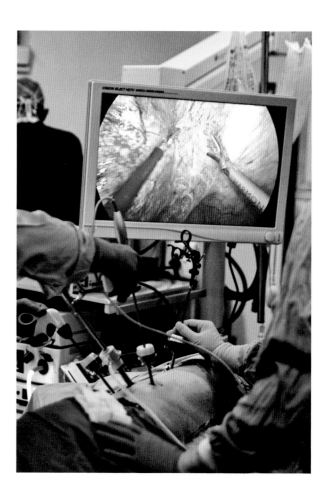

Above
Keyhole surgery: using the laparoscope, which is connected to a
camera linked to a screen and a range of miniature instruments,
surgeons no longer need to open up the body to see and work inside it.

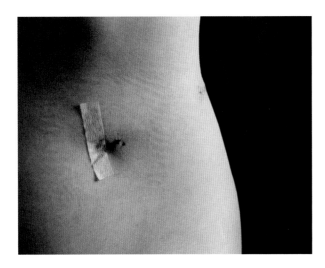

A significant new development came in the 1980s and 1990s when existing endoscopic and laparoscopic techniques were linked up with video technology. Doctors learnt that they could easily and effectively evaporate or excise diseased or troublesome tissues that they had diagnosed through their scopes using blades, heater probes, electrocautery or lasers. To the surprise of the surgical establishment, within a few years the numbers of procedures soared. In contrast to the usual pattern of surgical innovation, the rapid spread of keyhole surgery was largely driven by patient demand rather than surgeon interest.

Once minimally invasive surgery had been adopted on a large scale, the use of laparoscopy in surgical operations was explored in many different ways. The range of application of the technique now includes even the most routine, 'bread-and-butter' procedures of modern surgery, such as appendectomy and the repair of hernias. It turned out to be especially successful in the removal of gallstones, and by the 1990s began to challenge the role of open surgery in the management of the classic gall bladder case. The laparoscopic approach has also been applied to small bowel, colon and lung surgery, as well as the removal of spleens, adrenal glands, kidneys, uteruses and lymph glands, among other procedures. Often it is only after minimally invasive alternatives have been exhausted or ruled out that open surgery takes place today.

This trend has continued into the 21st century, with an even broader variety of instruments and techniques, including natural orifice transluminal endoscopic surgery (NOTES). In NOTES an endoscope, equipped with a tiny scalpel, is passed through a natural body orifice, such as the mouth, urethra or anus. The endoscope then cuts a hole, perhaps in the stomach wall, allowing surgeons to direct it to the organ needing removal. In this way, the gall bladder, for example, can be removed through the mouth.

Medical
TRIUMPHS

Nº 7.

People in the developed world now live longer, suffer less pain and are healthier than even their grandparents were two generations ago. Ironically, we also have less confidence in medicine and doctoring than our forebears.

The reasons for a healthier longevity are complex, and the real medical improvements that have been made during the past century are only a part of the story. Some of these advances are described in this final section, and they illustrate the variety of paths – technological, scientific, clinical, social – that can lead to a longer lifespan with an unimpeded quality of life.

Few things have improved infant survival rates more than vaccination programmes for the common scourges of early life. Vaccination can radically reduce the threat of measles, whooping cough, diphtheria and many other childhood diseases; it helped eliminate smallpox and promises to do the same for polio. Remarkably, vaccination could also have a dramatic influence on cervical cancer, which is frequently caused by a virus – a vaccine has been developed. The discovery of vitamins was also a major breakthrough, especially since germ theory (invasion from the outside) so dominated medical thinking in the early 20th century. That disease could be caused by the *absence* of something required another, new way of thinking about health and disease.

Two decades before penicillin became a wonder drug, insulin had already been hailed as such. Unlike penicillin, which sometimes could radically cure, insulin merely helped control a frequently fatal disease, diabetes. But it was an early example of what modern medicine actually does best: manage chronic illness. Without necessarily curing the underlying disorder, doctors can often prolong productive life, and with an ageing population throughout the developed world, that is exactly what they are called on to do. Insulin-dependent diabetics must themselves be methodical in their lives and personal care. For people with permanent kidney failure, dialysis with an artificial kidney can literally become a way of life. (For many, of course, a new transplanted kidney is the ultimate goal.)

In the early 20th century, cigarette smoking became a symbol of modernity, of liberated women and virile men. It also coincided with an epidemic of lung cancer, although it took a generation before the correlation was made. The early work – British and American – was done in the 1950s, but the campaign for tobacco control still goes on, an indication of how difficult it is to change habits, and how powerful multinational corporations are.

The relationship between smoking and health is at the heart of what is called 'lifestyle medicine' – no smoking, proper diet, exercise, moderate alcohol – and has given contemporary medicine a new moral role. So, too, has medicine's capacity sometimes to help couples have the baby they desire. Assisted reproduction relies on much science and even more technology, and can transform people's lives.

A medical triumph of a different sort was the remarkable discovery that a common complaint – peptic ulcer – was often caused by a germ, *Helicobacter pylori*, and could be cured by a course of antibiotics rather than merely managed by a lifetime of antacids. The description of its elucidation is written in the first person, by one of the two people who shared the Nobel Prize for proving that very important things can still be uncovered by traditional and relatively simple experiments.

A syringe being loaded with vaccine against H5N1 bird flu during a clinical trial in Hanoi, Vietnam, in 2008. Vaccines have changed the human experience of disease for the better, but must be rigorously tested – like any medical intervention – to ensure they do not cause more harm than good.

63. VACCINES
Preventing disease

John Ford

He is a better Physician that keeps diseases off us, than he that cures them being on us. Prevention is so much better than healing, because it saves the labour of being sick.
Thomas Adams, 1618

Immunization is a method of increasing the resistance of a human or animal to infectious agents so that they do not get a disease, or if they do, suffer from it in a much-reduced form. It has led to the eradication of smallpox worldwide and the control of potential killer diseases such as diphtheria and measles.

BEYOND JENNER

In the same way that Edward Jenner (1749–1823) used a different form of the disease to promote resistance to smallpox [**40**], Louis Pasteur (1822–95) injected an attenuated living bacterium successfully to immunize chickens against chicken cholera in 1880. The first use of this technique on a human was in 1885, when Pasteur used a series of different-strength rabies vaccines to save the life of Joseph Meister, a young boy who had been bitten by a rabid dog.

Live vaccines work by stimulating the body's immune system – this is known as active immunization. The vaccine used against tuberculosis [**38**], Bacille Calmette-Guérin (BCG), introduced in 1921, was another live vaccine. Some vaccines are produced using killed bacilli, such as that against plague [**34**], introduced by Waldemar Haffkine (1860–1930) and Alexandre Yersin (1863–1943). The germs of diphtheria and tetanus produce their effects by releasing a powerful toxin [**18**]. Administration of the relevant anti-toxin, modified chemically to a toxoid, protects the patient. This is passive immunization.

E. W. Goodpasture (1886–1960) introduced the use of fertile hen's eggs as a growing medium for viruses in 1931. Using this method, Jonas Salk (1914–95) developed an inactivated vaccine against poliomyelitis and Albert Sabin (1906–93) followed with a live one [**41**]. There was much discussion about their relative merits, with different countries favouring one or the other,

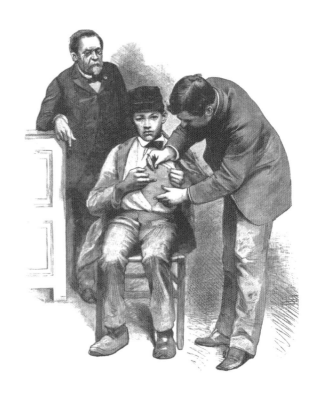

Above
Louis Pasteur looks on in 1885 as Joseph Meister is inoculated with anti-rabies vaccine after being bitten by a rabid dog. Pasteur was not a doctor and therefore could not administer the vaccine himself. Meister survived and went on to become the caretaker at the Pasteur Institute in Paris.

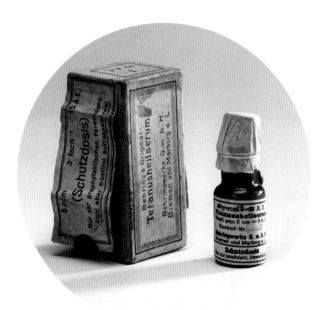

Above
A bottle of tetanus serum and its packaging, 1915, used to treat and provide a short-lived protection against tetanus or 'lockjaw'. The causative bacteria of tetanus, which release a powerful neurotoxin, multiply in low-oxygen conditions such as deep puncture wounds.

Below
Scanning electron micrograph of the coronavirus, which is linked to severe acute respiratory syndrome (SARS). The name of the virus (taken from the Greek for crown) refers to the ring of protein spikes rising from the surface of the viral envelope.

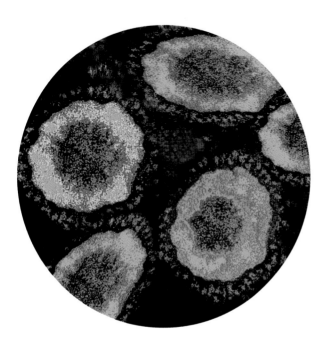

but their use has virtually eradicated the disease. The isolation of the viruses of measles, mumps and rubella (German measles) led to the production of vaccines against each of them. These were combined into a single vaccine, MMR, which was introduced into infant immunization schemes in the United Kingdom in 1988.

PREVENTION AND THERAPY

Live vaccines against influenza [39] were produced in the 1960s, but it was not until the 1990s that new techniques produced an attenuated product that produced longer immunity. Unfortunately, the virus mutates regularly so that a new vaccine has to be developed each year, based on a prediction as to which strain will be prominent that winter. The problems of forecasting and viral change make the production of vaccines difficult. Plans were drawn up for mass vaccination against bird flu (H5N1 strain of the virus), which caused its first human death in 1997, severe acute respiratory syndrome (SARS), which appeared in 2003, and swine flu (H1N1) in 2009, but they did not develop into pandemics and much of the vaccine was unused.

It has been known since the 1950s that viruses may produce tumours. Liver cancer can be a result of infection, so a vaccine against Hepatitis A has been in regular use since 1996 and against Hepatitis B since 1981. A strain of human papilloma virus [69] causes cancer of the cervix (neck of the womb), and in an attempt to eradicate it, HPV vaccine is offered to all girls in the UK aged between 12 and 13. Research into new vaccines, both for prevention and therapy, continues against other cancers such as that of the prostate. The potential of vaccines against addiction to nicotine and cocaine is also being studied.

NOT AS EASY AS IT SEEMS

Vaccines are not without their problems. Public anxiety about safety has often been based on prejudice or flawed science. The claim made by Andrew Wakefield in 1998 that MMR vaccine led to autism in some children produced a sharp decrease in immunization rates in the UK, which was followed by an increase of the diseases. It was feared that this would threaten the so-called 'herd immunity', a measure of natural defence in a population. After many clinical trials, Wakefield's hypothesis was finally discredited in 2010.

Other difficulties have arisen with contaminated products. In 1955 faulty production of the Salk polio

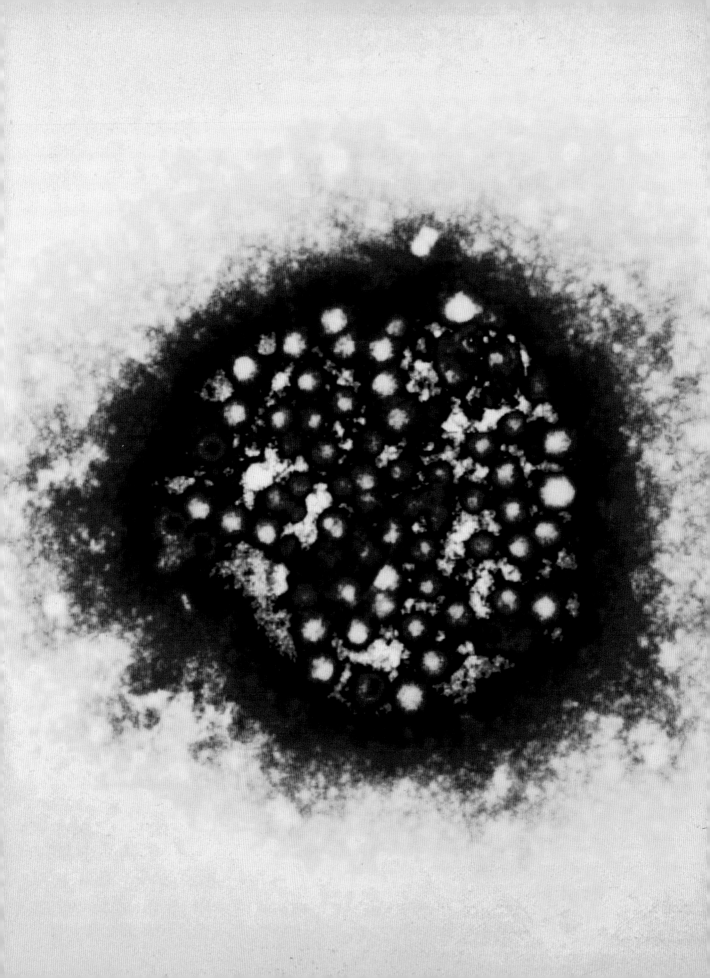

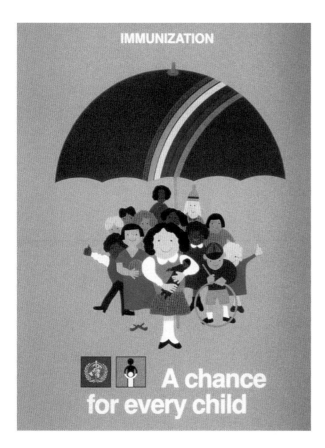

IMMUNIZATION

A chance for every child

vaccine manufactured by Cutter Laboratories of
Berkeley, California, produced paralytic poliomyelitis
in 56 patients from 120,000 doses. Five children died.

Because of the complexity of the human immune
mechanism, the length of immunity given by a vaccine
is variable. Some vaccines provide lifelong protection,
many require a course as a baby reinforced by boosters
as a teenager, and others need re-administering every
few years. Schedules for childhood immunizations
change with the introduction of new and improved
vaccines, and different interpretations of the data
mean that there is no international consensus of
administration. A few vaccines, such as for Hepatitis B,
may fail to produce immunity, while others need more
frequent boosters to produce their effect.

Many years of experiment have failed to produce
an effective vaccine for two of the most dangerous
diseases. The complex life cycle of the malaria mosquito
has prevented researchers designing an efficacious
vaccine against the disease, and although the Human
Immunodeficiency Virus [42] that causes AIDS was
discovered in 1983, it has been difficult to isolate and
grow it – necessary steps in vaccine development.

Schedules of protection for travellers are constantly
updated from information about the prevalence of
diseases worldwide and are vital for protecting health
and preventing the international spread of disease.
Certificates of immunization history may become
necessary before entry is allowed to some countries
and may also be requested by employers.

Immunization has always been associated with
government policy and regulation. Public health
campaigns that attempt to protect adults and children
have been successful in attenuating and abolishing
the scourge of infectious disease, both in human
medicine and animal husbandry. Other challenges
in immunology remain. These may be met by
new experimental techniques, such as the genetic
manipulation of causative organisms.

64. VITAMINS
Accessory food factors

Akihito Suzuki

A substance or substances present in normal foodstuffs (e.g. milk) can, when added to the dietary in astonishingly small amount, secure the utilization for growth of the protein and energy.
Frederick Gowland Hopkins, 1912

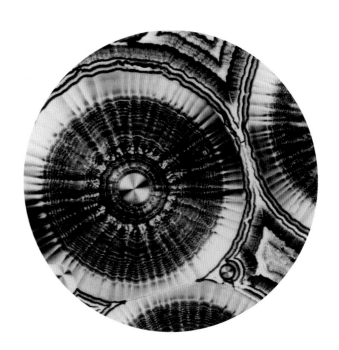

Vitamin C (ascorbic acid) is water-soluble and is thus excreted by the body. It has to be replaced by dietary intake as unlike most mammals we do not make our own vitamin C. Lack of this vitamin leads to scurvy, which can be fatal.

We call an organic compound a 'vitamin' when it is required by humans or animals as a nutrient obtained from the diet in a tiny amount; in excess they are damaging. Thirteen vitamins are now internationally recognized. Individual vitamins were typically discovered because they caused a disease through the *lack* of a specific nutrient in the diet; thus these are deficiency diseases.

Some vitamin-deficiency diseases were familiar for centuries, but it was only from the late 19th century that the major ones such as scurvy (resulting from the deficiency of vitamin C), beriberi (vitamin B1), pellagra (vitamin B3) and rickets (vitamin D) were formulated. Observations of the prevalence of the diseases among 'captive populations' (for instance soldiers, prisoners, those confined in lunatic asylums) played a major role in the study of these diseases. Experimental research using animal models was then crucial for establishing the exact causes. Once the role of vitamins was understood, mass-production and advertisement of supplements and pills popularized the notion of vitamins; our understanding of food has thereby been profoundly altered.

Principal Vitamin Deficiency Diseases

Vitamin	Chemical Name	Disease
A	Retinol	Xerophthalmia (nightblindness)
B1	Thiamine	Beriberi
B3	Niacin	Pellagra
B9	Folic acid	Anaemia
B12	Cobalamin	Pernicious anaemia
C	Ascorbic acid	Scurvy
D	Calciferol	Rickets
E	Tocopherol	Nerve damage

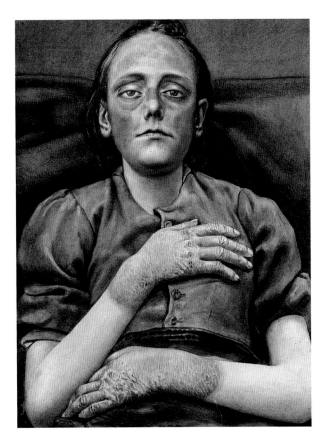

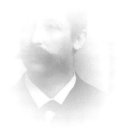

SCURVY

Scurvy became a major problem for Europeans when they regularly made long transoceanic voyages, typically to the Americas, Southeast Asia or the Pacific islands. Sailors developed spots on the skin and suffered from spongy gums and bleeding from mucous membranes. Though it was frequently fatal, it was soon realized that eating fresh fruits and vegetables brought about a quick recovery. In 1747 a Scottish naval surgeon, James Lind (1716–94), published the results of a sophisticated controlled experiment which showed that oranges and lemons in the diet successfully cured scurvy among sailors. This outcome, which seems so decisive today, was more ambiguous to Lind and his contemporaries because a number of other medicines and foods also appeared to have some effect on scurvy.

Ships of the celebrated expeditions of James Cook (1768–77) and of the British navy during the Napoleonic Wars (1799–1815) carried lemon juice, which prevented scurvy quite successfully, but no one was sure why it worked. Nor was its power always reliable, since vitamin C in lemons can be easily damaged by heat or long storage, and the limes that were often used contained variable amounts of the vitamin. Doubts over the use of lemons persisted, and even at the beginning of the 20th century theories were put forward denying their efficacy. Although experience and experiments had pointed in the right direction, the exact causation of scurvy was still unknown.

BERIBERI

An understanding of beriberi took a similar trajectory. Beriberi has long existed in East and Southeast Asia, where rice has been a staple food. In Japan in the 17th century, beriberi was called 'Edo-disease' or 'Osaka-disease' since, as we can now infer, people in large cities lived on white rice, which is pleasant to eat but lacks vitamin B1 because the thiamine-rich outer skin is removed during the milling process. In 1882–84 a Japanese naval surgeon, Takaki Kanehiro (1849–1920), changed the diet of seamen, replacing white rice with barley; the incidence of beriberi was dramatically reduced. Takaki, however, wrongly believed that protein in the Western-style diet held the key. Further progress was made by Christiaan Eijkman (1858–1930), a Dutch scientist in Batavia (now Jakarta).

Eijkman studied polyneuritis in fowls, comparable to human beriberi. He demonstrated that it occurred when chickens were fed only white rice, but that they recovered when their diet was supplemented with the outer skin of rice grains. Surveys of prisons and lunatic asylums revealed that human beriberi showed a similar dietary causation. Eijkman was close to the answer, but he theorized that white rice caused beriberi because it was toxic and the husk cured or prevented beriberi because it was an antidote.

THE SCIENCE OF NUTRITION

Animal experimentations introduced by a Norwegian bacteriologist, Axel Holst (1860–1931), in 1907 brought new rigour to the field. At Cambridge, Frederick Gowland Hopkins (1861–1947) conducted experiments in which he fed rats with mixtures of pure protein, carbohydrate, fat and salts. The rats did not grow properly on this supposedly essential mixture, but did when a very small amount of milk was added to their food. In a paper published in 1912 he named the key to the growth 'accessory food factors': if these were

lacking, animals would develop deficiency diseases such as scurvy or beriberi. In 1912 Casimir Funk (1884–1967) suggested that the active substance in rice bran was a 'vital amine' or 'vitamine', and he postulated that beriberi, scurvy, pellagra and rickets were caused by the lack of such substances in the diet. Once experiments on animals became possible and the theoretical basis was identified, the isolation of vitamins quickly followed from the 1920s on, and in 1932 vitamin C (ascorbic acid) was first synthesized.

As soon as science cracked the mystery of vitamins, they were aggressively popularized and commercialized. In developed countries every mother was expected to know about the vitamins in the food she cooked, and so vitamins brought science into the kitchen and on to the table. In 1925 wholesale vitamin sales were worth $343,000 in the USA, representing 0.1 per cent of all drug sales in that country. By 1939 the numbers were $41.6 million or 11.7 per cent. Around the mid-20th century, vitamins became firmly established in the landscape of our consumer-orientated health.

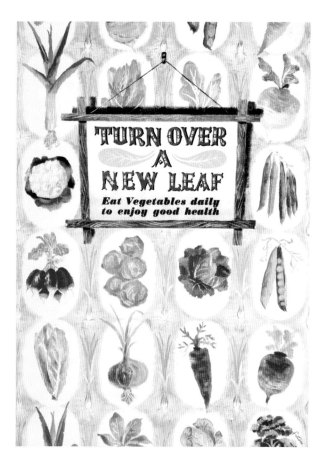

Right
A British Ministry of Food poster by James Fitton, *c.* 1951, showing a selection of vegetables. The poster was designed to encourage people to eat vegetables, which contain vitamins A, C and K as well as protein and the trace elements iron and zinc – all necessary in a healthy balanced diet.

Opposite
A multimillion-dollar industry: rows of dietary supplements in a modern pharmacy include a full range of vitamins. Many people prefer to obtain their vitamins in this highly processed form rather than at the 'grocery store' in fresh fruit and vegetables.

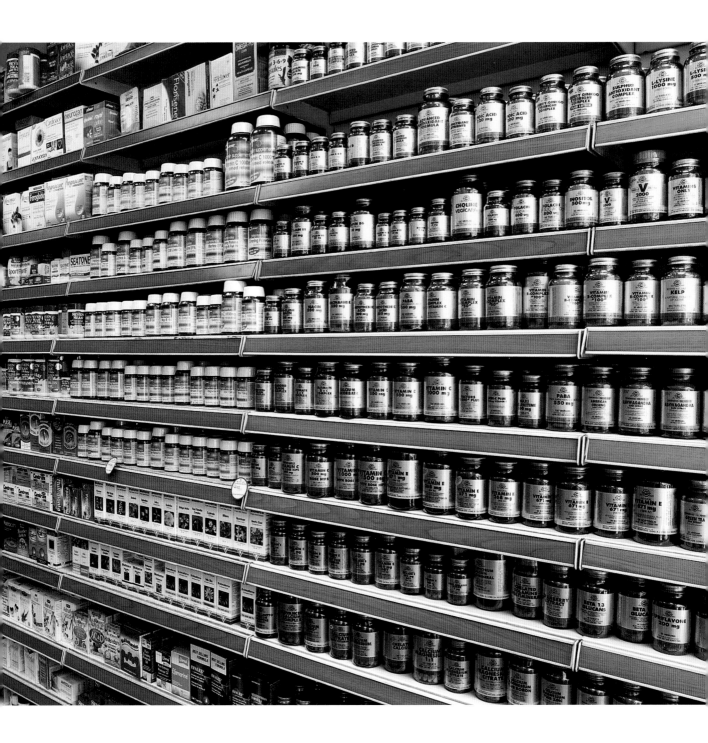

INSULIN
'A force of magical activity'

Robert Tattersall

Insulin is not a cure for diabetes, but it is a potent preparation,
alike for evil and for good ... insulin is a remedy which is primarily
for the wise and not for the foolish, whether they be patients
or doctors. Everyone knows it requires brains to live long with
diabetes, but to use insulin successfully requires more brains.
E. P. Joslin, H. Gray, H. F. Root, 1922

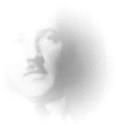

Diabetes had been recognized for over 2,000 years, but until the second half of the 19th century its cause was a mystery. In 1866 an English physician, George Harley (1829–96), suggested that there were two types of the disease. In those who were 'fat and ruddy', a condition he attributed to overproduction of glucose by the liver, the disease (now called type 2 diabetes) could be controlled by reducing carbohydrate intake and was compatible with many years of life. But the disease in young people (now called type 1) was much more serious, with relentless weight loss and death within a year; this type, in Harley's view, was due to 'defective combustion' of food.

The first clue to the cause of diabetes in the young was the discovery in 1889 by a German physician, Oskar Minkowski (1858–1931), that removal of the pancreas in dogs caused severe wasting diabetes. It was soon suggested that the small groups of cells scattered throughout the pancreas (the islands or islets of Langerhans) produced an internal secretion. The 1891 finding that thyroid extracts taken by mouth cured myxoedema (a condition caused by an underactive thyroid gland; [17]) raised hopes that pancreatic

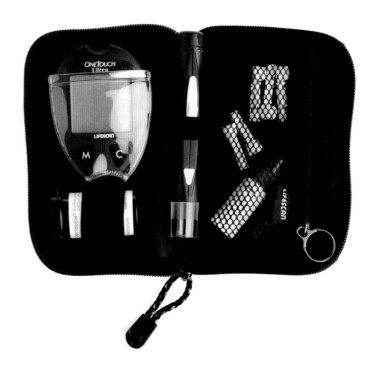

Above left
Charles Herbert Best was Fred Banting's student assistant in the isolation of insulin. Best was overlooked for the Nobel Prize; Banting, perceiving the inequity, shared his half of the prize money with Best, who became professor of physiology at the University of Toronto in 1929.

Above
Insulin is a hormone – a chemical messenger – that controls the uptake of glucose from the blood stream, allowing it to be stored until required. This testing kit allows diabetics to measure their blood glucose level and then regulate this by self-administering the appropriate amount of insulin. The kit includes a 'pen' to prick the finger and draw a drop of blood, test-strip papers and a digital reader.

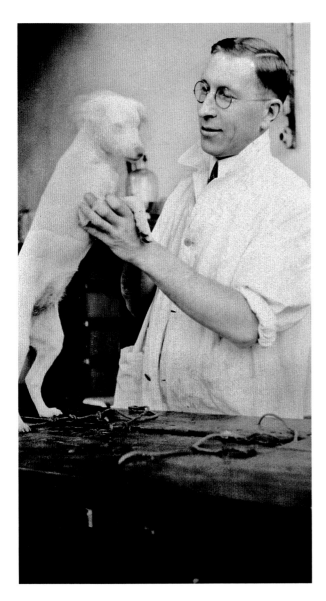

Above
Frederick Grant Banting with one of the dogs used in his insulin research in the physiology laboratories of the University of Toronto. Banting was subsequently elected to a professorship in the university and a research institute was established there named after him. He found the burden of being a Nobel laureate difficult to cope with.

extracts would have an equally miraculous effect for diabetics. Unfortunately, when swallowed they were ineffective. Sporadic efforts continued to isolate the hypothetical pancreatic hormone, which in 1909 a Belgian physiologist, Jean de Meyer (1878–1934), named insuline. Between 1900 and 1921 at least five investigators came close to discovering insulin, but most physicians gave up hope and treated their patients with starvation diets that prolonged life for up to five unpleasant years.

THE ISOLATION OF INSULIN

The eventual isolation of insulin came from an unlikely source. In Toronto in 1921 a young orthopaedic surgeon, Fred Banting (1891–1941), had the idea that others had failed because the hormone was digested by pancreatic enzymes during the process of extracting it. He would overcome this by tying the pancreatic duct so that the part of the pancreas that produced these enzymes degenerated, leaving the islets intact. The local professor of physiology, J. J. R. Macleod (1876–1935), was dismissive, but grudgingly gave Banting facilities and a student assistant, Charles Best (1899–1978). After showing that injections of extracts of islets could keep a diabetic dog alive, they made preparations from ox pancreas. Their first patient was treated for 10 days in January 1922 and showed a spectacular improvement in his clinical condition. Six others were treated and all responded. Blood sugar fell to normal levels and the patients gained weight and vigour. Banting and Macleod were awarded the 1923 Nobel Prize in Medicine.

SUBSEQUENT PROBLEMS

Publication of before-and-after photographs of skeletal children who had been resurrected by insulin left no doubt that it worked. Commercial production from ox pancreas followed rapidly and insulin was available throughout North America and Europe by 1923. Initially it was thought that it might cure diabetes, but it soon became apparent that it had to be given several times a day and only worked by injection. Also, the necessary dose varied according to how much the patient ate and exercised. Getting the dose wrong led to unpleasant and potentially fatal attacks of low blood sugar (hypoglycaemia).

In 1936/7 modified insulins, which worked for 24 hours, were welcomed by doctors and patients, and in their wake several doctors suggested that trying to keep blood sugar normal was unnecessary and that patients

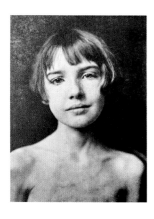
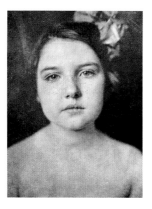

Left
An early success in the treatment of type 1 diabetes in a young girl. These before (left) and after (right) insulin therapy pictures from the *Journal of Metabolic Research* (1922) show why insulin was heralded as a 'force of magical activity'.

Below
A photomicrograph of a section through the pancreas of a patient with type 2 diabetes. Many of the special cells in the islands of Langerhans have been replaced by deposits of an amorphous amyloid (a starch-like protein) shown in pink. The islands are the regions of the pancreas that contain the hormone-producing cells, and their partial destruction means the body cannot make the insulin it requires.

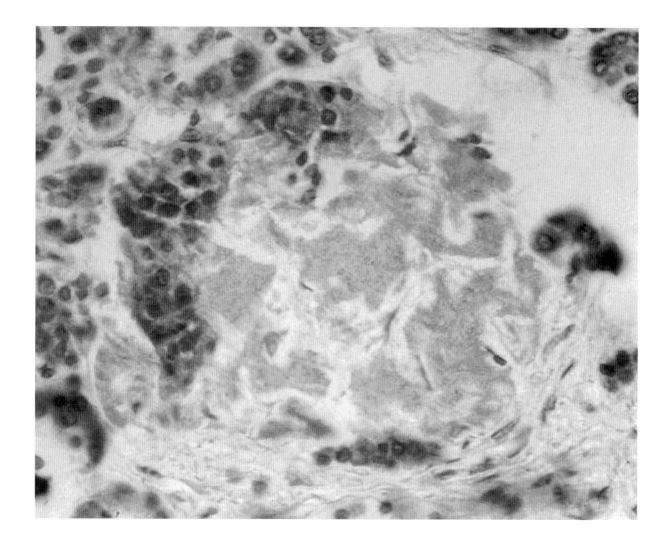

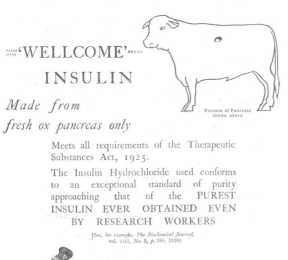

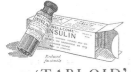

Left

An advertisement from the *British Medical Journal* (1929) for injectable insulin manufactured from ox pancreas by Burroughs Wellcome & Co., London. The advertisement emphasized the purity of the product; impurities could lead to allergic reactions.

Below

Dorothy Crowfoot Hodgkin was an expert X-ray crystallographer. She had already won the Nobel Prize in Chemistry (1964) for determining the structure of penicillin and vitamin B12 before leading the team that did the same for insulin.

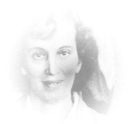

should eat what they liked (free diet). But by the 1940s it became apparent that young people whose lives had been saved by insulin in the 1920s were developing blindness, kidney failure and other unpleasant complications that had only previously been seen in type 2 diabetes. It was an unpalatable truth that insulin had transformed type 1 diabetes from an acute, rapidly fatal illness into a chronic one with long-term complications. Such effects are not inevitable, however, and the diabetes control and complications study published in 1993 proved that keeping blood sugar levels nearly normal prevented complications. This level of control is easier with regimens in which fast-acting insulin is injected before each meal, and this in turn became more convenient with the invention of pen injectors.

CONTINUED RESEARCH

Insulin is a protein and an important advance came in 1925 when John Jacob Abel (1857–1938) showed that it could be crystallized. This formed the basis for purification work for the next 60 years. In 1955 a Cambridge chemist, Frederick Sanger (1918–), worked out insulin's full amino acid structure, and in 1969

in Oxford Dorothy Crowfoot Hodgkin (1910–94) and an army of helpers worked out its three-dimensional structure. In the 1960s insulin was synthesized in the test tube in the USA, Germany and China, but the process was so laborious that it was clear it would not be commercially viable.

Then in 1974 the drug company Ciba Geigy produced enough synthetic human insulin for clinical tests and, although the results were not startling, there was a feeling that human must be better than beef or pork insulin. Production of human insulin became possible in the 1980s through genetic engineering, whereby an insulin gene was inserted into either a bacterium or yeast, which produced insulin in a process analogous to brewing beer. Small changes in the amino acid sequence led to synthetic insulins that were either faster- or longer-acting than native human insulin.

One downside of insulin treatment is the need for injections, and attempts have been made over the past 80 years to produce preparations that are active by mouth or when inhaled. Oral preparations have to date been unsuccessful. Inhaled insulin was marketed in 2006 but was a commercial flop.

Insulin **271**

66. DIALYSIS
The artificial kidney

John Turney & John Pickstone

What is man, when you come to think upon him, but a minutely set, ingenious machine for turning, with infinite artfulness, the red wine of Shiraz into urine?
Isak Dinesen (Karen Blixen), 1934

The most obvious function of the kidneys is to remove the waste products of digestion and metabolism from the blood and to excrete them as urine. Failure of the kidneys leads to accumulation of fluid and toxic substances, which may eventually cause death. Artificial dialysis replaces the excretory function of the kidneys, removing the toxic products and thus maintaining the patient's life. With its invention, the function of a whole organ was replaced by a machine for the first time – a new component in the technological revolution of the late 20th century.

THE PRINCIPLE

The principle underlying dialysis is the diffusion of toxins from the blood of the patient with kidney failure through a semipermeable membrane into a solution approximating to the chemical composition of blood. The phenomenon of osmosis through membranes was described in 1826 by the French physician and naturalist Henri Dutrochet (1776–1847); the diffusion of solutes was clarified by the London chemist Thomas Graham (1805–69), who in 1861 coined the term 'dialysis' (from the Greek, 'separate'). But no membrane was available that would allow the dialysis of flowing blood until cellophane was developed as a packaging material in 1910 and then spun into seamless sausage skins in 1929. One further requirement had to be satisfied before dialysis could be feasible as a treatment: an anticoagulant to prevent blood from clotting on contact with the artificial membrane surface. Early experiments with dialysis used an extract from leeches (hirudin), but heparin, developed for clinical use in the 1930s, was safer and more satisfactory, and indeed remains the anticoagulant used in clinical dialysis.

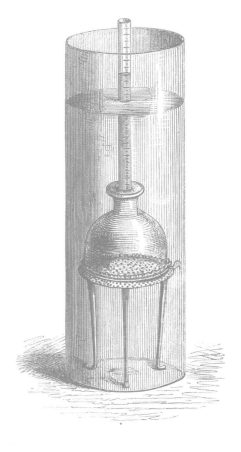

INVENTING THE MACHINE

Dialysis machines, or the artificial kidney, were invented more or less simultaneously in the mid-1940s by Willem (Pim) Kolff (1911–2009) in the Netherlands, Nils Alwall (1904–86) in Sweden and Gordon Murray (1894–1976) in Canada. Priority is given to Kolff, who performed the first treatments on patients in 1943 in German-occupied Holland. Kolff's story is one of ingenuity, perseverance and foresight: he worked as a physician, aided the Resistance movement and in his spare time constructed a dialysis machine using

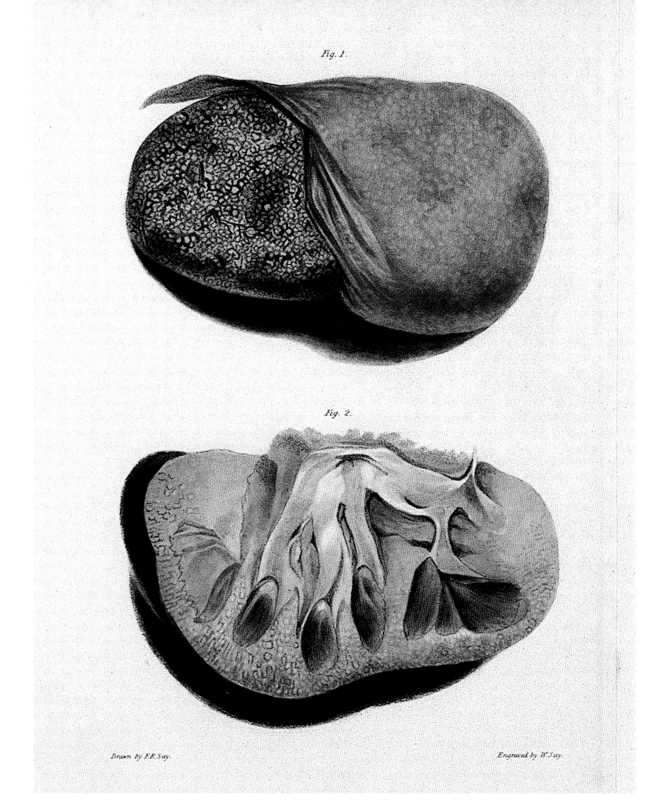

Fig. 1.

Fig. 2.

Drawn by F.R.Say.   Engraved by W.Say.

Opposite
Osmosis – the passage of small solutes and water across a
semipermeable membrane, from a high concentration to a low
concentration – underlies dialysis. This is a part of Thomas Graham's
experimental apparatus, *c.* 1854, for investigating the diffusion of
solutes.

Above
Two sections of diseased kidneys from Richard Bright's *Reports of
Medical Cases* (1827–31). Bright's correlation of symptoms and post-
mortem findings led him to conclude that oedematous (bloated with
excess water) patients who also had albumin in their urine were
suffering from renal failure.

aluminium from a shot-down bomber and parts from an old Ford engine. Kolff's machine comprised cellophane tubing wrapped round a slatted wooden drum. The rotation of the drum drew the blood along the tubing, which was partially immersed in a bath of solution into which the uraemic toxins could diffuse. The machine was large, cumbersome and difficult to operate, but it did achieve significant improvement in patients' blood tests and their symptoms. Kolff later emigrated to the United States, where he developed the first usable artificial heart and continued to refine haemodialysis machines, still using any available material, such as fruit cans, for the prototypes.

EARLY USE

Kolff's achievement, under extreme circumstances, cannot be overstated, but the early results were very mixed: although the condition of patients improved, it was only his 17th patient who survived. By the end of the Second World War, Kolff had made enough machines to donate to centres in the USA, Britain and elsewhere, but the reception of this radically new treatment was not generally enthusiastic. The mechanical substitution of function ran contrary to the physiological analyses and dietary treatments preferred by most of the physicians who had begun to specialize in kidney diseases. And

because of difficulties in getting a continuous blood flow from and to the patient's blood vessels, only a limited number of treatment sessions could be given to each individual. It was therefore used chiefly for patients with acute, potentially recoverable kidney failure.

Acute renal failure after trauma had become an issue in the Second World War, but interest then declined and over the next decade only a few enthusiasts persisted with dialysis, most notably John P. Merrill (1917–84) of Boston. During the Korean War, however, Merrill's students unarguably demonstrated the life-saving effect of dialysis, and its use then gradually spread, not least for obstetrical kidney failure.

RENAL UNITS

Dialysis, however, remained of little benefit to the more numerous patients with chronic renal failure until Belding Scribner (1921–2003) of Seattle, together with engineer Wayne Quinton, used a plastic tube coated with Teflon as a connection between an artery and a vein – a dialysis machine could be repeatedly connected to this 'shunt'. Once sufferers from terminal kidney failure could be kept in reasonable health indefinitely, Scribner explored the practical, ethical and financial aspects of running a 'renal unit'. Here was a new way of practising medicine, with staff and facilities

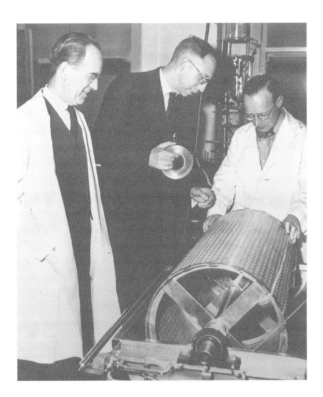

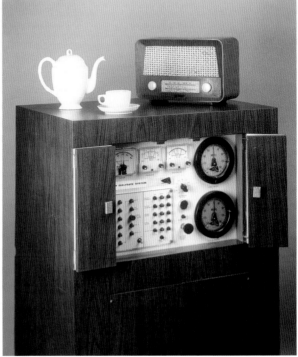

centred on a medical device to which independently living patients were attached three times a week. Treatment was managed by nurses, technicians and, most importantly, by the patients themselves, who thus became empowered as never before.

Some patients are dialysed in a different way: peritoneal dialysis, which utilizes the body's natural semipermeable membranes to effect the transfer of toxins, is a 'low-tech' procedure, also developed during the 1940s but little used until the 1980s, when technical developments sponsored by industry allowed its use for long-term treatment of ambulatory patients. From the 1960s, the expanding market for dialysis encouraged the commercial development of machines and services. Hundreds of thousands of patients are now maintained on machines that are safe, sleek, small, sophisticated and self-controlling – but they run on the same basic principle as Kolff's pioneering device.

Opposite left
Dutchman Willem Kolff (centre) demonstrates his dialysis machine, or artificial kidney, to Irvine Page (left), Research Director, and A. C. Corcoran (right) at the Cleveland Clinic, Ohio, USA in 1950, where he had moved after the Second World War.

Opposite right
A home dialysis machine, *c.* 1966: made by Milton Roy in the USA (manufacturers of metered pumps), this early automated machine was used by its owner for nine years. The machine and technical support cost £7,000, but this was infinitely preferable to attending a hospital for dialysis.

Below
A patient hooked up to a Kolff dialysis machine, 1947. The drum rotates in the salt bath while the blood flows through a cellophane tube which acts as the semipermeable membrane; the toxins pass through this into the bath, leaving the blood cleaner than before.

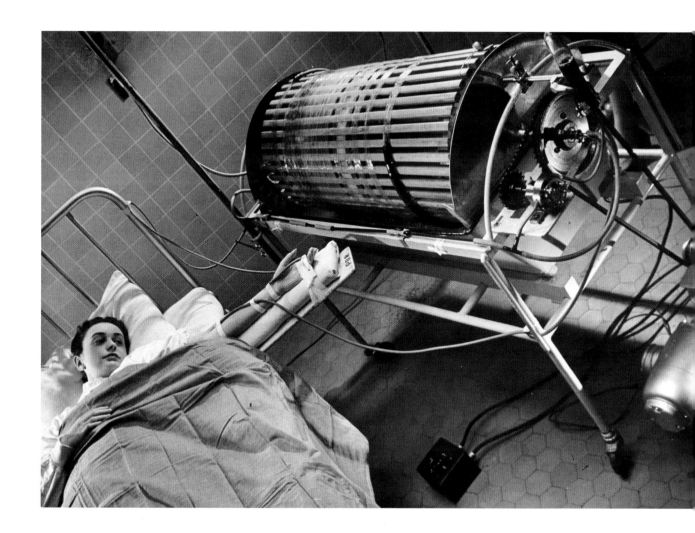

67. SMOKING & HEALTH

Lifestyle & medicine

Stephen Lock

The risk of developing carcinoma of the lung
increases steadily as the amount smoked increases.
Richard Doll & Austin Bradford Hill, 1950

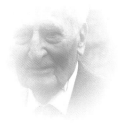

Left
Richard Doll traced the links between smoking and health for
50 years, following up his landmark 1950 paper (with Bradford Hill)
with another published in 2004 in the *British Medical Journal* giving
the results of five decades of observations of British male doctors.

Sixty years ago four-fifths of British men smoked; today
the proportion is only one-fifth. The reason for the
drop is the demonstration in 1950 of the link between
cigarette smoking and lung cancer, followed by the
discovery of links with many other serious conditions
– cancers, lung disease, coronary heart disease and
harm to the fetus. Spurred by voluntary pressure
groups, most Western countries eventually took action,
taxing tobacco highly, forbidding advertisements,
introducing warnings on packaging and banning
smoking in enclosed public spaces. Doctors, moreover,
then widened the research into links between other
lifestyles and health threats or premature death, such
as unbalanced diets, lack of exercise and alcohol abuse.

Europe encountered tobacco around 1600, using it
first as a medicine and then as an important source of
revenue both for the colonies who grew it and the home
governments who taxed it. Until the late 19th century
most tobacco was either chewed or smoked in pipes, but
two innovations led to the increasing predominance
of the cigarette. A new method of curing tobacco was
developed and a machine devised to replace hand
rolling, enabling five cigarettes to be sold for a penny.

The two world wars made cigarettes the preferred
form of smoking – in the First World War for men and
in the Second World War for women, who then started
smoking heavily.

DISCOVERING THE EPIDEMIC

To many older doctors in the 1940s lung cancer was still
the rarity their teachers had described. Nevertheless,
the British authorities became alarmed by reports of
a dramatic increase: between 1920/30 and 1940/44
there was a sixfold rise for men and a threefold one for
women. They asked a statistician, Austin Bradford Hill
(1897–1991), and a doctor, Richard Doll (1912–2005),
to investigate. Choosing 20 large London hospitals, they
compared the habits of 1,018 patients, half with lung
cancer and half with other conditions. The finding, that
the risk of lung cancer was 50 times greater in heavy
smokers than in lifelong non-smokers, was dramatic
and unexpected – so unexpected that before publishing
the team decided to repeat the study in other cities in
case there was some factor peculiar to London. Before
they could do this, however, two American researchers,
Ernst Wynder (1923–99) and Evarts A. Graham

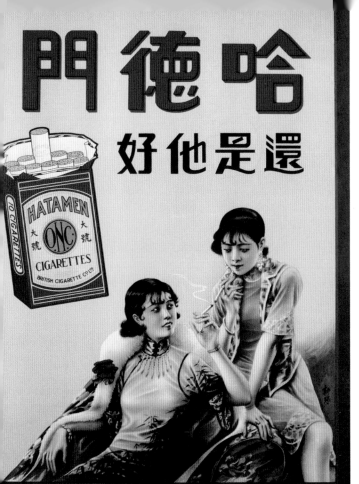

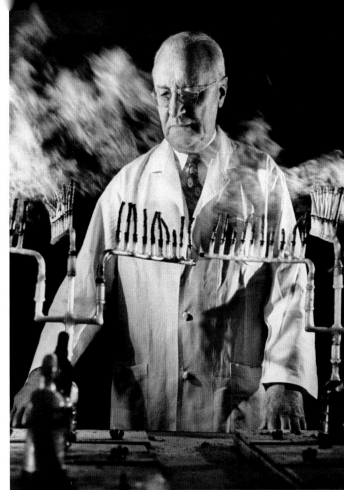

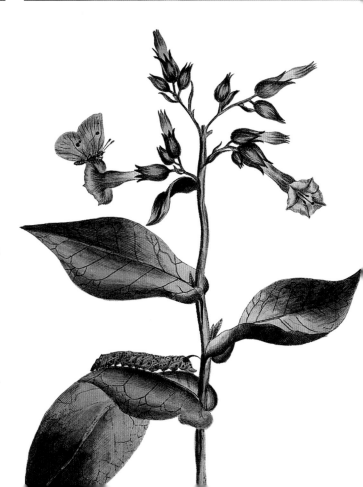

Above left
Cigarettes were marketed to women everywhere as a means of establishing their independence, liberation, sophistication and sexual allure – as in this advert for Hatamen cigarettes from China, *c.* 1932.

Above right
Evarts A. Graham was an American surgeon who had worked on surgical treatment for carcinoma of the lung and began to suspect there was a relationship between this disease and smoking. Graham was himself a smoker and died of lung cancer.

Right
A cultivated tobacco plant, *Nicotiana tabacum*, native to North and South America. Tobaccos contain a higher concentration of nicotine than other plants in their leaves. In nature nicotine acts as a powerful neurotoxin in insects and also deters the predations of herbivores.

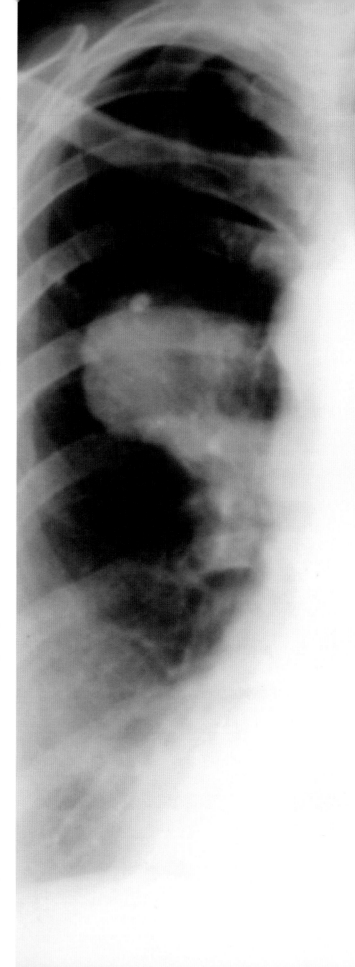

(1883–1957), reported similar findings from the USA. Doll and Hill then rushed their results into publication and soon further reports came from elsewhere. Even so, to address the serious implications, Doll and Hill now devised a different type of investigation.

This new, more rigorous study, called 'prospective', involved asking all registered British doctors about their smoking habits and then following them until their death. Even after a few years the results confirmed the original findings, but the researchers then found that it was feasible to prolong the study. The final report, presented by Doll himself 50 years later, showed that cigarette smoking doubles the death rate, with smokers dying on average 10 years younger than non-smokers, though stopping (even in middle age) increases the expectation of life.

As so often happens with 'new' discoveries, such findings were not the first. In the late 1930s, a German doctor had published relevant data, and Wynder himself had also theorized about a link, but the Second World War had prevented any dissemination of these ideas. In Britain in the previous century cigarettes had been identified as stunting growth in children, and, despite a lack of evidence, the 1908 Children's Act banned sales to youngsters under 16. But although certain lung diseases had long been recognized as associated with dusty occupations – pneumoconiosis with coal mining and byssinosis with cotton spinning, for example – smoking was so universal and apparently harmless (with cigarette advertisements appearing in medical journals) that even Doll started his study thinking that

Some Major Risks of Smoking

Respiratory tract
Cancer of the larynx, bronchus and lung; bronchitis and chronic obstructive lung disease
Digestive tract
Cancer of the oesophagus, stomach and pancreas; peptic ulcer
Urinary tract
Cancer of the kidney and bladder
Circulatory system
Myocardial infarction, peripheral vascular disease
Other
Impotence, stunted fetal growth, facial wrinkles

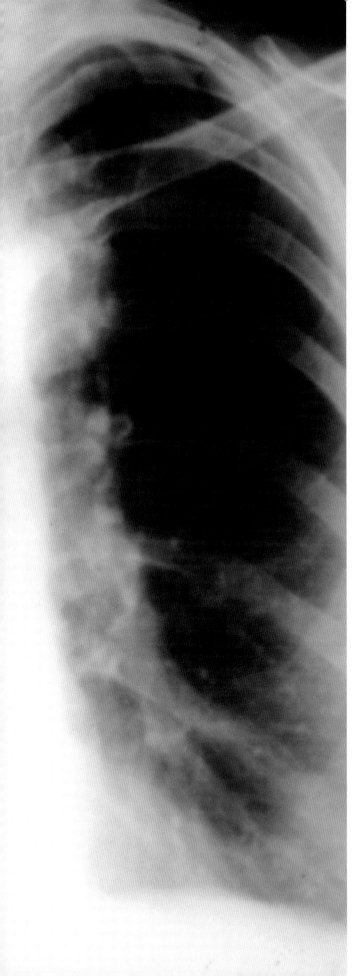

the lung cancer epidemic must be caused by something new in the atmosphere, such as road tar or diesel fumes.

A CONTINUING PROBLEM

Sixty years after the original published findings we know a lot more about the major hazards of cigarette smoking. Less well documented, but still proven, are the effects of secondary smoking, including lung cancer, childhood respiratory disease and sudden infant death syndrome. All this is hardly surprising, since tobacco smoke is now known to contain some 4,000 chemicals, 50 of them carcinogenic.

Today's statistics are stark. Every year in the USA smoking kills more people (400,000) than alcohol, car accidents, illegal drugs, murders and suicides put together – with health care costs put at $9.6 billion. In Britain 8.5 million people, 20 per cent of the population, smoke, and with over 80,000 deaths it is the main preventable cause of disease. In other developed countries an average 35 per cent of people smoke, the lowest proportion being in Sweden (19 per cent) and the highest in the Russian Federation (over 60 per cent) and China (with 300 million smokers).

But there remain the paradoxes: tobacco is the only known lethal product on sale to adults, and yet any government has health as a priority; the health costs of smoking are large, and yet society enjoys the profits and employment in the manufacture, promotion and taxation of tobacco; and there are limits to the extent to which any government can bully the population into healthy habits, a problem also seen with alcohol abuse and obesity. Tobacco smoking is a powerful addiction, but many people have been able to give it up, by willpower or methods such as nicotine patches or advice from their family doctor. Nevertheless, tobacco manufacturers have now switched their attention to emerging countries, where the population is less likely to know about the dangers; they would do well to remember that those who forget the lessons of history are destined to repeat them.

A chest X-ray of the lungs: on the right lung the shadow of a carcinoma is visible half way down the lung, towards the spine. Tobacco smoke contains numerous carcinogenic chemicals, which when inhaled can damage DNA in cells, making them grow and multiply abnormally.

68. ASSISTED REPRODUCTION
IVF & embryo transfer

Sarah Franklin & Martin H. Johnson

Human oocytes have been matured and fertilized by spermatozoa in vitro. *There may be certain clinical and scientific uses for human eggs fertilized by this procedure.*
R. Edwards, B. Bavister & P. Steptoe, 1969

Although *in vitro* fertilization (IVF) is predominantly associated with the birth of the world's first test-tube baby, Louise Brown, in 1978, its history, and that of embryo transfer (ET) with which it is inextricably linked, date back more than a century. The earliest embryo transfer experiments in mammals were conducted in the late 19th century by Walter Heape (1855–1929) as part of his investigations into the mechanism of heredity. Heape transferred embryos from a pair of white Angora rabbits into a black Belgian hare doe to demonstrate that gestation in the foster mother did not affect the pigmentation of the offspring.

UNDERSTANDING REPRODUCTION

In the 1930s, Gregory Pincus (1903–67) repeated Heape's experiments – this time in order to understand the mechanisms of reproduction. Pincus famously, but controversially, claimed to have induced parthenogenetic rabbit offspring (reproduction from an unfertilized ovum), as well as attempting lapine IVF. In 1944, after failing to gain tenure at Harvard, Pincus founded the Worcester Foundation for Experimental Biology in Shrewsbury, Massachusetts. He was joined by the Cambridge-trained zoologist Min Chueh Chang (1908–91), who specialized in the analysis of mammalian fertilization. In 1951 Chang discovered the phenomenon of capacitation – a uterus-mediated maturational change that sperm undergo before they are competent to fertilize eggs – as did, independently, C. R. 'Bunny' Austin. Together with the Harvard physician John Rock (1890–1984), Pincus and Chang developed the contraceptive pill [47] during the 1950s, in part by elucidating the role of hormones in ovulation and the development of ovulation induction, which later proved pivotal to successful IVF in humans.

Prior to this, Rock had focused his clinical work on infertility – its causes and possible treatments. With Miriam Menkin (1910–92), he experimented on fertilized and unfertilized eggs retrieved from patients during surgery, and in 1944 claimed the fertilization and cleavage (division of a fertilized egg cell) *in vitro*

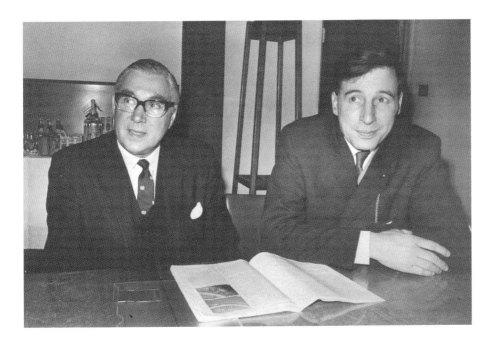

of three human ova. It was not until 1959, however,
that Chang provided definitive proof of the success of
IVF in mammals, by removing unfertilized ripe ova
from a rabbit, fertilizing them with capacitated sperm,
incubating them and then transferring the resultant
embryos to another rabbit, which gave birth to viable
offspring.

HUMAN IVF AND ET

A small number of scientists continued to pursue
the elusive and controversial goal of IVF in humans.
Landrum Shettles (1909–2003), a gynaecologist at
Columbia University, initiated a series of experiments
with retrieved human eggs during the 1960s. In 1973 he
agreed to attempt IVF and ET for a Florida couple, John
and Doris Del Zio. His experiment was discovered by
colleagues and terminated, leading to a lengthy court
case and much negative publicity.

In 1968, amid this heated public debate, the
Cambridge-based reproductive biologist Robert
Edwards (1925–) initiated a collaboration with the
gynaecologist Patrick Steptoe (1913–88), a consultant
in Oldham, northern England. Building on the methods
and knowledge developed by earlier investigators,
Edwards and Steptoe, and their assistant Jean Purdy,
developed novel techniques for studying human IVF.
Edwards allied his extensive experience and knowledge
of the timing of oocyte maturation (formation of an
egg cell) with a key technical innovation introduced
into the UK by Steptoe – namely the surgical use of the
laparoscope [62].

For his initial experiments leading up to the
first successful fertilization of a human egg *in vitro*,
in 1969, Edwards used oocytes recovered from the
biopsied ovaries of patients under anaesthesia. The
recovered eggs were cultured to maturity and fertilized
in vitro with capacitated sperm in a medium recently
developed by graduate student Barry Bavister for
his hamster fertilization studies. Afterwards, Edwards
and Steptoe successfully achieved laparoscopic
recovery of *in vivo* matured oocytes, followed by their
fertilization and cleavage, and blastocyst formation
(when the embryo has developed into a hollow sphere
of cells) *in vitro*. In 1974 they commenced the transfer
of embryos to volunteer female patients to try for
pregnancy.

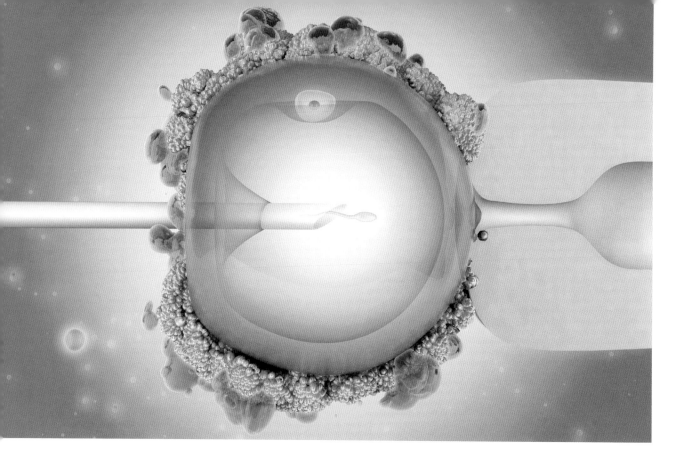

ADVANCES AND RISKS

Despite the long history of innovation preceding them, as well as their own advances, Edwards and Steptoe struggled to achieve the right hormonal conditions for successful implantation. Almost a decade separated the first successful fertilization of a human egg *in vitro* (1969) and the birth of Louise Brown (1978). Edwards and Steptoe also faced considerable ethical objections and worked under near constant media scrutiny.

Edwards and Steptoe's success in 1978 opened the door to the rapid clinical expansion of IVF and ET, enabling the birth of millions of IVF babies worldwide. Today it is the leading form of infertility treatment. It also formed a platform for basic and applied research in obstetrics and gynaecology, including in the 1980s Preimplantation Genetic Diagnosis (PGD: to prevent transmission of serious inherited disease), in the 1990s Intra-Cytoplasmic Sperm Injection (ICSI: to overcome certain forms of male infertility), and in the early 21st century the development and study of human embryonic stem cells.

However, despite significant advances in the hormonal control of ovulation, techniques of egg aspiration (removal of eggs by suction), embryo culture methods, as well as embryo selection and transfer and embryo freezing, IVF and ET is successful in only 25–30 per cent of treatment cycles. It thus remains a physically and psychologically demanding procedure for patients, particularly for women, who undergo a rigorous regime of hormonal stimulation as well as surgery, both carrying small but significant risks. Other risks of IVF and ET continue to cause concern. Trying to overcome low outcome rates by transferring several embryos has resulted in an epidemic of multiple pregnancies. Epidemiological studies have confirmed a slightly increased risk of congenital abnormality associated with IVF, although whether caused by the technology itself or a consequence of the sub-fertility that the technology has overcome is unclear.

Above
Intra-Cytoplasmic Sperm Injection (ICSI): a single sperm cell is directly injected into the egg cell (held by a micropipette) to assist fertilization. ICSI is used when the sperm count or sperm motility are low and fertilization is unlikely to occur naturally.

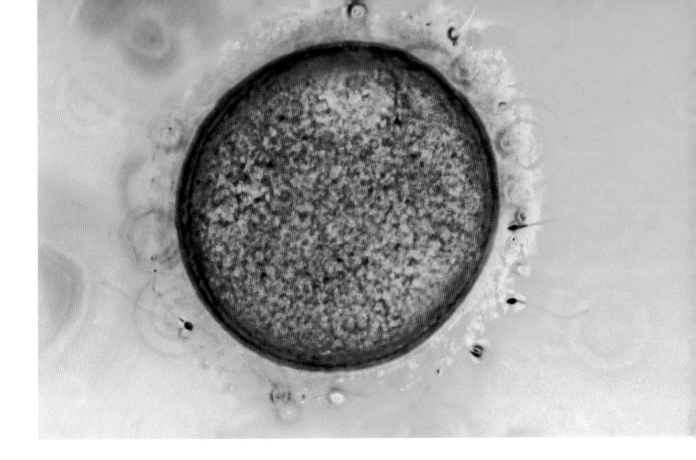

Above

Egg and sperm: the egg is surrounded by protective cumulus cells (yellow) beneath which is the membrane surrounding the egg, the zona pellucida (brown). The head of the sperm carries special enzymes to dissolve this membrane, which it must do in order to fertilize the egg.

Below

The laparoscopic approach (keyhole surgery) enables visualization of the inner abdomen. Using this method, the surface of the ovary can be clearly seen and the egg-containing follicles punctured with a thin hollow needle passed through the abdominal wall. Eggs are collected by aspiration (suction) of the follicle contents.

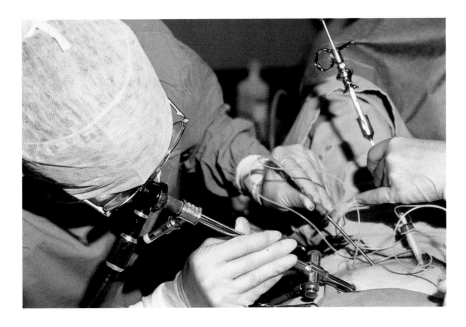

THE PAP SMEAR & HUMAN PAPILLOMA VIRUS
A preventable cancer

Ariane Dröscher

If by any chance a simple, inexpensive method of diagnosis could be developed which could be applied to large numbers of women in the cancer-bearing period of life, we would be in a position to discover the disease in its incipiency much more frequently than is now possible.
George N. Papanicolaou & Herbert Traut, 1941

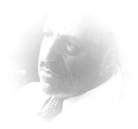

The Pap smear has transformed cervical cancer from being one of the most frequent forms of cancer in women to one of the most detectable and treatable. Furthermore, the Pap smear marks the beginning of gynaecological cytopathology: following the development of methods for detecting the cancer, the role of the papilloma virus in the cause of cervical cancer was also investigated from the late 1970s.

TWO NEW METHODS FOR DIAGNOSIS

In the late 1920s two new methods for the diagnosis of cervical cancer were developed contemporaneously but independently, by the Hungarian-Romanian pathologist and gynaecologist Aurel Babeş (1886–1961) and by Greek-American George Nikolas Papanicolaou (1883–1962). Babeş presented his findings to the Romanian Society of Gynaecology in Bucharest in January 1927. Using a platinum loop he had collected cells from a woman's cervix, which were then dried on a slide and stained; he demonstrated that the presence of cancer cells could be detected without prior indicators of disease and without recourse to invasive surgical biopsy. Several days earlier, Papanicolaou ('Dr Pap')

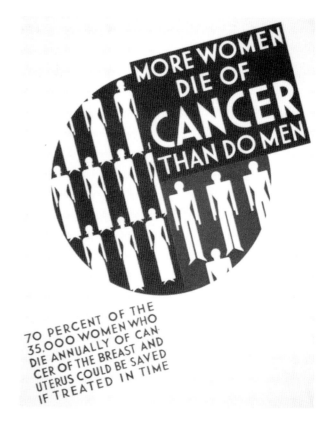

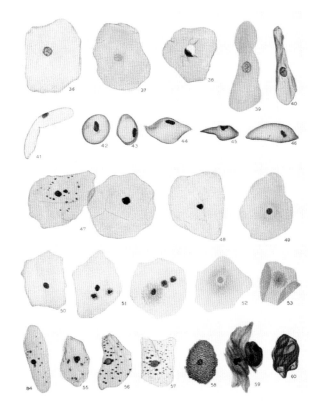

presented a different method at the Third Race Betterment Conference in Battle Creek, Michigan.

Papanicolaou had trained as a physician in Greece and had conducted studies of sex differentiation and determination with August Weismann and Richard Goldschmidt in Germany. Emigrating to the United States in 1913, he began work at the New York Hospital and then moved to Cornell Medical School. Here he developed a method to determine the ovulation time in guinea pigs, conducting a daily microscopic examination of the free-floating – 'exfoliative' as he called them – cells of the vagina obtained with the aid of a small nasal speculum. Excited by the results, he obtained the first human 'Pap' smear from his wife, and showed that it was an excellent tool to reveal endocrine changes. In 1925 he started systematically to study large numbers of vaginal smears, and, by chance, detected undiagnosed cancer cells in one of them.

Both presentations, Babeş's as well as Papanicolaou's, were met with great scepticism. However, they mark an epochal rethinking in cancer diagnosis. Most physicians were not convinced about exfoliative cell samples as potential indicators of cancerous changes that occur elsewhere. Moreover, they viewed the Pap test as both too time-consuming and unnecessary, because far too many normal samples had to be examined in order to find a pathological one, whereas diagnostic biopsy of the relatively accessible cervix furnished more certain results.

LARGE-SCALE SCREENING

To identify uterine precancerous cells and thus prevent malignancy, Papanicolaou first developed a new staining technique and then in 1948 a numeric cytological classification system. More important was the collaboration with his colleagues Herbert F. Traut and Andrew Marchetti, who persuaded every woman admitted to the gynaecological department of the New York Hospital to have a routine vaginal smear, thus providing Papanicolaou with the required database. An even larger-scale screening campaign began in 1945 when the Pap smear was enthusiastically promoted by the American Cancer Society, extending it as a preventive tool to an ever-greater proportion of the female population.

Yet large-scale screening is not that straightforward. Although the basic equipment consists simply of some kind of stick, swab or brush for obtaining the cells, a slide and a microscope to view them, the examination

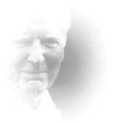

of the smear requires extensive training and continuous
concentration. Even for expert cytotechnicians and
pathologists the interpretation and classification of
'abnormal' cells remains ambiguous. Still today the
false-negative rate (the failure to detect such cells) is
rather high – in 1988 in the US it was an estimated
15–40 per cent – whereas a positive result might not
lead to invasive cancer and revert to normal at the
next smear. Therefore, efforts have concentrated first
on improving methods to identify precancerous cells;
secondly on elaborating cytological and morphological
criteria for a universal standard to distinguish between
normal, hyperplastic (excessive cell division) and
malignant cells; and thirdly on developing procedures
that lower costs and time in order to transform the Pap
smear into a preventive tool available for potentially
all women.

After the 1950s, James W. Reagan, Stanley Fletcher
Patten and others improved the methodology of
objective cell analysis and planimetry in formulating
reproducible cytological criteria, useful also for
automated screening. Yet, the smear reading has
remained resistant to automation efforts and furnishes
more secure results if integrated with other forms of
diagnosis. Also, the classification system has become
more diversified rather than standardized, and several
systems are used simultaneously.

THE HUMAN PAPILLOMA VIRUS

Driven by the suspicion that viruses might represent
the causative agents for cervical cancer, Harald zur
Hausen (1936–) and his team in the 1970s isolated many
different human papilloma viruses (HPV) from genital
warts. Then in 1983 and 1984 they isolated the DNA of
HPV16 and HPV18 and demonstrated their presence
in around 70 per cent of cervical cancer biopsies. In a
further step, they identified the two main viral genes
(E6 and E7) that are transcribed by cancer cells. For
this, zur Hausen shared the Nobel Prize in 2008.

In the 1980s several laboratories in the US and
Australia began work to develop cervical cancer
vaccines. In the early 1990s the first functional virus-
like particles (VLP) were generated, which gave birth
to the first commercial products around 2007.

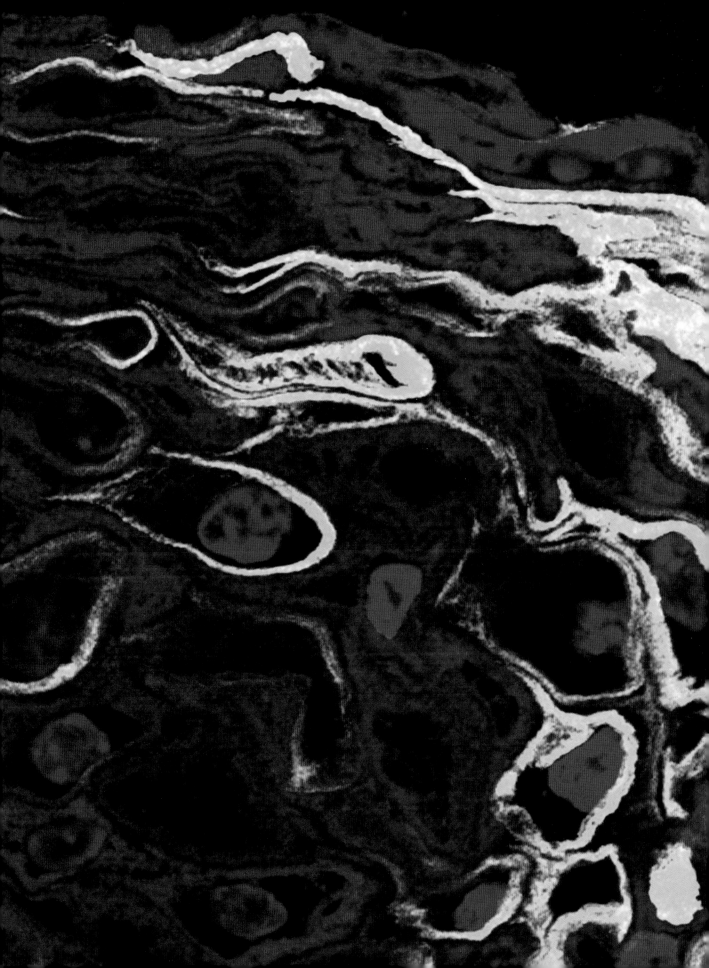

70. HELICOBACTER PYLORI & PEPTIC ULCER
Bacteria in an unexpected place

Barry Marshall

The greatest obstacle to discovering ... was not ignorance,
but the illusion of knowledge.
Daniel J. Boorstin, 1984

Peptic ulcer is an ulcer that occurs in a part of the gastrointestinal tract exposed to acid. Typically, a hole forms in the skin (the 'mucosa') in the wall of the lower stomach or in the first few centimetres of the intestine, in the duodenum. The hole is usually 1–2 cm in diameter and 5 mm deep, but generally does not penetrate all the way through the wall. It can exist for months or even years, coming and going unpredictably throughout the patient's life. At times, peptic ulcers can bore into an artery causing a major bleeding episode in which a patient might vomit blood and die. Ulcers can also penetrate through the wall so that intestinal contents leak out into the abdomen causing fatal peritonitis.

In the 20th century, about 10 per cent of people suffered from peptic ulcers at some stage in their life, and around 2–4 per cent of adults in the US or Britain were regularly taking antacid medication. The most commonly used acid-lowering drug was the H2 receptor blocker called cimetidine, costing $5 per day for the rest of the sufferer's life. Ulcers were so common that all doctors believed they were experts in ulcer treatment, and that stress was the cause.

THE GASTROENTEROLOGY ROTATION
In July 1981 I was 29 years old and mid-way through a three-year training programme at the Royal Perth Hospital, Western Australia. All being well, I could expect to be an internal medicine specialist at the end of 1983. I was doing gastroenterology for six months at the time and my boss told me that our pathologist, Dr Robin Warren, had come to him with a list of 20 patients who had curved bacteria and white cells on their stomach biopsies.

Dr Warren showed me what stomach tissue looked like under the microscope when normal, and then how it appeared when inflamed (i.e., many white cells were present), when he could see the curved

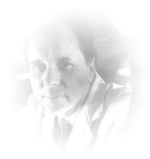

Above
Physician Barry Marshall, joint winner of the 2005 Nobel Prize for Medicine. Marshall's determination to prove that the bacterium *Helicobacter pylori* is the cause of most peptic ulcers involved collaboration and lone self-experimentation.

Below
Pathologist Robin Warren, who shared the Nobel Prize with Barry Marshall, had a long-standing interest in gastritis (inflammation of the lining of the stomach). Initially, microscopic examination of a stomach biopsy was the only way Warren could identify the bacterium. Today, a simple, non-invasive diagnostic test – the urea breath test developed by Marshall – is used to identify patients who are infected with *Helicobacter pylori*.

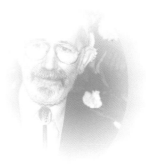

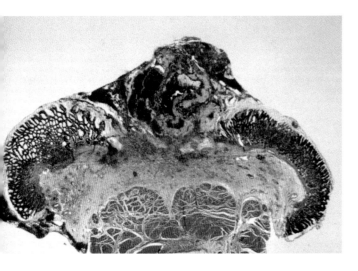

Left
Photomicrograph (magnified 50 times) of an acute perforating peptic ulcer breaking through the stomach lining; the contents of the stomach can then enter the abdominal cavity where the digestive acid and enzymes can destroy other tissues. Up to 90 per cent of these ulcers are caused by *Helicobacter pylori*.

Below
An X-ray of an ulcer on the lesser curve of the stomach taken after the patient has swallowed a barium meal. The shape of the stomach is unusual, being elongated, which could suggest infiltration with a tumour. In this case the ulcer was probably not directly caused by *Helicobacter pylori*, but lifelong *H. pylori* infection is the most common underlying cause of stomach cancer.

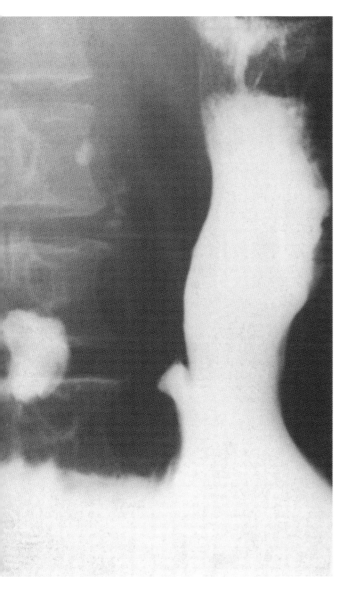

bacteria. The bacteria were apparently acid-tolerant, but preferred to live beneath the 0.2-mm thick gastric mucus layer, attached to the stomach mucus cells. The curved bugs were especially thick near the pyloric valve at the bottom of the stomach, so we called them *Campylobacter pyloridis* (curved pyloric bacteria); they were later renamed *Helicobacter pylori*.

After eight months of trying, we finally cultured them. The trick was to leave them in the incubator for five days, as they were slow to grow. They produced the enzyme urease, which allowed them to survive in acid by breaking down urea to form ammonia, an acid buffer.

Then, towards the end of 1982, Dr Warren and I made a breakthrough. The bacteria were present in almost every patient with a duodenal ulcer and in 80 per cent of those with gastric ulcers. Could it be that these bacteria caused ulcers? Were the bacteria harmful (pathogenic) or just there by chance (commensals)? Which came first, the bacteria or the ulcer? Few doctors believed our new theory, so we spent five years gathering more evidence.

THE HUMAN GUINEA PIG AND A CURE
First, I set about trying to infect animals with *Helicobacter* to see if ulcers developed. But maybe *Helicobacter* was a uniquely human bacterium only infecting people. So I decided I would be a human guinea pig. In July 1984 I drank some meat broth estimated to contain about 1,000,000,000 bacteria. After five days I began vomiting and after 10 days I underwent endoscopy and biopsy. The pathologist reported that my stomach was swarming with bacteria and inflammation (gastritis) was present. I had shown that the new bacterium was a pathogen, not a harmless commensal.

I proposed that if bacteria caused ulcers, then only treatment that eradicated the bacteria would permanently cure ulcers. A treatment called bismuth

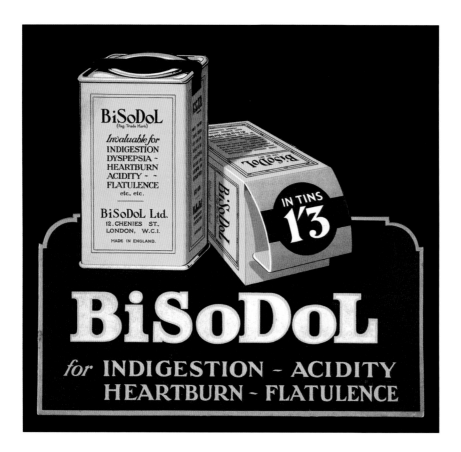

(actually bismuth subcitrate) could cure about 40 per cent. I placed some bismuth on a Petri dish of the bacteria. Sure enough, the bacteria were killed. When we looked at biopsies from patients taking bismuth, the bacteria were gone. Bismuth was not an antacid, but an antibacterial that could sterilize the stomach. Our hypothesis could predict the action of ulcer drugs.

Dr Warren and I treated 50 duodenal ulcer patients with the usual ulcer treatment plus antibiotics, and a second 50 with ulcer treatment plus placebo (fake antibiotics). After one year, 90 per cent of the patients cured of the bacteria were also cured of their ulcer. About five years later a Swedish discovery showed that a very strong new acid blocker – omeprazole – could assist ordinary antibiotics to cure 90 per cent of *Helicobacter* infections in just one week.

THE WORLD'S MOST COMMON INFECTION?

We now know that half the world's population is infected with *Helicobacter*. It spreads from mother to child, between siblings, in crowded unsanitary conditions and by drinking contaminated water. Most people with *Helicobacter* have few or no symptoms, but

10 per cent develop ulcers, 10 per cent have symptomatic gastritis and 1–2 per cent develop stomach cancer after many years. Treatment for *Helicobacter* cures most ulcers and probably also prevents future stomach cancer. *Helicobacter* can easily be diagnosed by family doctors with a blood test (for antibodies against the bacteria) or a breath test (which detects the urease enzyme of the bacteria inside the stomach).

Peptic ulcer, a disease which most people thought was hereditary or caused by stress, turned out to be a bacterial infection. Dr Warren and I won the Nobel Prize in 2005 for our discovery. Interestingly, Alfred Nobel always complained of stomach problems; he probably had an ulcer caused by *Helicobacter pylori*.

Above
A Bisodol advertisement from the 1930s. Bisodol, a proprietary mixture of antacid and bismuth, was used to neutralize the stomach's hydrochloric acid. At the time it became popular, many antacid formulations also contained bismuth subnitrate, a compound we now know could suppress *Helicobacter* infection, but not completely cure it.

Opposite
Helicobacter pylori: the bacteria move by tiny flagella at the tip and live beneath the gastric mucus layer in the stomach lining. Humans are the only known host; some 50 per cent of the world's population carries the bacteria.

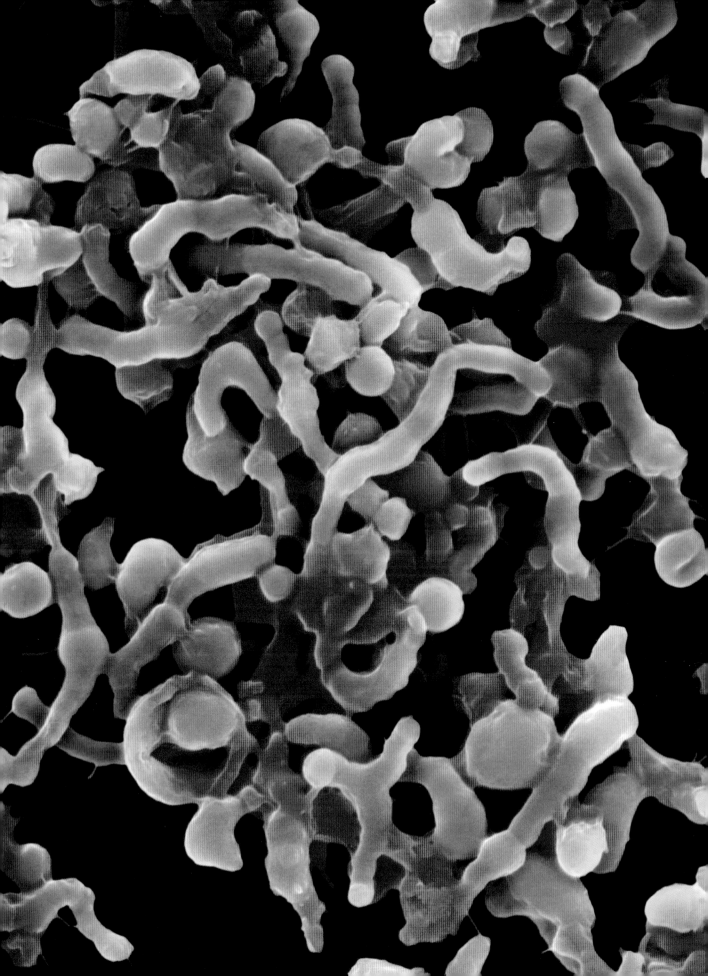

GLOSSARY

ablation Removal, usually surgically, of material from the surface of an organ or other tissue, for example by using a laser, although other means can be employed.

aetiology (also etiology) The cause or multiple causes of a disease or illness; for example infectious diseases are caused by invading bacteria, viruses, parasites or other microorganisms, while diabetes may be caused by a combination of factors including one's genetic makeup and lifestyle factors such as an inappropriate diet.

alkaloid Any of a group of organic chemicals containing nitrogen and other elements that have pronounced effects on the body, including such drugs as quinine and morphine.

analgesia The inability to feel pain; analgesics such as 'pain killers' or anaesthetics allow the body to achieve analgesia.

aneurysm An enlargement or out-pouching of an artery, filled with blood, resulting from a weakening in the muscle wall of the artery; should the weakened wall burst a potentially life-threatening haemorrhage can occur.

angiogenesis The development of new blood vessels.

antiretroviral Any of the class of drugs that work against retroviruses, especially the Human Immunodeficiency Virus (HIV) that causes AIDS, by inhibiting the life cycle of the retrovirus; when three or four drugs are taken in combination this is known as Highly Active Antiretroviral Therapy, or HAART.

auscultation Listening to sounds within the body, typically the heart and lungs but also other organs, and interpreting what is heard as normal or abnormal; immediate auscultation employs no technology to assist the ear, mediate auscultation uses a device, usually the stethoscope, to enhance the sounds.

base In the biochemistry of DNA a base is an organic nitrogen-containing compound with basic or alkaline properties. There are four bases or compounds in DNA: guanine and cytosine are always paired or joined together (with hydrogen bonds) and adenine with thymine (also with hydrogen bonds).

borreliosis The general name given to diseases (Lyme disease, relapsing fever) caused by members of the genus of bacteria known as borrelia, which are transmitted by the bites of ticks and lice.

cavitation The formation during the progress of a disease of an empty space in previously normal tissue, such as in the lungs or bones in tuberculosis.

chromosome The coiled threadlike structure of nucleic acids (DNA) and protein arranged in a double helix and found in the nucleus of cells; along its length are found the genes and regulatory sequences.

cytogenetics The study of inheritance at the level of the chromosome.

cytology The study of the structure and function of cells in plants and animals.

cytoplasm The liquid part of the cell, contained within the cell membrane – within the cytoplasm are found all the organelles of the cell except the nucleus, which is separated from the cytoplasm by its own membrane.

electrocardiogram or **ECG** The visualization of the electrical activity of the heart, which can be stored as a permanent record; electrocardiograms are produced by machines known as electrocardiographs.

endocrinology The medical and physiological discipline concerned with the production and use within the body of hormones – the chemicals that are part of the way the body regulates its functions.

epidemiology The statistical study of the incidence and distribution of diseases, and the factors that cause and might prevent and control them.

goitre A characteristic swelling of the neck caused by an enlarged thyroid gland, one of the endocrine glands, which produces the hormone thyroxine which regulates growth and development through its action on the body's metabolism.

histocompatibility The compatibility of tissues (including blood) of two different individuals; this must be matched as closely as possible to prevent the recipient's immune system rejecting the donated tissue, although such rejection can be modified by drugs. A specific region of chromosome 6 is known as the major histocompatibility complex and provides the genetic control for these functions.

histology Study of the tissues of the body using various techniques of microscopy and staining to enhance the images produced.

iatrogenic An illness caused by a medical intervention, an unwanted side effect of a diagnostic, surgical or medical procedure.

immunoproliferative Diseases or disorders of the immune system characterized by overproduction of the primary cells of the immune system such as B cells, T cells and Natural Killer cells, or overproduction of immunoglobulins (antibodies); in all cases the excess leads to illness.

inoculation A way of preventing disease, giving it in a mild form which will protect the inoculated individual by injecting living or dead organisms or their products.

in vitro In biology and medicine this is the duplication of processes that would normally occur within a living organism in artificial conditions outside the body in a culture dish or test tube.

in vivo Literally, within the living organism; the term is the opposite of *in vitro* and is applied to processes taking place within the body rather than artificially outside it.

'knockout' A term that applies to living organisms extensively used in medical and biological research such as mice or fruitflies; the knockout mouse or fly contains an artificially induced mutation of a specific gene(s) so that the gene(s) will not function correctly. The effects of this malfunction can be investigated and this can be used to mimic human diseases and in the testing of potential drugs to understand how they work.

lesion Characteristic damage to an organ or tissue caused by disease processes, for example the nodules or tubercles found in the lungs and elsewhere in tuberculosis or the fatty plaques found in the arteries in arteriosclerosis.

lymph The colourless fluid that bathes the tissues of the body; it contains white blood cells and drains through the lymphatic system into the bloodstream.

macular degeneration A condition (often associated with ageing) where the centre of the retina in the eye (the macula) is damaged, resulting in loss of the centre of the visual field so that reading or recognizing faces is impaired, but the peripheral vision is relatively unaffected.

metastases The development of a secondary cancerous growth away from the site of the original primary cancer but consisting of the same cancerous cells; for example a metastatic breast cancer tumour may be found as the disease develops in the bone, lung or liver.

microarray An automated laboratory procedure that allows the investigation of, for example, the role of specific sections of DNA from a gene to be conducted quickly and efficiently. Microarrays are part of the revolution in laboratory techniques beginning in the 1990s that combine molecular biology and microchip technology.

mitochondria Organelles found within the liquid cytoplasm in most cells. They are the powerhouse of the cell, where the biochemical processes of respiration and energy production take place; mitochondria have their own DNA, which is very useful in the study of molecular evolution.

myeloma A malignant tumour of the bone marrow.

myocardial infarction An MI or heart attack, when the blood supply to the heart is disrupted and cells in the heart's muscle walls die; most commonly caused by a blockage in the coronary arteries that supply the heart with oxygen-rich blood.

oncology The branch of medicine that deals with the study and treatment of cancerous tumours.

oocyte An immature egg cell, which will mature from a primary oocyte into a mature ovum or mature egg cell.

particulate In genetics, the inheritance of a specific trait from a single gene. Although Gregor Mendel did not know about genes, his famous experiments with the inheritance patterns of peas dealt with particulate characteristics – pea colour was either green or yellow, and never some colour halfway between; this kind of inheritance is still called 'Mendelian'.

pathogen Any microorganism, such as a bacterium, virus or parasite, that causes a disease; the Human Immunodeficiency Virus (HIV) is the cause of AIDS.

peptide/polypeptide A sequence of amino acids which are the building blocks of proteins; these chains are held together by specific chemical bonds called peptide bonds. A 'polypeptide' is simply a very long chain of amino acids.

plasma The fluid that surrounds the blood cells (red and white) in the body; it contains salts, proteins and other substances.

prosthesis An artificial body part, such as a limb or a hip-joint, to replace a natural one that is absent or does not function properly.

protoplasm A term introduced in the 19th century to describe the stuff of living matter; nowadays it refers more generally to the contents of the cell, including the formed structures such as the nucleus and mitochondria.

septum A partition separating two cavities. In the heart, the septum (part of the heart muscle) separates the right and left sides (both the atria and ventricles); when there is a hole in it more work is put on the heart, and correcting these 'septal defects' is part of modern heart surgery.

serology Literally, the scientific study of serum, which is the fluid left after the blood clots; it is rich in proteins and other organic substances.

soma/somaticism Technically, the 'soma' is the body apart from the reproductive cells (sperm and eggs); more generally, it simply refers to the body as opposed to the mind or soul, hence, 'somaticism' is a doctrine which puts emphasis on the physical body.

speculum A pronged instrument shaped to open body orifices, such as the nose or vagina, to allow them to be visualized more easily.

systolic The contraction of the heart is called systole and pumps the blood onwards, and its relaxation is diastole when the blood flows into the chambers of the heart; the systolic blood pressure is thus the maximum that occurs at the end of systole.

thermolysis The breakdown of molecules using a concentrated heat source, such as a laser.

thymus A small organ located in the neck, near the thyroid, which consists of lymph cells and is important in the development of immunity.

transgenic A laboratory animal, such as a mouse, in which genes from another species have been introduced at an early stage of the animal's development; it is an important technique for studying how genes function.

trypanosomiasis A disease caused by protozoan parasites called trypanosomes; in Africa, the disease is called sleeping sickness, and in South America a different kind of trypanosome causes Chagas' disease, named after the Brazilian doctor who first described it, Carlos Chagas.

uraemic One of the major waste products that is excreted through the kidneys is urea; when the kidneys fail, urea concentrations increase in the blood, and the patient is called uraemic, the symptoms include lethargy, headache and intense itching.

vaccination Originally, vaccination was applied to the procedure pioneered by Edward Jenner, which used cowpox (Vaccinia) to protect against smallpox; when Louis Pasteur and others introduced microorganisms that had been modified to make them less dangerous, but which still produced immunity, the term was applied more widely. The material used is called a vaccine.

LIST OF CONTRIBUTORS

William Bynum received his MD from Yale University and his PhD from the University of Cambridge. A Fellow of the Royal College of Physicians of London, he is professor emeritus of the history of medicine at University College London. He is the author of *Science and the Practice of Medicine in the Nineteenth Century* (1994) and *The History of Medicine: A Very Short Introduction* (2008), and the editor of numerous books, including (with Roy Porter), *Companion Encyclopedia of the History of Medicine* (1993) and *The Oxford Dictionary of Scientific Quotations* (2005). *45, 55*

Helen Bynum studied human sciences and the history of medicine at University College London and the Wellcome Institute for the History of Medicine, before lecturing in medical history at the University of Liverpool. Since then she has worked as a freelance lecturer, editor and writer. She is the author (as Helen Power) of *Tropical Medicine in the 20th Century* (1998), co-editor with William Bynum of the award-winning *Dictionary of Medical Biography* (2007) and co-editor of the Biographies of Disease series. *29, 38*

Michael Adler is Professor, Centre for Sexual Health & HIV Research, Research Department of Infectious Diseases & Population Health, University College London Medical School. He is the editor of *ABC of AIDS* (5th ed., 2001). *42*

Janette Allotey is Midwifery Lecturer at the School of Nursing, Midwifery and Social Work, University of Manchester, and Chair of the De Partu History of Childbirth Research Group. *58*

Cristina Álvarez Millán is in the Department of Medieval History in the Universidad Nacional de Educación a Distancia (UNED), Spain, and specializes in medieval Islamic medicine, particularly in the study of case histories, on which she has published several articles. *5*

Guy Attewell is a researcher at the French Institute of Pondicherry, India. He is the author of *Refiguring Unani Tibb: Plural Healing in Late Colonial India* (2007). *3*

Jeffrey Baker is Professor and Director, Program in the History of Medicine, Trent Center for Bioethics, Humanities & History of Medicine, Duke University and School of Medicine. He is the author of *The Machine in the Nursery: Incubator Technology and the Origins of Newborn Intensive Care* (1996). *32*

Linda L. Barnes is Associate Professor in the Department of Family Medicine at Boston University School of Medicine, and in the Division of Religious and Theological Studies at Boston University. She is the author of

Needles, Herbs, Gods, and Ghosts: China, Healing, and the West to 1848 (2005). *2*

Virginia Berridge is Professor of History, School of Hygiene and Tropical Medicine, University of London, and head of the Centre for History in Public Health. She is the author of *Opium and the People: Opiate Use and Drug Control Policy in Nineteenth and early Twentieth Century England* (1999) and co-author (with Alex Mold) of *Voluntary Action and Illegal Drugs: Health and Society in Britain since the 1960s* (2010). *43*

Sanjoy Bhattacharya is Reader in the History of Medicine, Department of History, University of York. He is the author of *Expunging Variola: The Control and Eradication of Smallpox in India 1947–1977* (2006) and co-author of *Fractured States: Smallpox, Public Health and Vaccination Policy in British India, 1800–1947* (2005). *40*

Michael Bliss is Professor Emeritus of History, University of Toronto. His books include *William Osler: A Life in Medicine* (1999) and *Harvey Cushing: A Life in Surgery* (2005). *56*

Robert Bud is Principal Curator of Medicine at the Science Museum, London, and Visiting Professorial Fellow, Queen Mary, University of London. He is the author of *Penicillin: Triumph and Tragedy* (2007). *46*

Douglas Chamberlain is Honorary Professor of Cardiology at the Brighton & Sussex Medical School and has been involved in resuscitation medicine since 1960. He was Editor in Chief of the journal *Resuscitation* from 1991 to 1997. *28*

Simon Chaplin is Head of the Wellcome Library, part of the Wellcome Collection, London. *6, 52*

Angus Clarke is Professor and Consultant in Clinical Genetics at Cardiff University. His interests include genetic screening, the genetic counselling process and the social and ethical issues around human genetics. He established and directs the Cardiff MSc course in Genetic Counselling. *19*

Gilberto Corbellini is professor of bioethics and the history of medicine at the faculty of medicine and pharmacy at Sapienza University of Rome. His interests include the rise and development of medical microbiology, malariology, immunosciences, neurosciences, medical genetics, evolutionary medicine and bioethics. *15, 18*

Dorothy Crawford is Robert Irvine Professor of Medical Microbiology and Assistant Principal, Public Understanding of Medicine, University of Edinburgh. She is the author of *The Invisible Enemy: A Natural History of Viruses* (2002) and *Deadly Companions: How Microbes Shaped our History* (2007). *34, 39* (with Ingo Johannessen), *41*

A. Rosalie David is Professor, Centre for Biomedical Egyptology, Faculty of Life Sciences, University of Manchester. She is the author of *The Experience of Ancient Egypt* (2000) and editor of *Egyptian Mummies and Modern Science* (2008). *1*

Ariane Dröscher works at the universities of Bologna and Bolzano. She is the author of *Die Zellbiologie in Italien im 19. Jahrhundert* (1996), *Le facoltà medico-chirurgiche italiane, 1860–1915* (2002) and *Biologia: storia e concetti* (2008). *8, 9, 23, 69*

John Ford is a medical historian and retired GP. He has served as President of the British Society for the History of Medicine and the Faculty of the History of Medicine of the Society of Apothecaries of London. His research interests include the history of primary care in the UK. *11, 25, 63*

Sarah Franklin is Professor of Social Studies of Biomedicine and Associate Director of the BIOS Centre, London School of Economics. She is the author of *Dolly Mixtures: The Remaking of Genealogy* (2007). *68* (with Martin H. Johnson)

Mel Greaves FRS is Professor of Cell Biology at the Institute of Cancer Research, London. He is the author of *Cancer: The Evolutionary Legacy* (2000) and editor of *White Blood: Personal Journeys with Childhood Leukaemia* (2008). *20*

Christine Hallett is Professor of Nursing History in the School of Nursing, Midwifery and Social Work, University of Manchester. She is the author of *Containing Trauma: Nursing Work in the First World War* (2009). *37*

Christopher Hamlin is Professor, Department of History, University of Notre Dame. He is the author of *Public Health and Social Justice in the Age of Chadwick* (1998) and *Cholera: The Biography* (2009). *36*

Mark Harrison is Professor of the History of Medicine and Director of the Wellcome Unit for the History of Medicine, University of Oxford. He is the author of *Medicine and Victory: British Military Medicine in the Second World War* (2004), *Disease and the Modern World: 1500 to the Present Day* (2004) and *The Medical War: British Military Medicine in the First World War* (2010). *35*

Mark Jackson is Professor of the History of Medicine and Director of the Centre for Medical History at the University of Exeter. He is the author of *Allergy: The History of a Modern Malady* (2006) and *Asthma: The Biography* (2009). *49*

Michael Jackson is a Specialist Registrar in Clinical Radiology working in the Southeast Scotland Deanery. He is a council member of the British Society for the History of Radiology, and has an interest in paediatric radiology. *26*

Ingo Johannessen is a member of the Department of Clinical Virology, the Royal Infirmary of Edinburgh. *39* (with Dorothy Crawford)

Martin H. Johnson is Professor of Reproductive Sciences, Department of Physiology, Development and Neuroscience, University of Cambridge. He is co-author of *Essential Reproduction* (7th ed. in prep.). *68* (with Sarah Franklin)

Stephen Lock is the former editor of the *British Medical Journal* and co-editor of *Ashes to Ashes: The History of Smoking and Health* (1998) and *The Oxford Illustrated Companion to Medicine* (2001). *67*

Lara Marks is Associate Lecturer at the Open University and Visiting Senior Scholar at Cambridge University and King's College, London. She is the author of *Sexual Chemistry, A History of the Contraceptive Pill* (2010, rev. ed.). *47*

Barry Marshall FRS is 2005 Nobel Prize winner in Physiology or Medicine and Professor of Clinical Microbiology at the University of Western Australia. He is the editor of *Helicobacter Pioneers: Firsthand Accounts from the Scientists Who Discovered Helicobacters 1892–1982* (2002). *70*

Malcolm Nicolson is Professor and Director of the Centre for the History of Medicine, University of Glasgow. He is the author of *Imaging and Imagining the Fetus: The Development of Obstetric Ultrasound* (2011). *7, 22, 31*

Vivian Nutton FBA is Emeritus Professor of the history of medicine at University College London, and the author of *Ancient Medicine* (2004). *4*

John Pickstone is Wellcome Research Professor, Centre for the History of Science, Technology and Medicine, University of Manchester. He is the author of *Ways of Knowing: A New History of Science, Technology and Medicine* (2000), editor of *Medical Innovations in Historical Perspective* (1992) and co-editor of *Medicine in the Twentieth Century* (2000). *57, 66* (with John Turney)

Andrew Robinson is an author, journalist and former Visiting Fellow of Wolfson College, Cambridge. His numerous books and articles include *The Story of Measurement* (2007), *The Last Man Who Knew Everything: Thomas Young* (2007) and *Sudden Genius: The Gradual Path to Creative Breakthroughs* (2010). *33*

Ana Cecilia Rodríguez de Romo is Professor in the Department of History of Medicine, NAUM (Mexico) and Head of the Laboratory of the History of Medicine, National Institute of Neurology and Neurosurgery. She is the author of papers and books on the history of medical scientific discovery, Mexican medicine in the 19th and 20th centuries and biographies of Mexican physicians. *13*

Thomas Schlich is Professor and Canada Research Chair in the History of Medicine, Department of Social Studies of Medicine, McGill University. He is the author of *Surgery, Science and Industry: A Revolution in Fracture Care, 1950s–1990s* (2002) and *The Origins of Organ Transplantation: Surgery and Laboratory Science, 1880s–1930s* (2010). *54, 60, 61, 62*

Andrew Scull is Distinguished Professor, Department of Sociology, University of California San Diego. He is the author of *Museums of Madness: The Social Organization of Insanity in Nineteenth-Century England* (1982), *Madhouse: A Tragic Tale of Megalomania and Modern Medicine* (2004) and *Hysteria: The Biography* (2009). *12, 16, 48*

Stephanie Snow is Wellcome Research Fellow, Centre for the History of Science, Technology and Medicine, University of Manchester. She is the author of *Operations Without Pain: The Practice and Science of Anaesthesia in Victorian Britain, 1846–1900* (2006) and *Blessed Days of Anaesthesia: How Anaesthetics Changed the World* (2008). *53*

Akihito Suzuki is Professor of History, Keio University, Japan, and the author of *Madness at Home* (2006). *51, 64*

Tilli Tansey is Professor of Modern Medical Sciences, Queen Mary, University of London. She is co-author of *Burroughs, Wellcome & Co.: Knowledge, Trust, Profit and the Transformation of the British Pharmaceutical Industry, 1880–1940* (2007) and co-editor of the Wellcome Witnesses to Twentieth Century Medicine series (1997–present). *44, 50*

Robert Tattersall is Emeritus Professor of Clinical Diabetes, Queen's Medical Centre, Nottingham. He is the author of *Diabetes: The Biography* (2009). *17, 24, 65*

Rodney Taylor is an academic gastroenterologist, former Professor of Medicine and now Visiting Professor of Bioethics, St Mary's University College; he is past-President of the Faculty of the History and Philosophy of Medicine and Pharmacy, Convenor of Examiners for the postgraduate Diploma in the History of Medicine and Junior Warden of the Worshipful Society of Apothecaries of London. *30*

Carsten Timmermann is a lecturer in the history of medicine and biomedical science at the University of Manchester. He has published on the histories of cardiovascular disease, lung cancer, pharmaceuticals, clinical trials and other topics in the history of recent medicine. *27*

Tom Treasure is Professor of Cardiothoracic Surgery, Clinical Operational Research Unit, University College London. *59*

John Turney is Consultant renal physician at Leeds General Infirmary, past-President of the British Renal Symposium and member of the Executive Committee of the Renal Association. *66* (with John Pickstone)

David Weatherall FRS won the 2010 Lasker-Koshlane Special Achievement Award in Medical Science and is Regius Professor of Medicine Emeritus and retired Honorary Director of the Weatherall Institute of Molecular Medicine at the University of Oxford. He is the Chancellor of Keele University, and Foreign Member of the US National Academy of Sciences. He is the author of *Science and the Quiet Art: Medical Research and Patient Care* (1995) and *Thalassaemia: The Biography* (2010). *10*

James Whorton is Professor Emeritus, Department of Bioethics and Humanities, University of Washington School of Medicine. He is the author of *Nature Cures: The History of Alternative Medicine in America* (2002) and *The Arsenic Century: How Victorian Britain was Poisoned at Home, Work and Play* (2010). *21*

Michael Worboys is Professor and Director, Centre for the History of Science, Technology and Medicine, University of Manchester. He is the author of *Spreading Germs: Disease Theories and Medical Practice in Britain, 1865–1900* (2000) and co-author (with Neil Pemberton) of *Mad Dogs and Englishmen: Rabies in Britain, 1830–2000* (2007). *14*

FURTHER READING

No. 1 Discovering the Body

01. Egyptian Medicine
Cockburn, A., Cockburn, E. & Reyman, T. A. (eds), *Mummies, Disease and Ancient Cultures* (Cambridge, 1998, 2nd ed.)

David, R. (ed.), *Egyptian Mummies and Modern Science* (Cambridge, 2008)

David, A. R., 'The art of medicine. The art of healing in ancient Egypt: a scientific appraisal', *Lancet*, 372 (2008), 1802–03

Ghalioungui, P., *Magic and Medical Science in Ancient Egypt* (Amsterdam, 1973, 2nd ed.)

Leitz, C., *Magical and Medical Papyri of the New Kingdom* (London, 2000)

Nunn, J. F., *Ancient Egyptian Medicine* (London & Norman, OK, 1996)

02. Chinese Medicine
Barnes, L. L., *Needles, Herbs, Gods, and Ghosts: China, Healing, and the West to 1848* (Cambridge, MA, 2005)

Hinrichs, T. J. & Barnes, L. L. (eds), *Chinese Medicine and Healing: An Illustrated History* (Cambridge, MA, in press)

Kaptchuk, T. J., *The Web that Has No Weaver* (Chicago, 2000)

Lu, Gwei-Djen & Needham, J., *Celestial Lancets: A History and Rationale of Acupuncture and Moxa* (London, 2002)

Scheid, V., *Chinese Medicine in Contemporary China: Plurality and Synthesis* (Durham, NC, 2002)

Unschuld, P., *Medicine in China: A History of Pharmaceutics* (Berkeley, CA, 1986)

03. Medicine in India
Attewell, G., *Refiguring Unani Tibb: Plural Healing in Late Colonial India* (Hyderabad, 2007)

Banerjee, M., *Power, Knowledge, Medicine: Ayurvedic Pharmaceuticals at Home and in the World* (Hyderabad, 2009)

Dash, B. & Kashyap, L., *Basic Principles of Ayurveda* (New Delhi, 1980)

Langford, J., *Fluent Bodies: Ayurvedic Remedies for Postcolonial Imbalance* (Durham, NC, 2002)

Wujastyk, D., *The Roots of Ayurveda: Selections from Sanskrit Medical Writings* (New Delhi, 1998)

Zimmermann, F., *The Jungle and the Aroma of Meats: An Ecological Theme in Hindu Medicine* (Berkeley, CA, 1987, 2nd ed.)

04. Humours & Pneumas
Arikha, N., *Passions and Tempers. A History of the Humours* (New York, 2007)

Filipczak, Z. Z., *Hot Dry Men, Cold Wet Women. The Theory of Humors in Western European Art, 1575–1700* (New York, 1997)

Jackson, S. W., *Melancholia and Depression: From Hippocratic Times to Modern Times* (New Haven, 1986)

Kagan, J., *Galen's Prophecy: Temperament in Human Nature* (New York, 1994)

Klibansky, R., Panowsky, E. & Saxl, F., *Saturn and Melancholy* (London, 1964)

Nutton, V., *Ancient Medicine* (London, 2004)

05. Islamic Medicine

Jacquart, D., *La médicine arabe et l'occident médiéval* (Paris, 1990)

Pormann, P. E. & Savage-Smith, E., *Medieval Islamic Medicine* (Edinburgh, 2007)

Savage-Smith, E., 'The practice of surgery in Islamic lands: myth and reality', in E. Savage-Smith & P. Horden (eds), *The Year 1000: Medical Practice at the End of the First Millennium* (Oxford, 2000), 307–21

– 'Europe and Islam', in I. Loudon (ed.), *Western Medicine: An Illustrated History* (Oxford, 1997), 40–53

– 'Attitudes toward dissection in medieval Islam', *Journal of the History of Medicine and Allied Sciences*, 50 (1995), 68–111

Ullmann, M., *Islamic Medicine* (Edinburgh, 1997)

06. Dissecting the Body

Carlino, A., *Books of the Body: Anatomical Ritual and Renaissance Learning* (Chicago, 1999)

Cunningham, A., *The Anatomical Renaissance: The Resurrection of the Anatomical Projects of the Ancients* (Aldershot, 1997)

– *The Anatomist Anatomis'd: An Experimental Discipline in Enlightenment Europe* (Farnham, 2009)

French, R., 'The anatomical tradition', in W. F. Bynum & R. Porter (eds), *Companion Encyclopedia of the History of Medicine* (London & New York, 1993)

– *Dissection and Vivisection in the European Renaissance* (Aldershot, 1999)

Payne, L., *With Words and Knives: Learning Medical Dispassion in Early Modern England* (Aldershot, 2007)

07. Pathological Anatomy

Hannaway, C. & La Berge, A. (eds), *Constructing Paris Medicine* (Amsterdam, 1998)

Long, E. R., *A History of Pathology* (New York, 1965)

Maulitz, R. C., 'The pathological tradition', in W. F. Bynum & R. Porter (eds), *Companion Encyclopedia of the History of Medicine* (London & New York, 1993), 169–91

– *Morbid Appearances: The Anatomy of Pathology in the Early 19th Century* (Cambridge & New York, 1987)

Moore, W., *The Knife Man: The Extraordinary Life and Times of John Hunter* (London, 2005)

Rodin, A. E., *The Influence of Matthew Baillie's Morbid Anatomy: Biography, Evaluation and Reprint* (Springfield, IL, 1973)

08. Cell Theory

Bechtel, W., *Discovering Cell Mechanisms. The Creation of Modern Cell Biology* (New York, 2006)

Duchesneau, F., *Genèse de la théorie cellulaire* (Montreal & Paris, 1987)

Harris, H., *The Birth of the Cell* (New Haven, 1999)

09. Neuron Theory

Barona, J. L., 'Ramón y Cajal, Santiago', in W. F. Bynum & H. Bynum (eds), *Dictionary of Medical Biography* (Westport, CT, & London, 2007), 1049–53

Mazzarello, P., *Golgi: A Biography of the Founder of Modern Neuroscience* (New York & Oxford, 2009)

Rubio, H., José, F. & López Piñero, J. M., *Filosofía y neuronismo en Cajal* (Murcia, 2008)

Shepherd, G. M., *Foundations of the Neuron Doctrine* (New York & Oxford, 1991)

10. Molecules

Brock, W. H., 'The biochemical tradition', in W. F. Bynum & R. Porter (eds), *Companion Encyclopedia of the History of Medicine* (London & New York, 1993), 153–69

Collins, F. S., *The Language of Life. DNA and the Revolution in Personalised Medicine* (New York, 2010)

Goertzel, T. & Goertzel, B., *Linus Pauling: A Life in Science and Politics* (New York, 1995)

Holmes, F. L., *Hans Krebs*. Vol. 1: *The Formation of a Scientific Life 1900–1933*; Vol. 2: *Architect of Intermediary Metabolism* (Oxford 1991, 1992)

Morage, M., *The History of Molecular Biology* (Cambridge, MA, 1998)

Wallace, D. C., 'Bioenergetics, the origins of complexity, and the ascent of man', *Proceedings of the National Academy of Sciences, USA*, 107 (2010), 8947–53

No. 2 Understanding Health & Disease

11. Circulation

Frank, R. G., *Harvey and the Oxford Physiologists* (Berkeley, 1980)

Harvey, W., *Circulation of the Blood and Other Writings*, trans. K. J. Franklin (London, 1963)

Keynes, G., *The Life of William Harvey* (Oxford, 1966)

Whitteridge, G., *William Harvey and the Circulation of the Blood* (London, 1971)

12. Bedlam & Beyond

Digby, A., *Madness, Morality and Medicine: A Study of the York Retreat, 1796–1914* (Cambridge, 1985)

Goldstein, J., *Console and Classify: The French Psychiatric Profession in the Nineteenth Century* (Chicago, 1987)

Scull, A., *Decarceration: Community Treatment and the Deviant* (Cambridge, 1984, 2nd ed.)

– *The Most Solitary of Afflictions: Madness and Society in Britain, 1700–1900* (London & New Haven, 1993)

Tomes, N., *A Generous Confidence: Thomas Story Kirkbride and the Art of Asylum Keeping* (Philadelphia, 1984)

13. The Milieu Intérieur

Bernard, C., *An Introduction to the Study of Experimental Medicine*, trans. H. C. Greene (New York, 1957)

Cannon, W. B., *The Wisdom of the Body* (New York, 1939)

Holmes, F. L., *Claude Bernard and Animal Chemistry* (Cambridge, 1974)

Lovelock, J., *The Revenge of Gaia* (London, 2006)

Rodríguez de Romo A. C., 'Bernard, Claude', in W. F. Bynum & H. Bynum (eds), *Dictionary of Medical Biography* (Westport, CT, & London, 2007), 194–96

14. Germs

Bynum, W. F., *Science and the Practice of Medicine in the Nineteenth Century* (Cambridge, 1994)

Tomes, N., *The Gospel of Germs: Men, Women and the Microbe in American Life* (Cambridge, MA, 1998)

Waller, J., *The Discovery of the Germ* (Cambridge & New York, 2002)

Worboys, M., *Spreading Germs: Disease Theories and Medical Practice in Britain, 1865–1900* (Cambridge & New York, 2000)

15. Parasites & Vectors

Chapin, C. V., *The Sources and Modes of Infection* (New York, 1910)

Kiple, K. F. (ed.), *Plague, Pox and Pestilence* (London, 1997)

Winslow, C.-E. A., *The Conquest of Epidemic Disease: A Chapter in the History of Ideas* (Princeton, 1944)

16. Psychoanalysis & Psychotherapy

Caplan, E., *Mind Games: American Culture and the Birth of Psychotherapy* (Berkeley, 1998)

Hale Jr, N. G., *Freud and the Americans: The Beginnings of Psychoanalysis in the United States, 1876–1917* (Oxford, 1971)

– *The Rise and Crisis of Psychoanalysis in the United States, 1917–1985* (Oxford, 1995)

Makari, G., *Revolution in Mind: The Creation of Psychoanalysis* (London, 2008)

Scull, A., *Hysteria: The Biography* (Oxford, 2009)

17. Hormones

Bliss, M., *Harvey Cushing: A Life in Surgery* (New York, 2005)

Cannon, W. B., 'Some conditions controlling internal secretion', *Journal of the American Medical Association*, 79 (1922), 92–95

Medvei, C., *The History of Clinical Endocrinology* (Carnforth, 1993)

18. Immunology

Mazumdar, P. M. H., *Species and Specificities* (Cambridge, MA, 1995)

Silverstein, A. M., *A History of Immunology* (New York, 2009)

Szentivany, A. & Friedman, H. (eds), *The Immunologic Revolution: Facts and Witnesses* (Boca Raton, FL, 1994)

Tauber, A., *The Immune Self* (Cambridge & New York, 1994)

19. The Genetic Revolution

Ashley, E. A. & others, 'Clinical assessment incorporating a personal genome', *Lancet*, 375 (2010), 1525–35

Gluckman, P. & Hanson, M., *The Fatal Matrix: Evolution Development and Disease* (Cambridge, 2005)

Jobling, M. A., Hurles, M. E. & Tyler-Smith, C., *Human Evolutionary Genetics: Origins, Peoples and Disease* (New York, 2004)

Weatherall, D., *Thalassemia: The Biography* (Oxford, 2010)

20. The Evolution of Cancer

Greaves, M., *Cancer. The Evolutionary Legacy* (Oxford, 2000)

Knowles, M. & Selby, P. (eds), *Introduction to the Cellular and Molecular Biology of Cancer* (Oxford, 2005, 4th ed.)

Weinberg, R. A., *The Biology of Cancer* (New York, 2007)

21. Complementary Medicine

Cooter, R. (ed.), *Studies in the History of Alternative Medicine* (New York, 1988)

Coulter, H., *Divided Legacy: A History of the Schism in Medical Thought* (Washington, DC, 1975)

Gevitz, N., *The D.O.s: Osteopathic Medicine in America* (Baltimore, 1982)

– *Other Healers: Unorthodox Medicine in America* (Baltimore, MD, 1988)

Moore, J. S., *Chiropractic in America: the History of a Medical Alternative* (Baltimore, MD, 1993)

Whorton, J., *Nature Cures. The History of Alternative Medicine in America* (Oxford & New York, 2002)

No. 3 Tools of the Trade

22. The Stethoscope

Bynum, W. F. & Porter, R. (eds), *Medicine and the Five Senses* (Cambridge & New York, 1993)

Duffin, J., *To See with a Better Eye: A Life of R. T. H. Laennec* (Princeton, NJ, 1998)

Reiser, S. J., *Medicine and the Reign of Technology* (Cambridge & New York, 1978)

– 'The science of diagnosis: diagnostic technology', in W. F. Bynum & R. Porter (eds), *Companion Encyclopedia of the History of Medicine* (London & New York, 1993), 826–51

23. The Microscope

Rasmussen, N., *Picture Control. The Electron Microscope and the Transformation of Biology in America 1940–1960* (Stanford, CA, 1997)

Schickore, J., *The Microscope and the Eye. A History of Reflections, 1740–1870* (Chicago, IL, 2007)

Wilson, C., *The Invisible World. Early Modern Philosophy and the Invention of the Microscope* (Princeton, NJ, 1995)

24. The Hypodermic Syringe

Howard-Jones, N., 'A critical study of the origins and early development of hypodermic medication', *Journal of the History of Medicine and Allied Sciences*, 1 (1947), 201–49

Mogey, G. A., 'Centenary of hypodermic injections', *British Medical Journal*, 2 (1953), 1180–85

25. The Thermometer

Allen, L. G., 'The history of clinical thermometry in the history of anaesthesia', *Royal Society of Medicine International Congress and Symposium Series* 134 (1989), 368–71

McGuigan, H. A., 'Medical Thermometry', *Annals of Medical History*, IX (1937), 148–54

Reiser, S. J., *Medicine and the Reign of Technology* (Cambridge, 1978), 110–21

26. X-Rays & Radiotherapy

Brecher, R. & E., *The Rays: A History of Radiology in the United States and Canada* (Baltimore, MD, 1969)

Burrows, E. H., *Pioneers and Early Years. A History of British Radiology* (Alderney, 1986)

Glasser, O., *Wilhelm Conrad Röntgen and the Early History of the Röntgen Rays* (London, 1933)

Thomas, A. M. K., Isherwood, I. & Wells, P. N. T., *The Invisible Light. 100 years of Medical Radiology* (Oxford, 1995)

27. The Sphygmomanometer

Crenner, C. W., 'Introduction of the blood pressure cuff into U.S. medical practice: technology and skilled practice', *Annals of Internal Medicine*, 128 (1998), 488–93

Evans, H., 'Losing touch: the controversy over the introduction of blood pressure instruments into medicine', *Technology and Culture*, 34 (1993), 784–807

Postel-Vinay, N., *A Century of Arterial Hypertension* (Chichester, 1996)

Roguin, A., 'Scipione Riva-Rocci and the men behind the mercury sphygmomanometer', *International Journal of Clinical Practice*, 60 (2006), 73–79

Swales, J. D., *Platt Versus Pickering: An Episode in Recent Medical History* (London, 1985)

Timmermann, C., 'A matter of degree: the normalisation of hypertension, c. 1940–2000', in W. Ernst (ed.), *Histories of the Normal and the Abnormal* (London, 2006), 245–61

28. Defibrillators

Eisenberg, M. S., Baskett, P. & Chamberlain, D., 'A history of cardiopulmonary resuscitation', in *Cardiac Arrest* (Cambridge, 2007, 2nd ed.)

29. Lasers

Bertolotti, M., *Masers and Lasers: An Historical Approach* (Bristol, 1983)

Bromberg, J. L., *The Laser in America, 1950–1970* (Cambridge, 1991)

Taylor, N., *Laser: The Inventor, the Nobel Laureate, the Thirty-Year Patent War* (New York, 2000)

Townes, C. H., *How the Laser Happened: Adventures of a Scientist* (Oxford, 1999)

30. The Endoscope

Andrews, C., Cosgrove, J. M. & Longo, W. E. (eds), *Minimally Invasive Surgery: Principles and Outcomes* (Newark, NJ, 1998)

Classen, M., Tytgat, G. N. J. & Lightdale, C. J., *Gastroenterological Endoscopy* (Stuttgart & New York, 2002)

DiMarino, A. J. & Benjamin, S. B. (eds), *Gastrointestinal Disease: An Endoscopic Approach* (Thorofare, NJ, 2002, 2nd ed.)

31. Imaging the Body

Blume, S., *Insight and Industry: On the Dynamics of Technological Change in Medicine* (Cambridge, MA, & London, 1992)

Kevles, B. H., *Naked to the Bone: Medical Imaging in the Twentieth Century* (New Brunswick, 1997)

McNay, M. B. & Fleming, J. E. E., 'Forty years of obstetric ultrasound 1957–1997: from A-scope to three dimensions', *Ultrasound in Medicine and Biology*, 25 (1999), 3–56

Webb, S., *From the Watching of Shadows: The Origins of Radiological Tomography* (Bristol, 1990)

Wolbarst, A. B., *Looking Within: How X-ray, CT, MRI, Ultrasound and Other Medical Images are Created* (Berkeley, CA, 1999)

32. The Incubator

Baker, J. P., *The Machine in the Nursery: Incubator Technology and the Origins of Newborn Intensive Care* (Baltimore, 1996)

Cone Jr, T. E., *History of the Care and Feeding of the Premature Infant* (Boston, MA, 1985)

MacFarquhar, D. M., *Newborn Medicine and Society: European Background and American Practice (1750–1975)* (Austin, 1998)

Meckel, R. A., *Save the Babies: American Public Health and the Prevention of Infant Mortality, 1850–1929* (Ann Arbor, MI, 1998)

Pernick, M. S., *The Black Stork: Eugenics and the Death of 'Defective' Babies in American Medicine and Motion Pictures Since 1915* (Oxford, 1996)

33. Medical Robots

Ichbiah, D., *Robots: From Science Fiction to Technological Revolution* (New York, 2005)

No. 4 Battling the Scourges

34. Plague

Benedictow, O., *The Black Death 1346–1353: The Complete History* (Woodbridge, 2004)

Crawford, D. H., *Deadly Companions: How Microbes Shaped our History* (Oxford, 2007)

Kiple, K. F. (ed.), *Plague, Pox and Pestilence* (London, 1997)

Sherman, I. W., *The Power of Plagues* (Washington, DC, 2006)

35. Typhus

Harrison, M., *Disease and the Modern World: 1500 to the Present Day* (Cambridge, 2004)

McNeill, W. H., *Plagues and Peoples* (New York, 1976)

Pelis, K., *Charles Nicolle, Pasteur's Imperial Missionary: Typhus and Tunisia* (Rochester, NY, 2006)

Weindling, P., *Epidemics and Genocide in Eastern Europe, 1890–1945* (Oxford, 2000)

Zinsser, H., *Rats, Lice and History* (New Brunswick, NJ, 2007 [1935])

36. Cholera

Barua, D. & Greenough III, W. B. (eds), *Cholera* (New York, 1992)

Briggs, C. & Mantini-Briggs, C., *Stories in the Time of Cholera: Racial Profiling During a Medical Nightmare* (Berkeley, CA, 2003)

Drasar, B. S. & Forrest, B. D. (eds), *Cholera and the Ecology of Vibrio Cholerae* (London, 1996)

Hamlin, C., *Cholera: The Biography* (Oxford, 2009)

Rosenberg, C. E., *The Cholera Years: The United States in 1832, 1849, and 1866* (Chicago, IL, 1962)

Wachsmuth, I. K., Blake, P. A. & Olsvik, Ø. (eds), *Vibrio Cholerae and Cholera: Molecular to Global Perspectives* (Washington, DC, 1994)

37. Puerperal Fever

Hallett, C., 'The attempt to understand puerperal fever in the eighteenth and early nineteenth centuries: the influence of inflammation theory', *Medical History*, 49 (1) (2005), 1–28

Holmes, O. W., 'The Contagiousness of Puerperal Fever', in *Medical Essays* (Cambridge, MA, 1883)

Loudon, I., *Death in Childbirth. An International Study of Maternity Care and Maternal Mortality, 1800–1950* (London, 1993)

– *The Tragedy of Childbed Fever* (Oxford, 2000)

Wilson, A., *The Making of Man-Midwifery: Childbirth in England, 1660–1770* (Cambridge, MA, 1995)

38. Tuberculosis

Dormandy, T., *The White Death: A History of Tuberculosis* (London, 1999)

Reichmann, L. B., *Timebomb: The Global Epidemic of Multi-drug Resistant Tuberculosis* (New York, 2002)

Roberts, C. A. & Buikstra, J. E., *The Bioarchaeology of Tuberculosis: A Global View on a Reemerging Disease* (Gainsville, FL, 2008)

Rothman, S. M., *Living in the Shadow of Death: Tuberculosis and the Social Experience of Illness in America* (New York, 1994)

39. Influenza A

Crawford, D. H., *The Invisible Enemy: A Natural History of Viruses* (Oxford, 2000)

– *Deadly Companions: How Microbes Shaped our History* (Oxford, 2007)

Honigsbaum, M., *Living with Enza: The Forgotten Story of Britain and the Great Flu Pandemic of 1918* (London, 2009)

Phillips, H. & Killingray, D. (eds), *The Spanish Influenza Pandemic of 1918–19: New Perspectives* (London, 2003)

40. Smallpox

Bhattacharya, S., *Expunging Variola: The Control and Eradication of Smallpox in India, 1947–1977* (Hyderabad & London, 2006)

Fenner, F., Henderson, D. A., Arita, I., Jezek, Z. & Ladnyi, I. D., *Smallpox and its Eradication* (Geneva, 1988)

Henderson, D. A., *Smallpox: The Death of a Disease* (New York, 2009)

Pead, P. J., *Vaccination Rediscovered: New Light in the Dawn of Man's Quest for Immunity* (Chichester, 2006)

41. Polio

Closser, S., *Chasing Polio in Pakistan: Why the World's Largest Public Health Initiative May Fail* (Nashville, TN, 2010)

Crawford, D. H., *The Invisible Enemy: A Natural History of Viruses* (Oxford, 2000)

Gould, T., *A Summer Plague: Polio and its Survivors* (New Haven, 1995)

Oshinsky, D., *Polio: An American Story* (Oxford & New York, 2005)

42. HIV

Iliffe, J., *The African AIDS Epidemic: A History* (Oxford, 2006)

Whiteside, A., *HIV/AIDS: A Very Short Introduction* (Oxford, 2008)

No. 5 'A Pill for Every Ill'

43. Opium

Berridge, V., *Opium and the People. Opiate Use and Drug Control Policy in Nineteenth and Early Twentieth Century England* (London, 1999)

Brook, T. & Wakabayashi, B. T. (eds), *Opium Regimes: China, Britain and Japan, 1839–1952* (Berkeley, CA, 2000)

Courtwright, D., *Forces of Habit. Drugs and the Making of the Modern World* (Cambridge, MA, 2001)

Dikotter, F., Laamann, L. & Zhou, X., *Narcotic Cultures: A History of Drugs in China* (London, 2004)

McAllister, W. B., *Drug Diplomacy in the Twentieth Century: An International History* (London & New York, 2000)

Musto, D., *The American Disease: Origins of Narcotic Control* (New York, 1987)

44. Quinine

Chininum: scriptiones collectae, Bureau tot Bevordering van het Kinine-Gebruik (Bureau for Increasing the Use of Quinine) (1924)

Honigsbaum, M., *The Fever Trail: The Hunt for the Cure for Malaria* (New York, 2001)

– & Willcox, M., 'Cinchona', in M. Willcox, G. Bodeker & P. Rasoanaivo (eds), *Traditional Medicinal Plants and Malaria* (Boca Raton, FL, 2004), 21–41

Markham, C. R., *Peruvian Bark. A popular account of the introduction of chinchona cultivation into British India* (London, 1880)

Taylor, N., *Plant Drugs that Changed the World* (London & New York, 1965), 72–100

45. Digitalis

Aronson, J. K., *An Account of the Foxglove and its Medical Uses, 1785–1985* (London, 1985)

Sheldon, P., *The Life and Times of William Withering: His Work, His Legacy* (Studley, 2004)

Worth Estes, J., *Hall Jackson and the Purple Foxglove: Medical Practice and Research in Revolutionary America, 1760–1820* (Hanover, NH, 1979)

46. Penicillin

Brown, K., *Penicillin Man: Alexander Fleming and the Antibiotic Revolution* (Stroud, 2004)

Bud, R., *Penicillin: Triumph and Tragedy* (Oxford, 2007)

Lax, E., *The Mould in Dr Florey's Coat* (New York, 2004)

Tansey, E. M. & Reynolds, L. A. (eds), *Post-Penicillin Antibiotics: From Acceptance to Resistance*, Wellcome Witnesses to Twentieth Century Medicine 6 (London, 2000)

47. The Pill

Asbell, B., *The Pill: A Biography of the Drug That Changed the World* (New York, 1995)

Marks, L. V., *Sexual Chemistry: A History of the Contraceptive Pill* (New Haven, 2010)

Marsh, M. S. & Ronner, W., *The Fertility Doctor: John Rock and the Reproductive Revolution* (Baltimore, MD, 2008)

May, E. T., *America and the Pill: A History of Promise, Peril and Liberation* (New York, 2010)

48. Drugs for the Mind

Healy, D., *The Anti-Depressant Era* (Cambridge, MA, 1998)

– *The Creation of Psychopharmacology* (Cambridge, MA, 2002)

Herzberg, D., *Happy Pills in America: From Miltown to Prozac* (Baltimore, MD, 2009)

Swazey, J., *Chlorpromazine in Psychiatry* (Cambridge, MA, 1974)

Tone, A., *The Age of Anxiety: A History of America's Turbulent Affair with Tranquilizers* (New York, 2009)

49. Ventolin

Brewis, R. A. L. (ed.), *Classic Papers in Asthma*, 2 vols (London, 1991)

Brookes, T., *Catching My Breath: An Asthmatic Explores His Illness* (New York, 1995)

Bryan, J., 'Ventolin remains a breath of fresh air for asthma sufferers, after 40 years', *Pharmaceutical Journal*, 279 (2007), 404–05

Jack, D., 'Drug treatment of bronchial asthma 1948–1995 – years of change', *International Pharmacy Journal*, 10 (1996), 50–52

Jackson, M., *Allergy: The History of a Modern Malady* (London, 2006)

– *Asthma: The Biography* (Oxford, 2009)

50. Beta-Blockers

Bylund, D. B., 'Alpha- and beta-adrenergic receptors: Ahlquist's landmark hypothesis of a single mediator with two receptors', *American Journal of Physiological Endocrinological Metabolism*, 293 (2007), E1479–E1481

McGrath, J. C. & Bond, R. A. (eds), Special issue celebrating the life and work of James Whyte Black, *British Journal of Pharmacology* 160, Supp. 1 (2010)

Obituary, Sir James Black: Nobel Prize winner who discovered beta-blockers *The Times*, 24 March, 2010

Quirke, V., 'Putting theory into practice: James Black, receptor theory and the development of the beta-blockers at ICI, 1958–1978', *Medical History*, 50 (2006), 69–92

51. Statins

Li, J. J., *Triumph of the Heart: The Story of Statins* (Oxford, 2009)

No. 6 Surgical Breakthroughs

52. Paré & Wounds

Drucker, C., 'Ambroise Paré and the birth of the gentle art of surgery', *Yale Journal of Biology and Medicine*, 81(4) (2008), 199–202

Dumaître, P., *Ambroise Paré: chirurgien de quatre rois de France* (Paris, 1986)

Malgaigne, J.-F., *Surgery and Ambroise Paré*, trans. & ed. W. B. Hamby (Norman, 1965)

Paré, A., *The Apologie and Treatise of Ambroise Paré*, ed. G. Keynes (London, 1951)

Shah, M., 'Premier Chirurgien du Roi: the Life of Ambroise Paré (1510–1590)', *Journal of the Royal Society of Medicine*, 85 (1992), 292–95

53. Anaesthesia

Dormandy, T., *The Worst of Evils* (New Haven & London, 2006)

Duncum, B. M., *The Development of Inhalation Anaesthesia* (London, 1994)

Pernick, M. S., *A Calculus of Suffering: Pain, Professionalism and Anesthesia in Nineteenth-Century America* (New York, 1985)

Rushman, M. S., Davies, N. J. H. & Atkinson, R. S., *A Short History of Anaesthesia: The First 150 Years* (Oxford, 1996)

Snow, S. J., *Blessed Days of Anaesthesia: How Anaesthetics Changed the World* (Oxford, 2008)

Sykes, K. & Bunker, J., *Anaesthesia and the Practice of Medicine: Historical Perspectives* (London, 2007)

54. Antisepsis & Asepsis

Crowther, A. & Dupree, M. W., *Medical Lives in the Age of Surgical Revolution* (New York & Cambridge, 2007)

Lawrence, C. (ed.), *Medical Theory, Surgical Practice: Studies in the History of Surgery* (London & New York, 1992)

Wangensteen, O. H. & Wangensteen, S. D., *The Rise of Surgery. From Empiric Craft to Scientific Discipline* (Folkestone, 1978)

Worboys, M., *Spreading Germs. Disease Theories and Medical Practice in Britain, 1865–1900* (Cambridge & New York, 2000)

55. Blood Transfusion

Diamond, L. K., 'A history of blood transfusion', in M. M. Wintrobe (ed.), *Blood, Pure and Eloquent* (New York, 1980)

Lederer, S. E., *Flesh and Blood: Organ Transplantation and Blood Transfusion in Twentieth-Century America* (Oxford, 2008)

Moore, P., *Blood and Justice* (Chichester, 2002)

Starr, D., *Blood: An Epic History of Medicine and Commerce* (New York, 1998)

56. Neurosurgery

Bliss, M., *Harvey Cushing: A Life in Surgery* (New York, 2005)

Greenblatt, S. H., *A History of Neurosurgery, in its Scientific and Professional Contexts* (Washington, DC, 1997)

Sachs, E., *The History and Development of Neurological Surgery* (New York, 1952)

Spencer, D. & Cohen-Gadol, A., *The Legacy of Harvey Cushing: Profiles of Patient Care*, American Association of Neurological Surgeons (2007)

Walker, A., *A History of Neurological Surgery* (New York, 1951)

57. Cataract Surgery

Apple, D. J., *Sir Harold Ridley and his Fight for Sight: He Changed the World So That We May Better See It* (Thorofare, NJ, 2006)

Kwitko, M. L. & Kelman, C. D., *The History of Modern Cataract Surgery* (The Hague, 1998)

Metcalfe, J. S., James, A. & Mina, A., 'Emergent innovation systems and the delivery of clinical services: the case of intraocular lenses', *Research Policy*, 34 (2005), 1285–1304

– & Pickstone, J., 'Replacing hips and lenses: surgery, industry and innovation in post-war Britain', in A. Webster (ed.), *New Technologies in Health Care* (Basingstoke, 2006), 146–60

58. Caesarean Section

Blumenfeld-Kosinski, R., *Not of Woman Born, Representations of Caesarean Birth in Medieval and Renaissance Culture* (Ithaca & London, 1990)

Churchill, H., *Caesarean Birth, Experience, Practice and History* (Hale, 1997)

Francome, C., Savage, W. & Churchill, H., *Caesarean Birth in Britain: 10 Years On. A Book for Health Professionals and Parents* (London, 2006)

Mander, R., *Caesarean, Just Another Way of Birth?* (London, 2007)

59. Cardiac Surgery

Tansey, E. M. & Reynolds L. A. (eds), *Early Heart Transplant Surgery in the UK*, Wellcome Witnesses to Twentieth Century Medicine 3 (London, 1999), 1–72

Treasure, T., 'Cardiac Surgery', in M. E. Silverman et al. (eds), *British Cardiology in the 20th Century* (London, Berlin & Heidelberg, 2000), 192–213

– & Hollman, A., 'The surgery of mitral stenosis 1898–1948: why did it take 50 years to establish mitral valvotomy?', *Annals of the Royal College of Surgeons of England*, 77(2) (1995), 145–51

Westaby, S., *Landmarks in Cardiac Surgery* (Oxford, 1997)

60. Transplant Surgery

Brent, L., *A History of Transplantation Immunology* (San Diego, CA, 1997)

Fox, R. C. & Swazey, J. P., *The Courage to Fail. A Social View of Organ Transplants and Dialysis* (Chicago, IL, 1974)

Küss, R. & Bourget, P., *An Illustrated History of Organ Transplantation. The Great Adventure of the Century* (Rueil-Malmaison 1992)

Lederer, S. E., *Flesh and Blood. Organ Transplantation and Blood Transfusion in Twentieth-Century America* (Oxford, 2008)

Nathoo, A., *Hearts Exposed. Transplants and the Media in 1960s Britain* (Basingstoke, 2009)

Schlich, T., *The Origins of Organ Transplantation: Surgery and Laboratory Science, 1880s–1930s* (Rochester, NY, 2010)

61. Hip Replacement

Anderson, J., Neary, F. & Pickstone, J. V., *Surgeons, Manufacturers and Patients. A Transatlantic History of Total Hip Replacement* (Basingstoke, 2007)

Klenerman, L. (ed.), *The Evolution of Orthopaedic Surgery* (London, 2002)

Reynolds, L. A. & Tansey, E. M. (eds), *Early Development of Total Hip Replacement*, Wellcome Witnesses to Twentieth Century Medicine 29 (London, 2007)

Schlich, T., *Surgery, Science and Industry: A Revolution in Fracture Care, 1950s–1990s* (Basingstoke, 2002)

Waugh, W., *John Charnley. The Man and the Hip* (London & Berlin, 1990)

62. Keyhole Surgery

Litynski, G. S., *Highlights in the History of Laparoscopy* (Frankfurt am Main, 1996)

Zetka, J. R., *Surgeons and the Scope* (Ithaca & London, 2003)

No. 7 Medical Triumphs

63. Vaccines

Parish, H. J., *A History of Immunization* (Edinburgh, 1965)

Plotkin, S. (ed.), *Vaccines* (Philadelphia, 2008, 5th ed.), 1–11

Silverstein, A. M., *A History of Immunology* (Amsterdam, 2009)

64. Vitamins

Apple, R., *Vitamania: Vitamins in American Culture* (New Brunswick, NJ, 1996)

Carpenter, K., *The History of Scurvy and Vitamin C* (Cambridge, 1988)

– *Beri-beri, White Rice, and Vitamin B*
(Berkeley, CA, 2000)

65. Insulin

Bliss, M., *The Discovery of Insulin* (Chicago, IL, 2009, new ed.)

Cox, C., *The Fight to Survive: A Young Girl, Diabetes and the Discovery of Insulin* (New York, 2009)

Ferry, G., *Dorothy Hodgkin. A Life* (London, 1998)

Straus, E., *Rosalyn Yalow, Nobel Laureate. Her Life and Work in Medicine* (New York, 1999)

Tattersall, R., *Diabetes: The Biography* (Oxford, 2009)

66. Dialysis

Cameron, J. S., *A History of the Treatment of Renal Failure by Dialysis* (Oxford, 2002)

Crowther, S. M., Reynolds, L. A. & Tansey, E. M. (eds), *History of Dialysis in the UK: c. 1950–1980*, Wellcome Witnesses to Twentieth Century Medicine 37 (London, 2009)

Heiney, P., *The Nuts and Bolts of Life* (Stroud, 2002)

Peitzman, S. J., *Dropsy, Dialysis, Transplant* (Baltimore, MD, 2007)

Van Noordwijk, J., *Dialysing for Life* (Dordrecht, 2001)

67. Smoking & Health

British Medical Association, *Smoking Out the Barons: The Campaign Against the Tobacco Industry,* Report of the British Medical Association Public Affairs Division (Chichester, 1986)

Hilton, M., *Smoking in British Popular Culture 1800–2000* (Manchester, 2000)

Lock, S., Reynolds, L. A. & Tansey, E. M. (eds), *Ashes to Ashes: The History of Smoking and Health* (Amsterdam, 1998)

Royal College of Physicians, *Health or Smoking?* (London, 1983)

Taylor, P., *Smoke Ring: The Politics of Tobacco* (London, 1984)

68. Assisted Reproduction

Edwards, R. G., 'The bumpy road to *in vitro* fertilization', *Nature Medicine*, 7 (2001), 1091–94

– & Steptoe, P. C., *A Matter of Life* (London, 1980)

Henig, R. M., *Pandora's Baby: How the First Test-Tube Babies Sparked the Reproductive Revolution* (New York, 2004)

Marsh, M. & Ronner, W., *The Fertility Doctor: John Rock and the Reproductive Revolution* (Baltimore, MD, 2008)

69. The Pap Smear & Human Papilloma Virus

Carmichael, E., *The Pap Smear: Life of George N. Papanicolaou* (Springfield, IL, 1973)

Clarke, A. E. & Casper, M. J., 'From simple technology to complex arena: classification of pap smears, 1917–90', *Medical Anthropological Quarterly*, 10 (4) (1996), 601–23

Diamantis, A., Magiorkinis, E. & Androutsos, G., 'What's in a name? Evidence that

Papanicolaou, not Babeș, deserves credit for the PAP Test', *Diagnostic Cytopathology* 38 (7) (2010), 473–76

Meisels, A., & Morin, C., *Modern Uterine Cytopathology: Moving to the Molecular Smear*, American Society of Clinical Pathologists (2007)

70. Helicobacter Pylori & Peptic Ulcer

Marshall, B. (ed.), *Helicobacter Pioneers: Firsthand Accounts from the Scientists Who Discovered Helicobacters 1892–1982* (Carlton & Oxford, 2002)

www.helico.com

SOURCES OF ILLUSTRATIONS

a-above; b-below; l-left; r-right; c-centre.
S&S – Science Museum, London/Science & Society Picture Library; WL – Wellcome Library, London/Wellcome Images.

1, 2–3, 5a, 5c WL; **5b** Anne Weston, LRI, CRUK/WL; **6al, 6bl, 6br** WL; **6ar** Private Collection; **7al** University of New Mexico, Albuquerque; **7b, 7r, 8, 10, 11, 12** WL; **14** New York Academy of Medicine; **15l** Science Museum, London/WL; **15r** Carole Reeves/WL; **16, 17, 18, 19** WL; **20a** Science Museum, London/WL; **20b** WL; **21a** Mark de Fraeye/WL; **21b** From San-ts'ai t'u-hui, 1607; **22, 23, 24–25a, 24b, 25b, 26, 27** WL; **28** British Museum, London; **29** Mark de Fraeye/WL; **30** From Colofón Libro de Medicina de Razi, 1250–60; **31** Freer Gallery of Art, Smithsonian Institution, Washington, D.C.; **32l** S&S; **32r, 33** WL; **34** Courtesy History of Science Collections, University of Oklahoma Libraries; **35, 36l, 36r, 37, 38l, 38r, 39, 40a** WL; **40b** Courtesy History of Science Collections, University of Oklahoma Libraries; **41a, 41b, 42, 43, 44, 45a** WL; **45b** From N. Grew, *Anatomy of Plants*, 1682; **46l, 46r** WL; **47** University of Edinburgh/WL; **48a** Private Collection; **48b** WL; **49a** Ludovic Collin/WL; **49b** Isabella Gavazzi/WL; **51l** From Joseph Priestley, *Experiments and Observations on Different Kinds of Air*, 1774; **51r** Underwood & Underwood/Corbis; **52** Peter Artymiuk/WL; **53l, 53r, 54** WL; **56l** John P. McGovern Historical Collections and Research Center, Houston Academy of Medicine, Texas; **56r, 57** WL; **58** Gordon Museum/WL; **59** S&S; **60, 61, 62, 63l, 63r** WL; **64a** Private Collection; **64b, 65, 66** WL; **67** Spike Walker/WL; **68, 69a, 69b** WL; **70a** From *The Graphic*, 1885; **70b** S&S; **71, 72, 73, 74, 75l, 75r, 76a, 76b** WL; **77l** U.S. National Library of Medicine, Maryland; **77r** U.S. National Archives and Records Administration, Maryland; **78, 79** WL; **80**

bpk; **81, 82, 84, 85l, 85r, 86, 87l, 87r, 88** WL; **89** R. Dourmashkin/WL; **91** Wessex Regional Genetics Centre/WL; **92** Nicoletta Baloyianni/WL; **93a** Sanger Institute/WL; **93b** Wessex Regional Genetics Centre/WL; **94** Professor Ott; **95** Anne Weston, LRI, CRUK/WL; **96l** Dr M.A. Konerding, Professor of Anatomy, Institute of Functional and Clinical Anatomy of the University Medical Centre, Johannes Gutenberg University, Mainz; **96r** Natural History Museum, London; **97l** Dr David Becker/WL; **97r** Dr Lyndal Kearney, Section of Haemato-Oncology, The Institute of Cancer Research, Sutton; **98, 99, 100, 101** WL; **102** D. D. Palmer, *Science, Art and Philosophy of Chiropractic*, Portland, 1910; **103** Kate Whitley, WL; **104** WL; **106** Private Collection; **107a, 107b, 108, 109a, 109b, 110** WL; **111** From Francesco Stelluti, *Melissographia*, 1625; **112** WL; **113a** M. Johnson/WL; **113b** S&S; **114** WL; **115a, 115bl** Science Museum, London/WL; **115br, 116l** WL; **116r** S&S; **117l** WL; **117r** Science Museum, London/WL; **118, 119, 120, 121a** WL; **121b** S&S; **122l, 122r, 123** WL; **124a** S&S; **124b** WL; **125** S&S; **126, 127l, 127r** WL; **128** Bettmann/Corbis; **129a** medicalpicture/Alamy; **129b** Yang Yu/iStockphoto.com; **130l, 130r, 131a, 131b, 132, 133, 134l** WL; **134r** Private Collection; **135** Mark Lythgoe & Chloe Hutton/WL; **136** WL; **137** Visuals Unlimited/Corbis; **138** WL; **139** Stefano Bianchetti/Corbis; **140** Library of Congress, Washington, D.C.; **141a** Intuitive Surgical, Inc.; **141b** Oliver Burston/WL; **142** WL; **144a** CDC/PHIL/Corbis; **144b, 145, 146** WL; **147** British Library, London; **148, 149** WL; **150l** Library of Congress, Washington, D.C.; **150r** U.S. National Archives and Records Administration, Maryland; **151, 152, 153, 154a** WL; **154b** Science Museum, London/WL; **155a** WL; **155b** Science Museum, London/WL; **156l** Kunsthistorisches Museum, Vienna; **156r** National Portrait Gallery, London; **157** Kunsthistorisches Museum, Vienna; **158, 159a** WL; **159b** Science Museum, London/WL; **160** Time Life Pictures/Getty; **161a** C.N.R.I./Photolibrary; **161b, 162** WL; **163** Library of Congress, Washington, D.C.; **164** Dr Terrence Tumpey/Centers for Disease Control and Prevention; **165l** Office of Public Health Service Historian, Maryland; **165r** U.S. Army; **166** Anna Tanczos/WL; **167** Wang Ying/EPA/Corbis; **168, 169a, 169b, 170** WL; **171l** S&S; **171r** WL; **172a** Visuals Unlimited/Corbis; **172b** Library of Congress, Washington, D.C.; **173** Bettmann/Corbis; **174l, 174r** WL; **175** Bettmann/Corbis; **176a** R. Dourmashkin/WL; **176b** Alfredo Aldai/EPA/Corbis; **177** Carole Morgane/Corbis; **178a, 179a, 178–79b** WL; **180** Worden Sports College/WL; **182** Royal Botanic Gardens, Kew/WL; **183** S&S; **184** WL; **185l** Library of Congress, Washington, D.C.; **185r** S&S; **186, 187a** WL; **187b** Science Museum, London/WL; **188** S&S; **189, 190l, 190r, 191a, 191b** WL; **192** NMeM Daily Herald Archive/S&S; **193al, 193ar** WL; **193b** David Gregory & Debbie Marshall/WL; **194a, 194b** WL; **195l** U.S. National Archives and Records

Administration, Maryland; **195r** S&S; **196** Bettmann/Corbis; **197** Annie Cavanagh/WL; **198** George Grantham Bain Collection/Library of Congress, Washington, D.C.; **199l** S&S; **199r** Henry Diltz/Corbis; **200l** S&S; **200r** Pfizer Inc.; **201** NMeM Daily Herald Archive/S&S; **202, 203, 204l** WL; **204r** Private Collection; **205** Spike Walker/WL; **206** WL; **207a** Annie Cavanagh/WL; **207b** WL; **208** Anne-Katrin Purkiss/WL; **209** WL; **210** Arran Lewis/WL; **211l** Reid Parham; **211r** WL; **212** Tokyo University of Agriculture and Technology; **213** WL; **214** Biblioteca Casanatense, Rome; **216a** Courtesy History of Science Collections, University of Oklahoma Libraries; **217a** Universitätsbibliothek Basel; **216–17b, 218l** WL; **218r** From John Snow, *On Chloroform*, London, 1858; **219a, 219b, 220, 222, 223, 224a, 224b, 225** WL; **226** Bettmann/Corbis; **227, 228, 229a** WL; **229b** W.G. Purmann, *Lorbeerkrantz oder Wundartzney*, 1685; **230l, 230r** WL; **231a** Harvey Cushing/John Hay Whitney Medical Library, Yale University; **231b** S&S; **232** Harvey Cushing/John Hay Whitney Medical Library, Yale University; **233** Library of Congress, Washington, D.C.; **234, 235l** WL; **235r** Joe McNally/Getty Images; **236** Bibliothèque Nationale, Paris; **237, 238, 239, 240, 241** WL; **242** Johns Hopkins School of Medicine, Baltimore; **243, 244l, 244r** WL; **245** S&S; **246l** Pictorial Press Ltd/Alamy; **246r** WL; **247** From Theodor Kocher, *Chirurgische Operationslehre*, 1907; **248** WL; **250** From Borst Enderlen, *Beitrage zur Gefässchirurgie und zur Organtransplantation*, 1910; **251** Bettmann/Corbis; **252l** Private Collection; **252r** WL; **253** S&S; **254** Photomorgana/Corbis; **255** WL; **256** Gallo Images/Getty Images; **257a** Tessa Oksanen/WL; **257b** WL; **258** Kham/Reuters/Corbis; **260** From *Harper's Weekly*, 1885; **261a** S&S; **261b, 262** WL; **263** U.S. National Library of Medicine, Maryland; **264** Gwyneth Thurgood/WL; **265l** WL; **265r** Museum Boerhaave, Leiden; **266** S&S; **267, 268l, 268r, 269, 270a** WL; **270b** Anne Clark, University of Oxford/WL; **271l** WL; **271r** NMeM Daily Herald Archive/S&S; **272, 273** WL; **274l** Bettmann/Corbis; **274r** S&S; **275** Fritz Goro/Time Life Pictures/Getty Images; **276** C.J. Dub; **277al** Swim Ink 2, LLC/Corbis; **277ar** Fritz Goro/Time Life Pictures/Getty Images; **277b, 278–79** WL; **280** K. Hardy/WL; **281** Trinity Mirror/Mirrorpix/Alamy; **282** Maurizio de Angelis/WL; **283a** Spike Walker/WL; **283b** WL; **284a** Bettmann/Corbis; **284b** Library of Congress, Washington, D.C.; **285** WL; **286** Bob Strong/Reuters/Corbis; **287** MRC NIMR/WL; **288a** Tony McDonough/EPA/Corbis; **288b** Oliver Berg/EPA/Corbis; **289a, 289b, 290** WL; **291** Dennis Kunkel Microscopy, Inc./Visuals Unlimited/Corbis.

SOURCES OF QUOTATIONS

p. 14 J. F. Nunn, *Ancient Egyptian Medicine* (London & Norman, OK, 1996); p. 30 Abu Marwan 'Abd al-Malik b. Zuhr, *Kitab al-Taysir fi al-mudawat wa-l-tadbir*; ed. M. Khouri (Damascus, 1983), 290; p. 34 William Hunter, *Two Introductory Lectures...* (London, 1784); p. 40 François Xavier Bichat *Anatomie générale* (Paris, 1801); p. 44 Robert Hooke, *Micrographia* (London, 1665), Observation XVIII; p. 48 W. von Waldeyer-Hartz, *Über einige neuere Forschungen im Gebiete der Anatomie des Centralnervènsystems* (Berlin, 1891); p. 50 Claude Bernard, *Introduction to the Study of Experimental Medicine*, trans. H. C. Green (New York, 1957 [Paris, 1865]), 65; p. 56 William Harvey, *De motu cordis et sanguinis in animalibus* (Frankfurt, 1628); p. 60 Samuel Tuke, *Description of the Retreat, an Institution near York ...* (York, 1813); p. 64 Walter B. Cannon, 'Organization for physiological homeostasis', *Physiological Reviews*, 9, 1929, pp. 399–431; p. 64 Claude Bernard, *Lectures on the Phenomena of Life*, trans. H. E. Hoff, R. Guillemin & L. Guillemin (Springfield, IL, 1974); p. 68 Charles Singer, *A History of Biology. A General Introduction to the Study of Living Things* (New York, 1950); p. 74 Charles Chapin, *The Sources and Modes of Infection* (New York, 1910); p. 78 Richard C. Cabot, *Psychotherapy and its Relation to Religion* (Boston, 1908); p. 82 Walter B. Cannon, 'Some conditions controlling internal secretion', *Journal of the American Medical Association*, 79 (1922), 92–95; p. 86 Frank Macfarlane Burnet, 'Immunology as a scholarly discipline', *Perspectives in Biology and Medicine* 16 (1972), 1–10; p. 90 A. E. Garrod, 'The incidence of alkaptonuria: a study in chemical individuality', *Lancet* ii (1902), 1616–30; p. 94 J. Ewing, 'Pathological aspects of some problems of experimental cancer research', *Journal of Cancer Research* (1916), 1, 71, citing Virchow; p. 98 A. A. Erz, *The Medical Question. The Truth About Official Medicine...* (Butler, NJ, 1914); p. 106 René Laennec, *Traité de l'auscultation médiate et des maladies des poumons et du cœur...* (1826); p. 110 Robert Hooke, *Micrographia* (London, 1665), preface, sig. A2v; p. 114 Arthur Conan Doyle, *The Sign of the Four* (London, 1890); p. 116 Carl Wunderlich, *Medical Thermometry and Human Temperature* (New York, 1871); p. 118 Dr Henry W. Cattell, *The New York Times*, Feb. 15, 1896; p. 122 G. W. Pickering, *High Blood Pressure* (New York, 1955); p. 126 W. B. Kouwenhoven, J. R. Jude, G. G. Knickerbocker, 'Introducing the modern age of resuscitation', *Journal of the American Medical Association* 178 (1960), 1064; p. 128 Thomas Gray, 1757, *The progress of Poesy*, line 101; p. 158 Dr Pierre Budin, *The Nursling* (London, 1900); p. 140 Dr A. Menciassi, Associate Professor of Biomedical Robots, Scuola Superiore Sant'Anna, http://www.rcseng.ac.uk/museums/exhibitions/

archive/sci-fi-surgery/sci-fi-surgery-medical-robots; pp. 144–45 in O. J. Benedictow, *The Black Death 1346–1353* (Woodbridge, 2004), 143; p. 148 Hans Zinsser, *Rats, Lice and History* (London, 1935); p. 152 Richard L. Guerrant, Benedito A. Carneiro-Filho & Rebecca A. Dillingham, 'Cholera, diarrhea, and oral rehydration therapy: triumph and indictment', *Clinical Infectious Diseases* (2003), 398–405; p. 156 Alexander Gordon, *The Treatise on the Epidemic Puerperal Fever of Aberdeen* (London, 1795); p. 160 John Bunyan, *The Life and Death of Mr Badman*, (London, 1680); p. 164 C. Creighton, *History of Epidemics in Britain*, 3 (London, 1965), 308; p. 168 http://www.who.int/mediacentre/news/notes/2010/smallpox_20100517/en/index.html; p. 186 Bernardo Ramazzini, *Opera omnia, medica et physica*, 1717; p. 190 William Withering, *An Account of the Foxglove and some of its Medical Uses* (Birmingham, 1785); p. 192 Ritchie Calder, *Medicine and Man. The History of the Art and Science of Healing* (London, 1958), 204; p. 202 Peter D. Kramer, *Listening to Prozac* (New York, 1993), 300; p. 206 Sir David Jack, 'Drug treatment of bronchial asthma 1948–1995: years of change', *International Pharmacy Journal*, 10 (1996), 50–52; p. 212 *New England Journal of Medicine*, 304 (1981); p. 216 Ambroise Paré, *The Apologie and Treatise, containing the Voyages made into Diverse places*, ed. Geoffrey Keynes, (1951 [1585]), 88; p. 218 Charles Darwin, Letter 1293 to J. S. Henslow, 17 January 1850; p. 222 Charles Barrett Lockwood, *Aseptic Surgery* (Edinburgh, 1896), 193; p. 228 Goethe, *Faust*, part 1 (1808); p. 230 William Osler, quoted in M. Bliss, *Harvey Cushing: A Life in Surgery* (New York, 2005), 126; p. 234 http://www.who.int/blindness/causes/priority/en/index1.html; p. 236 M. Stephen, *Domestic midwife; or, the best means of preventing danger in child-birth* (London, 1795), 23; p. 240 Stephen Paget, *The Surgery of the Chest* (Bristol, 1896); p. 246 Otto Lanz, *Zur Schilddrüsenfrage* (Leipzig, 1894–97), 55; p. 256 David L. Nahrwold, 'The surgeon and biliary lithotripsy', *Archives of Surgery* 124 (1989), 780; p. 260 Thomas Adams, *The Happiness of the Church* (1618); p. 264 F. Gowland Hopkins, 'Feeding experiments illustrating the importance of accessory food factors in normal dietaries', *Journal of Physiology*, 44 (1912), 425; p. 268 *The Times* 7 August 1923; p. 268 E. P. Joslin, H. Gray & H. F. Root, 'Insulin in hospital and home', *Journal of Metabolic Research* 2 (1922) 651–99; p. 272 Isak Dinesen (Karen Blixen), *Seven Gothic Tales* (London, 1934); p. 276 Richard Doll & Austin Bradford Hill, 'Smoking and Carcinoma of the Lung', *British Medical Journal* (1950), 746; p. 280 R. G. Edwards, B. D. Bavister & P. Steptoe, 'Early stages of fertilization *in vitro* of human oocytes matured *in vitro*', *Nature*, 221 (1969), 632; p. 284 G. N. Papanicolaou & H. F. Traut, 'The diagnostic value of vaginal smears in carcinoma of the uterus', *American Journal of Obstetrics and Gynecology* 42 (1941), 193; p. 288 Daniel J. Boorstin, *The Discoverers* (New York, 1984).